The Handbook of Language Assessment Across Modalities

Perspectives on Deafness

Series Editors
Stephanie Cawthon
Harry Knoors

Innovations in Deaf Studies: The Role of Deaf Scholars
Annelies Kusters, Maartje De Meulder, Dai O'Brien

Educating Deaf Learners: Creating a Global Evidence Base
Edited by Harry Knoors and Marc Marschark

Evidence-Based Practices in Deaf Education
Edited by Harry Knoors and Marc Marschark

Teaching Deaf Learners: Psychological and Developmental Foundations
Harry Knoors and Marc Marschark

The People of the Eye: Deaf Ethnicity and Ancestry
Harlan Lane, Richard C. Pillard, and Ulf Hedberg

Deaf Cognition: Foundations and Outcomes
Edited by Marc Marschark and Peter C. Hauser

How Deaf Children Learn: What Parents and Teachers Need to Know
Marc Marschark and Peter C. Hauser

Research in Deaf Education: Contexts, Challenges, and Considerations
Edited by Stephanie Cawthon and Carrie Lou Garberoglio

Diversity in Deaf Education
Edited by Marc Marschark, Venetta Lampropoulou, and Emmanouil K. Skordilis

Bilingualism and Bilingual Deaf Education
Edited by Marc Marschark, Gladys Tang, and Harry Knoors

Early Literacy Development in Deaf Children
Connie Mayer and Beverly J. Trezek

The World of Deaf Infants: A Longitudinal Study
Kathryn P. Meadow-Orlans, Patricia Elizabeth Spencer, and Lynn Sanford Koester

Approaches to Social Research: The Case of Deaf Studies
Alys Young and Bogusia Temple

Deaf Education Beyond the Western World
Edited by Harry Knoors, Maria Brons, and Marc Marschark

Co-Enrollment in Deaf Education
Edited by Marc Marschark, Shirin Antia, and Harry Knoors

The Handbook of Language Assessment Across Modalities

Edited by
Tobias Haug,
Wolfgang Mann,
and Ute Knoch

OXFORD
UNIVERSITY PRESS

OXFORD
UNIVERSITY PRESS

Oxford University Press is a department of the University of Oxford. It furthers the University's objective of excellence in research, scholarship, and education by publishing worldwide. Oxford is a registered trade mark of Oxford University Press in the UK and certain other countries.

Published in the United States of America by Oxford University Press
198 Madison Avenue, New York, NY 10016, United States of America.

Library of Congress Cataloging-in-Publication Data
Names: Haug, Tobias, 1971– editor. | Mann, Wolfgang, 1970– editor. |
Knoch, Ute, editor.
Title: The handbook of language assessment across modalities /
edited by Tobias Haug, Wolfgang Mann, and Ute Knoch.
Description: New York, NY : Oxford University Press, [2022] |
Series: Perspectives on deafness |
Includes bibliographical references and index.
Identifiers: LCCN 2021034887 (print) | LCCN 2021034888 (ebook) |
ISBN 9780190885052 (hardback) | ISBN 9780190885076 (epub) |
ISBN 9780197609378 (digital-online)
Subjects: LCSH: Children—Language—Evaluation. |
Children with disabilities—Language—Evaluation. |
Language disorders in children. | LCGFT: Essays.
Classification: LCC RJ496.L35 H337 2021 (print) |
LCC RJ496.L35 (ebook) | DDC 618.92/855—dc23
LC record available at https://lccn.loc.gov/2021034887
LC ebook record available at https://lccn.loc.gov/2021034888

DOI: 10.1093/oso/9780190885052.001.0001

The manufacturer's authorised representative in the EU for product safety is Oxford University Press España S.A. of El Parque Empresarial San Fernando de Henares, Avenida de Castilla, 2 – 28830 Madrid (www.oup.es/en or product.safety@oup.com). OUP España S.A. also acts as importer into Spain of products made by the manufacturer.

Contents

Contributors

Sara Pivac Alexander
School of Linguistics and Applied Language Studies
Victoria University of Wellington
Wellington, NZ, USA

Lisa M. Bedore
Department of Communication Sciences and Disorders
Temple University
Philadelphia, PA, USA

Eveline Boers-Visker
Institute for Sign, Language and Deaf Studies
Utrecht University of Applied Sciences
Utrecht, NL, USA

Patrick Boudreault
Graduate School, Research and Continuing and Online Education
Gallaudet University
Washington, DC, USA

Richard Bowden
Centre for Vision Speech and Signal Processing
University of Surrey
Guildford, UK

Necati Cihan Camgöz
Centre for Vision, Speech and Signal Processing
University of Surrey
Guildford, UK

Bernard Camilleri
Division of Language and Communication Science
University of London
London, UK

Carol A. Chapelle
English and Applied Linguistics
Iowa State University
Ames, IA, USA

Shula Chiat
Division of Language and Communication Science
University of London
London, UK

Kathryn Crowe
Schools of Health Sciences and Education
University of Iceland
Reykjavík, Iceland
School of Teacher Education
Charles Sturt University
Canberra, Australia

Hilary Dumbrill
Hamilton Lodge School and College for Deaf Learners
Brighton, UK

Kathleen Durant
Speech Pathology and Audiology Program
Kent State University
Kent, OH, USA

Kathrin Eberharter
Department of Subject-Specific Education
University of Innsbruck
Innsbruck, Austria

Sarah Ebling
Department of Computational Linguistics
University of Zurich
Zurich, Switzerland

Charlotte Enns
Department of Educational Administration, Foundations and Psychology
University of Manitoba
Manitoba, Canada

Amy Kissel Frisbie
Department of Audiology, Speech and Learning
Children's Hospital Colorado
Denver, CO, USA

Pauline Frizelle
Department of Speech and Hearing Sciences
University College Cork
Cork, Ireland

Kellie Frost
School of Languages and Linguistics
University of Melbourne
Melbourne, Australia

Annemiek Hammer
Vrij University
Faculteit der Letteren
Amsterdam, Netherlands

Luke Harding
Linguistics and English Language
Lancaster University
Lancaster, UK

Natalie Hasson
Independent Speech and Language Therapist and Registered Intermediary, UK

Tobias Haug
Institute of Language and Communication in Special Needs
University of Teacher Education in Special Needs (HfH)
Zurich, Switzerland

Peter C. Hauser
NTID Research Center on Culture and Language
Rochester Institute of Technology
Rochester, NY, USA

Volker Hegelheimer
Department of English
Iowa State University
Ames, IA, USA

Jonathan Henner
Specialized Education Services
University of North Carolina
Greensboro, NC, USA

Rosalind Herman
Division of Language and Communication Science
University of London
London, UK

Joanna Hoskin
Division of Language and Communication Science
University of London
London, UK

Ute Knoch
Language Testing Research Centre
University of Melbourne
Melbourne, Australia

Benjamin Kremmel
Department of Subject-specific Education
University of Innsbruck
Innsbruck, Austria

Hye-won Lee
Research and Thought Leadership
Cambridge Assessment English
Cambridge, UK

Susy Macqueen
School of Literature, Languages and Linguistics
Australian National University
Canberra, Australia

Wolfgang Mann
School of Education
University of Roehampton
London, UK

Cristina McKean
Professor of Child Language Development and Disorders
Newcastle University
Honorary Fellow
Murdoch Children's Research Institute
Victoria, Australia
Adjunct Fellow
Griffith University
Queensland, Australia

Rachel McKee
School of Linguistics and Applied Language Studies
Victoria University of Wellington
Wellington, NZ, USA

Stephanie McMillen
Department of Communication Sciences & Disorders
Syracuse University
Syracuse, NY, USA

Deborah Mood
Department of Pediatrics, Developmental Behavioral Pediatrics
University of Colorado
Aurora, CO, USA

Carol-Anne Murphy
School of Allied Health and Health Research Institute
University of Limerick
Limerick, Ireland

Phuong Nguyen
Language Center
University of Chicago
Chicago, IL, USA

Elizabeth D. Peña
School of Education
University of California
Irvine, CA, USA

Geoffrey Poor
American Sign Language Training and Evaluation
National Technical Institute for the Deaf, Rochester Institute of Technology
Rochester, NY, USA

David Quinto-Pozos
Department of Linguistics
University of Texas
Austin, TX, USA

Christian Rathmann
Department of Deaf Studies and Interpreting
Humboldt-Universität
Berlin, Germany

Katherine Rowley
Deafness, Cognition and Language Research Centre
University College London
London, UK

Penny Roy
Division of Language and Communication Science
University of London
London, UK

Nicole Salamy
Otolaryngology/Center for Communication Enhancement; Deaf and Hard of Hearing Program
Boston Children's Hospital
Boston, MA, USA

Krister Schönström
Department of Linguistics
Stockholm University
Stockholm, Sweden

Aaron Shield
Speech Pathology and Audiology
Miami University
Cincinnati, OH, USA

Beppie van den Bogaerde
Amsterdam Center for Language and Communication
University of Amsterdam
Amsterdam, Netherlands

Wenda Walton
Victoria University
Wellington, Netherlands

Introduction

Why an Edited Volume on Signed and Spoken Language Assessment?

Tobias Haug, Wolfgang Mann, and Ute Knoch

The first part of this chapter provides an overview of how the idea of this edited volume on spoken and signed language assessment came about. The chapter also gives an insight into the different histories of spoken and signed language assessment and test research with their different backgrounds and contexts. It shows that very little interaction between signed and spoken language assessment communities exist so far. The second part of this chapter outlines the structure and the 12 themes that are addressed in this volume. While themes 1–6 focus one the assessment of young learners, the themes 7–12 focus on the assessment of adult learners.

Why is it important to publish a volume of paired chapters written by contributors from the signed and spoken language assessment communities? Signed language test research can be considered a fairly young subdiscipline that emerged from the fields of deaf education and signed language linguistics. In comparison, spoken language test research represents a well-established area that emerged from the well-established field of applied linguistics and second language education. To this day, there has been little interaction between both fields. Traditionally, most publications on signed language testing have been published in specialized journals within their "own" scientific community, including the *Journal of Deaf Studies and Deaf Education*, *Deafness & Education International*, or *Sign Language Studies*, while journals like *Language Assessment Quarterly* or *Language Testing* publish research almost exclusively on spoken languages. Only in recent years have the lines become "blurred," with several journal articles on signed language assessment being published in peer-reviewed journals of the spoken language testing community (e.g., Bochner et al., 2016; Haug, 2011; Haug et al., 2020; Mann et al., 2015). Similarly, researchers from the signed language assessment community started presenting at conferences that had been less likely to include research on signed language assessment in the past. Examples include the 2014 conference of the Association of Language Testing in Europe (ALTE) in Paris; the

Tobias Haug, Wolfgang Mann, and Ute Knoch, *Introduction* In: *The Handbook of Language Assessment Across Modalities.* Edited by: Tobias Haug, Wolfgang Mann, and Ute Knoch, Oxford University Press. © Oxford University Press 2022. DOI: 10.1093/oso/9780190885052.003.0001

2014 Language Testing Research Colloquium, the annual meeting of the International Language Testing Association (ILTA) in Amsterdam, and the 2018 European Association of Language Testing and Assessment (EALTA) meeting in Bochum, Germany. These presentations were received with considerable interest.

When discussing the idea of bringing together colleagues from signed and spoken language assessment for the purpose of this volume, we (the editors) realized that there are, perhaps unsurprisingly, quite a few aspects that are relevant to both fields. At the same time, some undeniable differences exist. Our aim was to explore both similarities as well as differences and identify the "common ground." We believed that pairing experts from each field would offer both sides an opportunity to learn from each other, not just from a purely academic point of view, but also on a more practical level, for instance in the areas of training of raters/assessors or test development.

This book is in the form of an edited volume with 36 chapters organized under 12 different topics. Each topic is addressed in three chapters, the first two of which are written from a spoken and signed language assessment perspective, respectively. The third chapter takes on the format of a joint discussion written collaboratively by the authors of the paired contributions.

The original idea of an edited volume on signed and spoken language assessment was developed by Tobias Haug in 2013, following several casual conversations at conferences with colleagues from the field of spoken language testing. This resulted in some handwritten notes on the back of a napkin which were tossed back and forth via email for a while between Tobias and colleagues from spoken language testing, without further follow up. The book idea was finally picked up again at the Language Testing and Research Colloquium (LTRC) in Amsterdam, in summer 2014, where the three editors of this volume presented on topics related to signed (Haug and Mann) and spoken (Knoch) language assessment. Over the course of the next two years the idea was developed further as (additional) key issues in signed/spoken language assessment came to light following a short survey distributed to researchers from both scientific communities. In the survey, colleagues were asked to raise topics they considered of relevance for and in their work on signed and spoken language assessment. Their responses and comments helped to shape the current form and structure of this book.

RESEARCH IN LANGUAGE TESTING

The assessment of speaking ability is the youngest subbranch of language testing (Fulcher, 2003). This is because, especially in the United States before the Second World War, spoken tasks were generally not included in language assessments because they were not deemed to be sufficiently reliable when compared to more objectively scored test tasks. During the Second World War, it was recognized that spoken competence was important, in particular for foreign service personnel due to be stationed in other countries, and this led to a subsequent focus on assessing speaking. This led to interlocutors and raters being trained.

In recent years, the research foci have broadened considerably, including concerns about rater cognitive processes (see, e.g., Brown, 2000) and questions related to which aspects of speaking to measure to best represent the construct of spoken language in different settings (e.g., academic vs. professional contexts; see e.g., Elder et al., 2013; Frost et al., 2012), how to best administer spoken assessments (directly or indirectly using computers; e.g., O'Loughlin, 2001), and whether speaking can be measured validly in pairs or groups of students (May, 2011). More recently, there has been an increased focus on the inclusion of technology in spoken assessment, including automated scoring of spoken assessment (Xi et al., 2008).

Research on signed language assessment can be considered a rather young field, one that was mainly driven by studies carried out in the United States in the late 1990s (e.g., Hoffmeister, 2000; Strong & Prinz, 1997). In most cases, the development of signed language tests has been influenced by (1) a practical need by schools that serve deaf children (e.g., Herman et al., 1999) or by tertiary institutions that offer signed language teaching and learning (e.g., signed language interpreter training programs) and (2) a specific research purpose, for example, learning more about the morpho-syntactic structures of a signed language (for American Sign Language: Supalla et al., 1995) or addressing issues related to late learning of a (signed) language, including the possible effects on language processing (e.g., Boudreault & Mayberry, 2006; Mayberry et al., 2002). Although the number of signed language tests has increased considerably over the course of the past decade, including tests for other signed languages (e.g., British Sign Language [BSL; Herman et al., 1999], German Sign Language [Haug, 2006], Sign Language of the Netherlands [Hermans et al., 2007]), very few signed language tests, for both young and adult learners, are commercially available and/or can be used in an applied context.

Many of the research studies that have been carried out over the past 20 years and that involved signed language tests utilized these assessments as means to explore the link between deaf children's proficiency in signed language as first language (L1) and their literacy skills (e.g., Hoffmeister, 2000; Mann, 2007). In other studies, signed language tests were designed exclusively for research purposes (e.g., the Test Battery for Australian Sign Language (Auslan) Morphology and Syntax) to gather data on specific linguistic structures (e.g., Schembri et al., 2002). As a consequence, there have been very few publications that specifically addressed methodological issues in the development of signed language tests (e.g., Haug, 2011; Haug & Mann, 2008; Mann, 2007). This has changed only in recent years following the growing interest in and awareness of these issues.

In addition to the aforementioned need for tests as research tools to investigate signed languages, there is an equal demand for signed language assessments for use in applied contexts, such as schools or universities. For instance, assessing the language abilities of signing deaf children is essential to identifying particular needs when specific language milestones are not met (Enns et al., 2016). Such assessments need to be carried out regularly over time to successfully monitor a child's development. However, this requires assessments that address or measure specific linguistic domains and features of a child's signed language. *Language Assessment Across Modalities* uses the existing research on signed language assessment as a starting point for a series of cross-disciplinary discussions on different issues related to language assessment with specialists in the field of spoken language assessment. Some of these issues are considered shared, whereas others may be considered unique to each discipline. For instance, one critical difference between signed and spoken language assessment is that most of the research on signed language focuses on children acquiring a signed language as L1 or delayed L1. In comparison, the majority of studies on spoken language tests tend to target adult L2/foreign language learners of English (although this focus has changed in recent years with much more work being undertaken on the assessment of young learners). The resulting consequences (i.e., first vs. second/foreign language learning and a minority [signed] vs. majority [spoken] language) are an integral part of the interdisciplinary discussions in this book.

SIGNED LANGUAGES AND DEAF COMMUNITIES

Just like spoken languages, signed languages are complex linguistic systems, including features of all subsystems, such as phonetics, phonology, morphology, syntax, semantics, and discourse (Pfau et al., 2012; Sandler & Lillo-Martin, 2006). Signed languages are used by deaf people around the world to communicate with one another. For instance, it is a widely recognized convention to use the uppercase *Deaf* to describe members of the linguistic community of signed language users and, in contrast, the lowercase *deaf* to describe the audiological state of a hearing impairment (Morgan & Woll, 2002). Linguistic communities of signers have been the focus of a growing number of studies over the past 30 years, in part because the visual/spatial modality of their language presents "structural possibilities unseen in spoken languages" (Senghas & Monaghan, 2002, p. 84). Findings from this research have contributed to the discussion of general theoretical issues in multiple disciplines (e.g., anthropology, linguistics, and education). In addition, signed language teaching and assessment and their link to the Common European Framework of Reference (CEFR) have gained more attention in recent years (e.g., Haug et al., 2019; Leeson & van den Bogaerde, 2020).

LANGUAGE ASSESSMENT WITHIN THE CONTEXT OF THE COMMON EUROPEAN FRAMEWORK OF REFERENCE

The CEFR was developed by the Council of Europe in an attempt to provide common reference levels for teaching and learning for all languages in Europe (Council of Europe, 2001, 2020). Since its inception, the CEFR has become hugely influential in language assessment circles. In fact, the CEFR was designed with language testing in mind. The manual states that "one of the aims of the Framework is to help partners to describe the levels of proficiency required by existing standards, tests and examinations in order to facilitate comparisons between different systems of qualification" (Council of Europe, 2001, p. 21). The influence of the CEFR has been felt not only in Europe but also more globally. The scales have become a set of standards adhered to across the world, and most major language testing agencies have already, are in the process of, or are feeling pressure to link their tests to the CEFR (see, e.g., Martyniuk, 2010). To help practitioners in the linking process, the Council of Europe piloted a set of procedures for linking tests to the CEFR in 2003. and a formal manual on the process was published entitle *Relating Language Examinations to the Common European Framework of Reference for Languages: Learning, Teaching, and Assessment in 2009* (Council of Europe, 2009). While many institutions have conducted linking studies, most of these are unpublished or published only as an internal report. One notable exception is the edited collection of linking studies "Aligning Tests with the CEFR: Reflections on Using the Council of Europe's Draft Manual" (Martyniuk, 2010). This collection is particularly useful because it provides an insight into the range of projects that have taken place and reflections on some of the problems encountered by different practitioners and researchers.

Only in the past 10 years has the CEFR become a matter of interest for many institutions in higher education that train signed language interpreters or teachers for the deaf across Europe. This includes a number of projects carried out to develop CEFR-aligned curricular, for example in Ireland (Leeson & Grehan, 2009) and the Netherlands (Van den Bogaerde et al., 2015). Other European projects included ProSigns 1 (2012–2015) and ProSign 2 (2016–2019), which were carried out at the European Centre for Modern Languages in Graz, Austria. As a result of the growing awareness for the learning of a signed language as a second/foreign language in adults, assessment for adult learners has become more prominent in the discussion of the scientific community.

AIMS AND STRUCTURE OF THIS BOOK

The aim of the current volume is to address 12 timely issues in the fields of signed and spoken language assessment and provide thoughtful insights from researchers and practitioners working in these fields. The first six topics (Topics 1–6) focus on the assessment of young learners/children (mono-/bi-/multilingual children), and the remaining six topics (Topics 7–12) were written by authors mostly focusing on the assessment of adult L2 learners. Each topic is addressed sequentially by contributors from spoken language followed by contributors from signed language. The two chapters are complemented by a joint discussion between the authors of each companion chapter.

All chapters in this book are meant as cross-disciplinary dialogues or conversations between colleagues. By including authors from different disciplines and backgrounds, the volume combines the rich experience established in the field of spoken language assessment, including some of the lessons learned from previous mistakes, with a more current perspective represented by deaf and hearing authors from signed language research which, in comparison, is still a very young field. This unconventional approach makes it possible for questions that are relevant to the field of signed language assessment to be discussed and commented on by experts and specialists with long-standing experience in testing of spoken languages. Similarly, it offers spoken language assessment specialists an opportunity to engage with and learn from relevant issues revolving around signed language assessment. To our knowledge, this type of interdisciplinary discussion has never taken place before in this format.

What makes the collaboration particularly exciting is that, aside from all the obvious differences between signed and spoken language assessment (e.g., different modality, different population), there are also many shared interests across both fields. Some of these include issues related to the assessment of (small) non-mainstream populations, the development of robust psychometric values, and the use of new technologies (e.g., web-based testing, mobile-assisted language testing, automatic speech or sign recognition). To those who come to the field of signed language assessment as researchers developing a test or as practitioners looking for a test to use, this volume will serve as a (stimulating) introduction to some of the key issues in signed and spoken language assessment. Specifically, those interested in developing a test for signed language will find the volume helpful to familiarize themselves with the many challenges inherent in this process. To those coming from a background in spoken language assessment, the book offers some fascinating insights into the world of signed language research along with a glimpse at widening the construct with other aspects (such as body language, gestures) and the use of technologies to capture these aspects not commonly assessed in spoken assessment.

The first topic examines issues related to the development of tests for signed or spoken language. Representing the field of spoken language, Penny Roy and Shula Chiat provide insights into the criteria that inform test developers' decisions in Chapter 1.1. These insights are complemented by Rosalind Herman and Katherine Rowley, who present views from the signed language assessment perspective in Chapter 1.2.

The next three chapters (Topic 2) focus on issues related to the use and interpretation of test scores. Starting things off in Chapter 2.1, Bernard Camilleri focuses on the way in which scores and other data obtained from standardized tests for spoken language are interpreted and used for clinical decision-making and highlights both advantages and limitations of these procedures. In Chapter 2.2, Charlotte Enns and Patrick Boudreault then examine critically the different uses of signed language test scores by educators and researchers.

The next three chapters (Topic 3) examine dynamic assessment, a lesser researched area within the language-learning context. In Chapter 3.1, Natalie Hasson reviews multiple models and methods of dynamic assessment that have informed the development of tools to assess language skills in L1 learners. This narrative is picked up in Chapter 3.2 by Wolfgang Mann, Joanna Hoskin, and Hilary Dumbrill, who present rare insights from a signed language (dynamic) assessment perspective.

The assessment of children with autism spectrum disorder/condition (ASD/C), another understudied area, is addressed in Chapters 4.1–4.3 (Topic 4). Starting with Amy Frisbie, Chapter 4.1 describes and critiques the use of standardized measures to evaluate different elements of spoken language with children diagnosed with ASD/C. This is followed by Aaron Shield, Deborah Mood, Nicole Salamy, and Jonathan Henner's Chapter 4.2, in which the authors take a closer look at assessing signed language development in deaf/signing children with ASD/C.

Topic 5 focuses on the assessment of individuals with developmental language disorder (DLD), formerly referred to as specific language impairment (SLI). Particularly for young language users, this is an area where researchers have relied heavily on the judgments of language professionals. In Chapter 5.1, Carol-Anne Murphy, Pauline Frizelle, and Cristina McKean outline recent changes in diagnostic criteria and core features of DLD and discuss how these changes affect assessment. David Quinto-Pozos outlines in Chapter 5.2 some of the challenges related to assessing signing deaf children who are suspected of exhibiting

DLD. This chapter provides much needed insights given that deaf and hard-of-hearing (D/HH) children have been excluded for a long time from consideration for DLD because they did not meet the criteria traditionally used to diagnose hearing children.

Moving on to another understudied population, Chapters 6.1–6.3 (Topic 6) shifts the focus to bi-/multilingual language learners. In Chapter 6.1, Lisa M. Bedore, Elizabeth D. Peña, Kathleen Durant, and Stephanie McMillen review how best practices in the development of assessment can be applied to bi-/multilingual children; specifically, how language history questionnaires can be used to inform the assessment process to make decision about the language(s) of assessment. This is followed by Kathryn Crowe who explores in Chapter 6.2 how areas of assessment that are relevant to bi-/multilingual DHH children can be used to guide practitioners' decisions on selecting and using appropriate assessment materials and approaches. Particular attention is given to assessment considerations that can inform practice when assessment resources for a particular (signed) language are not available.

Susy Macqueen addresses in Chapter 7.1 different notions of an assessment construct (Topic 7) by first considering the nature of speaking and how it is represented in assessment. In Chapter 7.2, Tobias Haug addresses the issue of how constructs in signed language assessment are represented—in most cases implicitly, which is not surprising in a discipline that is just emerging.

In Topic 8, the validation of assessments for second language learners, Carol Chapelle and Hye-won Lee, in Chapter 8.1, address a range of validation practices used to evaluate the degree to which interpretations and uses of test scores are justified in particular contexts. This is followed by Peter Hauser, Krister Schönström, and Christian Rathmann who, in Chapter 8.2, apply an argument-based approach to validate a sample of signed language tests developed for adult language users.

In Chapter 9.1, Ute Knoch reviews research on scoring second language spoken assessments, examining issues related to both human raters and automated scoring. Some of these issues are picked up by Tobias Haug, Eveline Boers-Visker, Wolfgang Mann, Geoffrey Poor, and Beppie Van den Bogaerde in Chapter 9.2, which explores scoring issues of signed language tests that assess adult L2 learners' proficiency.

For Topic 10, test-takers discourse analysis, in Chapter 10.1, Kellie Frost provides an overview of ways discourse analytic methods have informed speaking task and assessment design and explores new approaches to discourse analysis that have emerged in relation to the incorporation of listening and reading to speaking tasks in second language assessment contexts. In Chapter 10.2, Rachel McKee, Sara Pivac Alexander, and Wenda Walton focus on the ways in which interlocutors co-construct communication in the context of the Sign Language Proficiency Interview (SLPI). This chapter breaks new grounds by examining a micro-level aspect of discourse between fluent deaf interviewers and non-native (L2) SLPI candidates.

Focusing on language assessment literacy (LAL), Luke Harding, Benjamin Kremmel, and Kathrin Eberharter discuss in Chapter 11.1 the broad elements of language assessment literacy that might be considered of core importance across different language modalities. More specifically, the authors focus on the specific type of LAL that would need to be developed with respect to the construct of spoken language and present methods for developing and improving construct knowledge related to spoken language among language teachers and other stakeholders. While LAL is a very new concept in signed language assessment, Eveline Boers-Visker and Annemiek Hammer, in Chapter 11.2, address one of the key issues raised in Chapter 11.1: How does modality change the construct-related LAL required of signed language teachers?

The final topic discussed in this book addresses issues related to the use of technology in L2 assessment. In Chapter 12.1, Phuong Nguyen and Volker Hegelheimer provide an overview of the use and usefulness of new technologies in the assessment of L2 speaking in the language-learning classroom and in high-stakes testing. The authors review synchronous and asynchronous technologies employed to assess L2 speaking and outline inherent challenges and opportunities presented by these technologies. In Chapter 12.2, Sarah Ebling, Necati Cihan Camgöz, and Richard Bowden discuss different kinds of signed language technologies and provide examples of how these technologies can be used within the language assessment context.

The epilogue draws together some of the key topics that emerge from this volume and discusses possible opportunities of collaboration between researchers and practitioners interested in signed and/or spoken language assessment.

The chapters in this volume constitute a state-of-the-art view of the key topics and issues central to work in both signed and spoken language assessment. The volume is relevant to practitioners engaged in the development of language assessments and researchers in academic institutions as well as graduate students learning for the first time about their respective disciplines. The breadth of topics covered from the view of authors from different disciplinary backgrounds and schools of thought offers much to our endeavor to develop more appropriate, accurate, and valid language assessments. The breadth of background of the contributors is a real strength of this volume—we hope that this shines through to readers and starts a rich, enduring dialogue that will continue into the future.

REFERENCES

Bochner, J. H., Samar, V. J., Hauser, P. C., Garrison, W. M., Searls, J. M., & Sanders, C. A. (2016). Validity of the American Sign Language Discrimination Test. *Language Testing*, *33*(4), 473–495. https://doi.org/10.1177/0265532215590849

Boudreault, P., & Mayberry, R. (2006). Grammatical processing in American Sign Language: Age of first-language acquisition effects in relation to syntactic structure. *Language and Cognitive Processes*, *21*(5), 608–635. https://doi.org/10.1080/01690960500139363

Brown, A. (2000). An investigation of the rating process in the IELTS oral interview. *IELTS Research Reports Volume 3*. IELTS Australia Pty. Ltd.

Council of Europe. (2001). *Common European Framework of Reference for Languages: Learning, Teaching, Assessment*. Cambridge University Press.

Council of Europe. (2009). *Relating language examinations to the Common European Framework of Reference for Languages: Learning, teaching, assessment. A manual.* http://www.coe.int/t/DG4/Portfolio/documents/Manual%20Revision%20-%20proofread%20-%20FINAL.pdf

Council of Europe. (2020). *Common European Framework of Reference for languages: Learning, teaching, assessment. Companion volume.* Council of Europe Publishing.

Elder, C., McNamara, T., Woodward-Kron, R., Manias, E., McColl, G., Webb, G., Pill, J., & O'Hagan, S. (2013). Developing and validating language proficiency standards for non-native English speaking health professionals. *Papers in Language Testing and Assessment*, *2*(1), 66–70.

Enns, C., Haug, T., Herman, R., Hoffmeister, R. J., Mann, W., & Mcquarrie, L. (2016). Exploring signed language assessment tools in Europe and North America. In M. Marschark, V. Lampropoulou, & E. K. Skordilis (Eds.), *Diversity in Deaf Education* (pp. 171–218). Oxford University Press.

Frost, K., Elder, C., & Wiggleworth, G. (2012). Investigating the validity of an integrated listening-speaking task: A discourse-based analysis of test takers' oral performances. *Language Testing*, *29*(3), 345–369. https://doi.org/10.1177/0265532211424479

Fulcher, G. (2003). *Testing second language speaking*. Pearson.

Haug, T. (2006). *Deutsche Gebärdensprache Verständnistest (DGS-VT)*. Unpublished test.

Haug, T. (2011). Methodological and theoretical issues in the adaptation of sign language tests: An example from the adaptation of a test to German Sign Language. *Language Testing*, *29*(2), 181–201. https://doi.org/10.1177/0265532211421509

Haug, T., Batty, A. O., Venetz, M., Notter, C., Girard-Groeber, S., Knoch, U., & Audeoud, M. (2020). Validity evidence for a sentence repetition test of Swiss German Sign Language. *Language Testing*, *37*(3), 412–434. https://doi.org/10.1177/0265532219898382

Haug, T., Ebling, S., Boyes Braem, P., Tissi, K., & Sidler-Miserez, S. (2019). Sign language learning and assessment in German Switzerland: Exploring the potential of vocabulary size tests for Swiss German Sign Language. *Language Education & Assessment*, *2*(1), 20–40. https://doi.org/10.29140/lea.v2n1.85

Haug, T., & Mann, W. (2008). Adapting tests of sign language assessment to other sign languages: A review of linguistic, cultural, and psychometric

problems. *Journal of Deaf Studies and Deaf Education, 13*(1), 138–147. https://doi.org/10.1093/deafed/enm027
Herman, R., Holmes, S., & Woll, B. (1999). *Assessing BSL development: Receptive Skills Test*. Forest Books.
Hermans, D., Knoors, H., & Verhoeven, L. (2007). *An assessment instrument for Sign Language of the Netherlands*. Saint-Michielsgestel.
Hoffmeister, R. (2000). A piece of puzzle: ASL and reading comprehension in deaf children. In C. Chamberlain, J. P. Morford, & R. Mayberry (Eds.), *Language acquisition by eye* (pp. 143–163). Lawrence Erlbaum.
Leeson, L., & Grehan, C. (2009). A Common European Framework for Sign Language Curricula? D-Sign(ing) a curriculum aligned to the Common European Framework of Reference. In M. Mertzani (Ed.), *Sign language teaching and learning: Papers from the 1st Symposium in Applied Sign Linguistics* (vol. 1, pp. 21–33). Centre for Deaf Studies, University of Bristol.
Leeson, L., & van den Bogaerde, B. (2020). (What we don't know about) Sign languages in higher education in Europe: Mapping policy and practice to an analytical framework. *Sociolinguistica, 34*(1), 31–56. https://doi.org/10.1515/soci-2020-0004
Mann, W. (2007). German deaf children's understanding of referential distinction in written German and German Sign Language. *Educational and Child Psychology, 24*(4), 59–76.
Mann, W., Roy, P., & Morgan, G. (2015). Adaptation of a vocabulary test from British Sign Language to American Sign Language. *Language Testing, 33*(1), 3–22. https://doi.org/10.1177/0265532215575627
Martyniuk, W. (Ed.). (2010). *Aligning tests with the CEFR: Reflections on using the Council of Europe's draft manual*. Cambridge University Press.
May, L. (2011). *Interaction in a paired speaking test: The rater's perspective*. Peter Lang.
Mayberry, R. I., Lock, E., & Kazmi, H. (2002). Linguistic ability and early language exposure. *Nature, 417*, 38. https://doi.org/10.1038/417038a
Morgan, G., & Woll, B. (Eds.). (2002). *Directions in sign language acquisition: Trends in language acquisition research*. John Benjamins.
O'Loughlin, K. J. (Ed.). (2001). *The equivalence of direct and semi-direct speaking tests. Studies in Language Testing*. Press Syndicate of the University of Cambridge.
Pfau, R., Steinbach, M., & Woll, B. (Eds.). (2012). *Sign language: An international handbook*. DeGruyter.
Sandler, W., & Lillo-Martin, D. (2006). *Sign language and linguistic universals*. Cambridge University Press.
Schembri, A., Wigglesworth, G., Johnston, T., Leigh, G., Adam, R., & Baker, R. (2002). Issues in development of the Test Battery for Australian Sign Language Morphology and Syntax. *Journal of Deaf Studies and Deaf Education, 7*(1), 18–40. https://doi.org/10.1093/deafed/7.1.18
Senghas, R. J., & Monaghan, L. (2002). Signs of their times: Deaf communities and the culture of language. *Annual Review of Anthropology, 31*(1), 69–97. https://doi.org/10.1146/annurev.anthro.31.020402.101302
Strong, M., & Prinz, P. M. (1997). A study on the relationship between American Sign Language and English literacy. *Journal of Deaf Studies and Deaf Education, 2*(1), 37–46.

Supalla, T., Newport, E., Singleton, J. L., Supalla, S. J., Metlay, D., & Coulter, G. (1995, April). *An overview of the Test Battery for American Sign Language Morphology and Syntax*. presented at the Annual Meeting of the American Educational Research Association (AERA), San Francisco, CA.

Van den Bogaerde, B., Boers, E., & Hammer, A. (2015, July). *Sign language teaching: An assessment in higher education: Didactic use and effectiveness of the CEFR*. Paper presented at the International Congress on the Education of the Deaf, Athens.

Xi, X., Higgins, D., Zechner, K., & Williamson, D. M. (2008). *Automated scoring of spontaneous speech using SpeechRater v1.0*. Educational Testing Service.

Topic 1

Design of First Language Assessments

1.1

Design of Spoken Language Tests for Hearing L1 Children

Penny Roy and Shula Chiat

The identification of language problems and subsequent evaluation of interventions depend in part on the availability of useful and psychometrically robust assessments to determine their nature and severity and monitor progress. The purpose of these assessments may be to measure a child's language proficiency—that is, how they perform relative to other children and whether they have the language level expected and needed for schooling—or they may have a specifically clinical purpose in identifying the occurrence and nature of a disorder. The purpose of assessment is key to the aspects of language targeted in an assessment and the methods used to target these. In the case of spoken English, there are many language assessments ranging from broad language tests to more narrowly focused measures, reflecting the complexity of the language system and its use.

Test developers are in general agreement that crucial early steps in developing a test are to clarify the purpose of the test and to provide a clear definition of the concept to be measured (Streiner et al., 2015). In considering the development of spoken language tests, the starting point should therefore be a definition of language and its functions. For the purposes of this chapter, we take language to be a representational system that uses forms (phonology) and structures, combining these into words (morphology) and sentences (syntax) to convey meanings and meaning relations (semantics) (Chiat, 2000; Dockrell & Marshall, 2015). In the case of spoken language, *forms* consist of sequences of sound that are produced orally and perceived aurally (rather than graphic forms which are produced manually and perceived visually, as in written language, or signs, which are produced gesturally and perceived visually, as in a signed language). These definitions of language, and specifically spoken language, highlight the complexity of the construct and hence the many aspects that might be measured, collectively or individually, when assessing children's language. They also distinguish *language*

Penny Roy and Shula Chiat, *Design of Spoken Language Tests for Hearing L1 Children* In: *The Handbook of Language Assessment Across Modalities*. Edited by: Tobias Haug, Wolfgang Mann, and Ute Knoch, Oxford University Press.
 DOI: 10.1093/oso/9780190885052.003.0002

from *communication*, the transmission of information. While communication is a key function of language, as defined, it is not the only function, and, conversely, communication does not necessarily involve language. Nonlinguistic communication, for example, may be used for certain types of communication, as exemplified in preverbal infants who are highly attuned and sensitive to the expressions of others and engage in "proto" conversations with caregivers (Bateson, 1975; Trevarthen, 1979) and in adults' use of gestures and facial expressions with language or in their own right. Conversely, while interpersonal communication is the most obvious function of language, as a system that encodes complex meanings and meaning relations language is also used intrapersonally for thinking.

ISSUES IN SPOKEN LANGUAGE TESTS

The tests available for spoken English vary in scope, content, and methods depending on their purpose. Most are direct, eliciting and scoring children's behaviors in response to test items, but some are indirect, eliciting ratings of children's behaviors from adults who know the children well (see Law & Roy, 2008, for discussion). They may target recognition and production of phonology (the sounds and sound combinations that make up word forms); recognition, understanding, and production of vocabulary (lexicon) and syntax (combination of words in sentences); understanding and production of narrative or discourse; or social communication (i.e., understanding and use of language in context). Some are comprehensive, with subtests or subscales targeting a wide range of language skills using a variety of methods, while others target a particular aspect of language using a particular method of elicitation.

The most widely used language assessments in the English-speaking world are direct, composite tests that have been standardized on an English-speaking population. Their purpose is to evaluate a child's broad language skills in relation to peers, and they are particularly appropriate for indicating whether and how well the child is prepared to cope with the language demands of the classroom and whether the child needs language support. Examples of composite tests are the Clinical Evaluation of Language Foundation (CELF; Semel et al., 2017; and CELF-Preschool, Wiig et al., 2006), New Reynell Developmental Language Scales (NRDLS; Edwards et al., 2011), and Preschool Language Scales (PLS; Zimmerman et al., 2014), which target some or most of the structural aspects of language just identified. These typically yield individual subtest (or subscale) scores and composite scores for receptive and expressive language (comprehension and production) that combine subtest scores (see Dockrell & Marshall, 2015, for full a discussion of measurement issues).

Other tests target a specific aspect of language more comprehensively and systematically. They not only indicate the child's performance relative to peers, but also reveal particular areas of difficulty and need, providing a guide for intervention to support the child's language development. The Test for Reception of Grammar (TROG; Bishop, 2003b), for example, assesses children's comprehension of morphology and syntax. The method it uses is picture selection, where the child is asked to identify which of four pictures corresponds to a spoken sentence. One picture matches the morphological or syntactic structure in the sentence, and the other three are distractors differentiated from the target to varying degrees. Success in this test indicates that the child recognizes the morphological or syntactic form targeted and is able to retrieve the meaning it conveys; low performance indicates some difficulty with recognizing or understanding the target structure or processing the pictures to identify the one matching the meaning of the sentence. Sentence repetition tests such as the Sentence Imitation Test (Seeff-Gabriel et al., 2008) also target morphology and syntax. In this case, children are presented with sentences containing particular morphological and syntactic structures and asked to repeat these. Success in sentence repetition tests again indicates that the child recognizes the morphological or syntactic form targeted, while low performance points to difficulties with recognizing or producing the target structures. In contrast to picture-pointing tasks, sentence repetition provides no evidence that the child understands the meaning conveyed by the target forms (see Polisenska et al., 2015). The advantage is that it enables us to assess knowledge of morphological and syntactic structures whose meaning cannot be depicted visually (e.g., determiners, auxiliary verbs) or that are difficult to elicit using pictures (e.g., negative and question structures, relative clauses), and it allows us to sample a wide range of these structures in a task that is quick to administer and score. This example of two different tests that assess the same domain of language illustrates the ways in which choice of test method affects the type of targets that can be tested and the information that the test provides about the child's knowledge of those language domains.

Other spoken language tests focus on skills needed to deal with the spoken forms that convey morphology and syntax. The Diagnostic Evaluation of Articulation and Phonology (DEAP; Dodd et al., 2002), for example, tests speech production and indicates whether children's speech is as expected for their age or is delayed or disordered relative to peers. Other tests target cognitive processes hypothesized to underpin language, such as phonological short-term memory and working memory, which are needed to store and manipulate verbal information, and nonverbal social understanding, which is needed to interpret the meanings behind what people say, taking into account the context in which it is said. While all targets are amenable to various methods of testing, they may be more amenable to some methods than others. For example, direct, highly structured test methods are well suited to testing vocabulary knowledge and sentence comprehension. In contrast, they are not well suited to assessing understanding of language in context or social understanding and behavior. For this reason, indirect methods are commonly used for these targets, with parents/caregivers or teachers asked to rate the appropriateness of children's verbal and nonverbal responses and behaviors, as exemplified by the Children's Communication Checklist (CCC-2; Bishop, 2003a) and the Social Responsiveness Scale (SRS; Constantino & Gruber, 2005).

The preceding examples of spoken language and language-related assessments are just a handful of the many available for English-speaking children, and these serve to illustrate the choice of purpose, targets, and methods to be made in test development. Where existing assessments are psychometrically robust (reliable and valid; see later discussion), widely used in clinical practice, and generally subject to revisions and updated norms, the questions to be asked by anyone considering developing a new test of spoken language are: Do we need it? Does it serve a new purpose? Do the scope and methods of the new test better achieve or supplement the information provided by existing tests?

ISSUES IN TEST DEVELOPMENT

There is general agreement in the field of test development that developing a new assessment or test for spoken language or any other area is a challenging, time-consuming, and costly task (Rust & Golombok, 2009; Streiner et al., 2015). It follows that the rationale for a new test needs to be strong, and a clear "gap" in the market or clinical toolbox must be identified. New tests need in some way to go beyond those tests that are already available. This requires a thorough and exhaustive search not only of clinically relevant catalogues, but also the research literature to ensure that no comparable measure or instrument exists that could be used or modified for use to address the identified need in question. An additional reason for a literature search is to learn more about the nature of the target structure to inform any subsequent selection of components or items for the new test in the event no comparable measure is found. It is argued that, providing a test is valid, successful test development results from a combination of a theoretical advance, an empirical advance, and a practical (market/clinical) need. To illustrate the process, we refer to two preschool assessments of very early processing skills (VEPS) we developed as part of a longitudinal study of early predictors of later language and communication problems: the Preschool Repetition test (PSRep) and the Early Sociocognitive Battery (ESB) (Chiat & Roy, 2008). Both are now fully standardized and published measures: the PSRep is part of the Early

Repetition Battery (ERB), co-normed with the PLS-4[UK] on a stratified sample of children in the United Kingdom (Seeff-Gabriel et al., 2008), and, more recently, the ESB was standardized on a sample of children in the United Kingdom, aged 2;0–4;11, which included bilingual children (Roy et al., 2019).

The motivation for a new test provides the impetus, but not the formal starting point, of test development (Irwing & Hughes, 2018). This may be broad-based, as for example the development of language assessments in countries such as Saudi Arabia, where few if any formal pediatric assessments of language existed (AlKadhi, 2015). In contrast, our motivation for the development of the VEPS measures was narrower and concerned with issues around the unreliability of existing language measures as long-term predictors of outcomes in late-talkers and children with language delay (Bishop et al., 2017; Chiat & Roy, 2008), together with the view that measures of skills that underpin early language development would be better indicators of the reasons for language delay and indicators of longer-term outcomes. Although the development of a test is often in response to a practical problem or, as in our case, a theoretically motivated response to clinical issues, the formal start of test development is to generate a theoretically driven construct and provide a clear definition of what is to be measured. The flow diagram in Figure 1.1.1, taken from Streiner et al. (2015), provides a "road map" (p. 3) of the process and shows the early positioning of construct definition. As indicated earlier, our VEPS measures were theoretically driven and developed as predictors of long-term language and communication skills for clinically referred preschoolers (Chiat, 2001; Chiat & Roy, 2008, 2013; Roy & Chiat, 2014). The PSRep is a word and nonword repetition test of early phonological and memory skills known to relate to later morphosyntactic skills, and the ESB measures early developing sociocognitive skills known to be related to normal language acquisition and impaired in children with autistic spectrum disorders (ASD) (see Chiat & Roy, 2008, 2013, and Roy et al., 2019, for full discussion of the theoretical and empirical evidence underpinning these tests). Our literature searches at the time revealed that no comparable preschool measures existed, and the remainder of the chapter focuses primarily on the left-hand side of the flow chart. As is the case in any clinical test development, in devising our items and subtests/scales we drew on clinical observations and theoretical models and looked at research literature and existing scales. We also needed to specify our target population. Our original target population was preschoolers aged 2;6–<4;0 years who had been referred to speech and language therapy services with concerns about language and communication skills. Most were "late talkers" (Chiat & Roy, 2008), and none had a clinical diagnosis of ASD. Subsequent standardization of both measures has extended the target age range to 2;0–<5;0 years (Seeff-Gabriel et al., 2008; Roy et al., 2019).

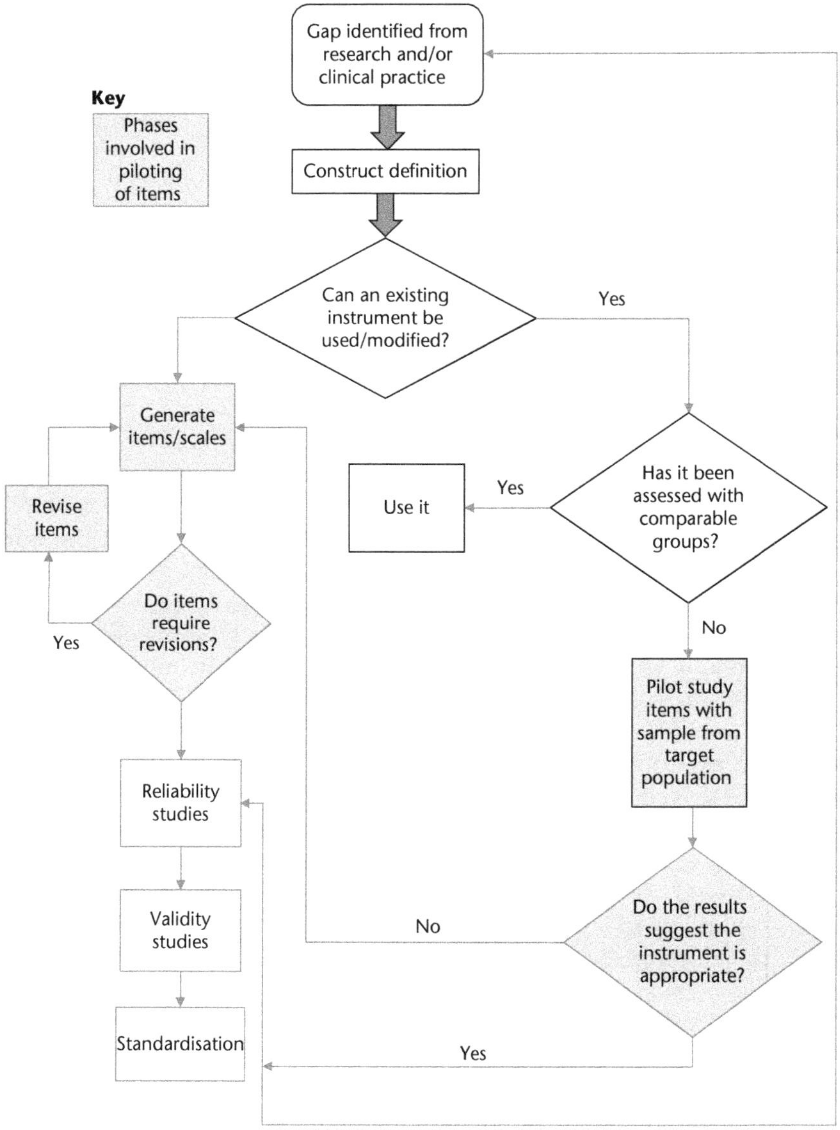

Figure 1.1.1 Flowchart showing stages involved in test development.
Figure adapted from D. L. Streiner, G. R. Norman, and J. Cairney (2015), *Health Measurement Scales* (5th ed.). Oxford University Press. Reproduced with permission of the Licensor through PLSclear.

Once the construct under consideration has been clearly defined, the test's purpose and target population specified, and the components to be included identified, further decisions are required. These include questions around the nature of the task, the number and type of items to be included, and administration and scoring methods. In "criterion-referenced" tests, performance is judged against some external criterion (e.g., the individual's ability to carry out a task), whereas in "norm-referenced" tests an individual's performance is judged against the average performance of a given population (e.g., typically developing children of the same age; see the later discussion on standardization). In reality, although separable, the two approaches have much in common. Not least, reference to external criteria (concurrent or future outcomes) is a necessary part of test validation (see Chapters 8.1–8.3 in this volume). Item selection involves review by experts for face validity/suitability and a pilot study, with a population of individuals similar to those for whom the test is intended. As shown in the flow diagram in Figure 1.1, an early stage of item selection includes the identification and removal of any potentially biased, inappropriate items and redundant/uninformative items (undiscriminating items that are passed or failed by all participants) by referring to group(s) of experts or users and running initial pilot studies with groups similar to but smaller than anticipated target populations. Classical item analysis concentrates on two statistics: *item facility* (redundancy of items, the ratio of the number of respondents who give the right response to the whole number of respondents) and *item discrimination* (extent to which each item correlates with the overall total score) (see Rust & Golombok, 2009). In case of scale development, this may also include the statistical identification of subscales and profiles using, for example, confirmatory factor analysis (CFA); this topic is beyond the scope of the current chapter (but see Irwing & Hughes, 2018). More generally, Rust and Golombok (2009) provide a note of caution, arguing that more sophisticated models drawing on advances in statistics and computing need to be used knowledgeably because high-level statistical analysis does not necessarily make these models problem-free.

Test items can be objective where scoring is objective (criteria provided) or open-ended where scoring is subjective (more reliant on individual judgment). One clear advantage of an objective measure is reliability of scoring. Scoring for both VEPS measures is objective, with scoring criteria provided to support testers' decision-making on whether any given repetition in the PSRep is correct or incorrect (p. 15, Chiat & Roy, 2008; Roy & Chiat, 2004; Seeff-Gabriel et al., 2008) or sociocognitive behavior is present or absent in the case of the ESB (Chiat & Roy, 2008, 2013; Roy et al., 2019). In addition, because respondents are required to attempt all items in an objective test (or to an agreed discontinuation point), objective measures provide information about what individuals don't know as well as what they do know, and this can be clinically informative. For example, children's scores on the ESB subscales, which tap different sociocognitive skills, provide targets for intervention by providing profiles of their strengths and difficulties. On the whole, the development process of objective measures is substantially longer, but, once constructed, scoring is quicker as well as more reliable.

For a test to address a clinical need it should be technically sound (in terms of theoretical grounding and psychometric properties) and useful (Irwing & Hughes, 2018), of which perhaps the most important component is that the results from the test can be shown to correlate with one or more key outcome measures. No measure is entirely error-free, and any test of children's skills and competences is subject to random errors that can affect an individual's performance at any one time. However, test developers have a responsibility to minimize any systematic error inherent in the test and establish its reliability by demonstrating that the test measures something in a reproducible way. While a test can be reliable but not valid, it is impossible for an unreliable test to be valid, and reliability places an upper limit on validity. Although we talk about the reliability of a test as if it were a characteristic of the test in question, Streiner et al. (2015) see reliability as inherently linked to the results of the test *with any one population*. Accordingly, as can be seen from their road map, any test used or modified for use in different populations requires further reliability and validation studies to confirm its psychometric robustness, as was the case with the ESB when used with young Saudi children (AlKadhi, 2015). Likewise, Rust and Golombok (2009) note the importance of human judgment when using published data on reliability. They highlight the need to interpret such information, taking into account the samples used and types of reliability coefficient obtained, as well as the intended use of the test. All published tests are required to report details of reliability and how it was calculated.

According to Irwing and Hughes (2018), three conceptually different estimates of reliability can be described: internal consistency of items, test-retest, and coefficients of equivalence. In many language and language-related tests, including our VEPS measures, total scores are obtained by summing items, implying that items are to some extent measuring the same thing or construct. *Internal consistency* refers to how consistently individual items on a test sample the overall performance and can be statistically calculated using Cronbach's coefficient alpha (see, e.g., Roy & Chiat, 2004). *Test-retest* is appropriate for tests where the focal construct is hypothesized to have some stability across time. It involves administering the test twice to the same group of respondents, separated by a time interval between administrations, generally between 2 and 14 days, although opinions vary on the optimal length of the interval. Test-retest can be seen as an example of *intrarater reliability* (consistency of scores by the same administrator across different occasions), as distinct from *interrater* reliability, which provides a measure of scoring consistency achieved between different raters. Two of the most commonly used statistical coefficients of equivalence are *Pearson's product correlation* and *Cronbach* (see Streiner et al., 2015, for a discussion of their relative merits). Both produce coefficients that are based on rank ordering (not absolute values) of scores and range from

0 (indicative of no relation between two sets of scores) to 1 (perfect and positive relation). Opinions vary on what values are considered acceptable or optimal, and interpretation may depend in part on how the test is used. Nunnally (1978), for example, argued that .7 is acceptable for scales used for group or research purposes and that .9 should be achieved for scales used for judging individuals or clinically. Finally, the production of parallel forms of a test provides another option to assess reliability by looking at the consistency of scores achieved across two equivalent measures of the same construct. However, as Rust and Golombok (2009) point out, in practice this is rarely used, partly because it is time-consuming, but also pragmatically: test developers' preference to select "the best" items is not well served by producing two parallel tests drawing on the same pool of items.

Although reliability gives us some idea of consistency, measures of validity provide information on the degree of confidence we can have on inferences we make based on scores on any one scale (also see Chapters 8.1–8.3 in this volume). Irwing and Hughes (2018) refer to the *3 C's*: content validity, criterion validity, and construct validity. *Content* and *face validity* generally rely on subjective judgments, typically those of one or more experts in the field, on whether or not the test or items of the test sample relevant domains and, on the face of it, if the instrument looks to be assessing what it was designed to measure. Beyond content validity, validation of a new measure can be seen as series of hypothesis testing. *Criterion validity* is perhaps the most common form of validation and arguably clinically the most important. It refers to how well scores on the new measure predict scores on another measure of interest (i.e., the criteria), made either at the same time (concurrent validity) or at a later point (predictive validity). Clearly this process depends on both the quality of existing measures and the theoretical underpinnings of any predicted relationship. Existing measures that are well-established are sometimes referred to as "gold standards," and correlations between at least .4 and .8 are typically required. Although there are more or less well-established language assessments for children that are frequently used for evaluation of concurrent validity, none has been nor—given the complexity of the language system—is likely to be identified as *the* "gold standard," the choice of which varies from study to study (e.g., Law & Roy, 2008). If, on the other hand, no other measures exist, then test developers are reliant on *construct validity*, which rests more on hypothetical constructs and predicted relations and looks at how the measure relates (or does not relate) to other variables in theoretically predicted ways.

Standardization is the last box in the flow chart and is a prerequisite for norm-referenced tests (see earlier discussion). Standardization has two aspects. First, detailed instructions (e.g., in the test manual and record sheets) are provided to ensure that the measure is administered and scored in the same way to all children, to provide all children with an equal opportunity of understanding and responding to test items. Second, scores (norms) are obtained from administering the measure to a large and representative group of respondents. What constitutes "representative" may vary but needs to be specified in full so test users can interpret individuals' results in a meaningful way. Apart from age, most UK standardized developmental language assessments for children include data on key child and demographic factors such as gender, ethnicity, parental educational qualifications (as a measure of socioeconomic status [SES]; Roy & Chiat, 2013), and, if appropriate, distributions may be compared with national statistics. What is meant by a "large" sample size varies and is subject to the nature of the test and availability of funds, but Bishop (1997) recommended a minimum normative sample size of 50 children per age group for language assessments. Apart from defining what is meant by "typical" in a normative sample and determining the extent to which the standard scores are valid, analysis of demographic factors is informative about potential performance bias in any test. For example, recent analyses of ESB standardization data revealed that, in contrast to a measure of receptive vocabulary, scores were unaffected by bilingualism and less affected by SES, supporting its use with children from diverse language and cultural backgrounds.

A long-term objective in the development of the VEPS, and arguably many language measures for young children, was how accurately these preschool measures predicted long-term outcomes measured 7–8 years later. These kinds of evaluations draw on measures of clinical accuracy including sensitivity, specificity, and likelihood ratios (Chiat & Roy, 2013; Roy & Chiat, 2019). This entails identifying cases and non-cases (those with or without a disorder) by selecting cutoffs for predictors and outcome measures. In other words, the distinction between criterion- and norm-referenced tests and between categorical scores (medical diagnosis, the presence or absence of a disorder) or dimensional or continuous scores (proficiency) may be more apparent than real, with the boundary between case and non-case depending on the cutoffs adopted for clinical classification in the continuum of scores on norm-referenced tests. Both categorical and dimensional measures may be involved in validating new tests.

FUTURE DIRECTIONS

Arguably, test development is a process, not a one-off event, that continues as we establish the properties of the test across time. It is both dependent on and contributes to the process of hypothesis testing, hypothesis generating, and theory building with the aim of supporting clinical practice and extending the understanding of young children who struggle to acquire language. For example, a recent report of an intervention study with children with a diagnosis of autism, aged 2–11 years, using the ESB as a baseline measure added to existing evidence in a number of ways (Taylor et al., 2020). Firstly, a high compliance rate established the ESB as a suitable measure for use with older children with complex needs. Second, although our evidence to date had looked at the long-term risks associated with low performance on the battery as a whole, this study took the three subscale scores as outcome measures. The results showed that subscale scores were significantly and *differentially* associated with ASD symptom domains and receptive and expressive language. These findings, in turn, raise questions about how associations between ESB subscale scores, separately and together, and measures of spoken language in different groups, including typically developing children and those with developmental language disorder (DLD; see Chapters 5.1–5.3 in this volume), might add to our theoretical understanding of language development.

REFERENCES

AlKadhi, A. (2015). *Assessing early sociocognitive and language skills in young Saudi children*. PhD thesis, City, University of London (unpublished). https://openaccess.city.ac.uk/id/eprint/13675/

Bateson, M. C. (1975). Mother-infant exchanges: The epigenesis of conversational interaction. *Annals of the New York Academy of Sciences, 263*, 101–113. https://doi.org/10.1111/j.1749–6632.1975.tb41575.x

Bishop, D.V.M. (1997). *Uncommon understanding: Development and disorders of language comprehension in children*. Psychology Press.

Bishop, D. V. M. (2003a). *The Children's Communication Checklist (CCC-2)*. Pearson Assessment.

Bishop, D. V. M. (2003b). *Test for Reception of Grammar (TROG)*. Pearson Assessment.

Bishop, D. V. M., Snowling, M. J., Thompson, P. A., Greenhalgh, T., & the CATALISE-2 consortium. (2017). Phase 2 of CATALISE: A multinational and multidisciplinary Delphi consensus study of problems with language development: Terminology. *Journal of Child Psychology and Psychiatry, 58*(10), 1068–1080. https://doi.org/10.1111/jcpp.12721

Chiat, S. (2000). *Understanding children with language problems*. Cambridge University Press.

Chiat, S. (2001). Mapping theories of developmental language impairment: Premises, predictions and evidence. *Language and Cognitive Processes, 16*(2–3), 113–142. https://doi.org/10.1080/01690960042000012

Chiat, S., & Roy, P. (2008). Early phonological and sociocognitive skills as predictors of later language and social communication outcomes. *Journal of Child Psychology and Psychiatry, 49*(6), 635–645. https://doi.org/10.1111/j.1469-7610.2008.01881.x

Chiat, S., & Roy, P. (2013). Early predictors of language and social communication impairments at ages 9-11 years: A follow-up study of early-referred

children. *Journal of Speech, Language, and Hearing Research, 56*(6), 1824–1836. https://doi.org/10.1044/1092-4388(2013/12-0249)
Constantino, J. N., & Gruber, C. P. (2005). *Social Responsiveness Scale* (SRS). Western Psychological Services.
Dockrell, J., & Marshall, C. R. (2015). Measurement issues: Assessing language skills in young children. *Child and Adolescent Mental Health, 20*(2), 116–125. https://doi.org/10.1111/camh.12072
Dodd, B., Crosbie, S., Zhu Hua, Holm, A., & Ozanne, A. (2002). *The diagnostic evaluation of articulation and phonology*. Psychological Corporation.
Edwards, S., Letts, C., & Sinka, I. (2011). *New Reynell Developmental Language Scales (NRDLS)*. GL Assessment.
Irwing, P., & Hughes, D. J. (2018). Test development. In P. Irwing, T. Booth, & D. J. Hughes (Eds.), *Wiley handbook of psychometric testing* (pp. 1–47). Wiley-Blackwell. https://doi.org/10.1002/9781118489772.ch1
Law, J., & Roy, P. (2008). Parental report of infant language skills: A review of the development and application of the Communicative Development Inventories. *Child and Adolescent Mental Health, 13*(4), 198–206. https://doi.org/10.1111/j.1475-3588.2008.00503.x
Nunnally, J. C. (1978) *Psychometric theory*. 2nd ed. New York: McGraw-Hill.
Polišenská, K., Chiat, S., & Roy, P. (2015). Sentence repetition: What does the task measure? *International Journal of Language & Communication Disorders, 50*, 106–118.
Roy, P., & Chiat, S. (2004). A prosodically controlled word and nonword repetition task for 2- to 4-year-olds: Evidence from typically developing children. *Journal of Speech, Language, and Hearing Research, 47*(1), 223–234. https://doi.org/10.1044/1092-4388(2004/019)
Roy, P., & Chiat, S. (2013). Teasing apart disadvantage from disorder: The case of poor language. In Marshall, C. R. (Ed.), *Current issues in developmental disorders* (pp. 125–150). Routledge.
Roy, P., & Chiat, S. (2014). Developmental pathways of language and social communication problems in 9-11 year olds: Unpicking the heterogeneity. *Research in Developmental Disabilities, 35*(10), 2534–2546. https://doi.org/10.1016/j.ridd.2014.06.014
Roy, P., & Chiat, S. (2019). The Early Sociocognitive Battery: A clinical tool for early identification of children at risk for social communication difficulties and ASD? *International Journal of Language and Communication Disorders, 54*(5), 794–805. https://doi.org/10.1111/1460-6984.12477
Roy, P., Chiat, S., & Warwick, J. (2019). *The Early Sociocognitive Battery*. Hogrefe.
Rust, J., & Golombok, S. (2009). *Modern psychometrics: The science of psychological assessment* (3rd ed.). Routledge.
Seeff-Gabriel, B., Chiat, S., & Roy, P. (2008). *Early Repetition Battery* (ERB). Pearson Assessment.
Semel, E., Wiig, E. H., & Secord, W. (2017). *Clinical Evaluation of Language Fundamentals—Fifth Edition (CELF-5)*. London: Pearson Assessment.
Streiner, D. L., Norman, G. R., & Cairney, J. (2015). *Health Measurement Scales*. (5th ed.). Oxford University Press.
Taylor, L. J., Charman, T., Howlin, P., Slonims, V., Green, J., & The PACT-G Consortium. (2020). Brief report: Associations between preverbal social communication skills, language and symptom severity in children with

autism: An investigation using the Early Sociocognitive Battery. *Journal of Autism and Developmental Disorders, 50*(4), 1434–1442. https://doi.org/10.1007/s10803-020-04364-z
Trevarthen, C. B. (1979). Communication and cooperation in early infancy: A description of primary intersubjectivity. In M. Bullowa (Ed.), *Before speech.* Cambridge University Press.
Wiig, E. H., Secord, W., & Semel, E. (2006). *Clinical Evaluation of Language Fundamentals—Preschool 2 (CELF Preschool 2).* Pearson Education/PsychCorp.
Zimmerman, I. L., Pond, R. E., & Steiner, V. G. (2014). *Pre-school Language Scale—Fifth Addition (PLS-5UK).* Pearson Assessment.

1.2

Design of Signed Language Tests for Deaf L1 Children

Rosalind Herman and Katherine Rowley

Signed languages have been used with deaf children in educational contexts for many years (Bouvet, 1990; Mahshie, 1995; Pickersgill, 1998; Strong & Stuckless, 1995). For signing deaf children, mastery of signed language as a first language (L1) is crucial because it paves the way to communication, with consequences for cognition, socialization, and mental health. It also provides the basis for the development of spoken language, in either its oral or written form, as a second language (L2).

Recent changes in the earlier diagnosis of deafness and earlier use of improved amplification options in the United Kingdom and elsewhere have had a major impact on the deaf population. According to recent UK figures by the Consortium for Research into Deaf Education (CRIDE, 2017), 67% of severely and profoundly deaf children use oral communication, and outcomes for spoken language have improved, with some deaf children achieving near age-appropriate scores on speech and language measures (e.g., Yoshinaga-Itano et al., 2010). However, as Yoshinaga-Itano and colleagues (2010) point out, deaf children with cochlear implants also have access to early intervention initiatives that emphasize spoken language and contribute to improved outcomes. Nevertheless, a significant proportion of children (around 20,000 in the United Kingdom; British Deaf Association, 2019) continue to use signed language as an L1, either because their families are deaf and signed language is the language of the home or because hearing parents choose to learn signed language to communicate with their deaf child.

It is important to deaf children who use signed language and their families that language development proceeds in an age-appropriate manner because delays in language development have an impact on cognitive development (Botting et al., 2017), academic achievement (Mayberry et al., 2010), and socioemotional well-being (Humphries et al., 2014). To ensure appropriate development, professionals who work with deaf signing children need to assess and monitor children's language levels. While a wide variety of tests are used to assess

Rosalind Herman and Katherine Rowley, *Design of Signed Language Tests for Deaf L1 Children* In: *The Handbook of Language Assessment Across Modalities.* Edited by: Tobias Haug, Wolfgang Mann, and Ute Knoch, Oxford University Press. © Oxford University Press 2022. DOI: 10.1093/oso/9780190885052.003.0003 developmental outcomes in spoken language, very few assessments exist for deaf children who are signed language users. Consequently, making decisions about appropriate educational placements or recommending interventions for deaf children is challenging, and such decisions has historically been based on assessments of spoken or written language skills, with only impressionistic assessments being made of signed language skills (Herman, 1998b).

However, the development of effective tests of signed language acquisition is not without challenges. While the general principles of test development that apply to developing spoken language tests (Irwing, Booth, & Hughes, 2018) apply equally to the assessment of signed language development, there are additional issues that test developers face when the language is signed (Woolfe et al., 2010). These include the *limited research base* (only a small minority of deaf children, approximately 5–10% [Mitchell & Karchmer, 2004], have deaf parents and can therefore be considered native users of a signed language) that is available for signed language acquisition, which is important in determining which features of signed language to measure; the *necessary knowledge and skills of those involved* in test development, test administration, and analysis of signed language samples; the most *appropriate test methodology* to use; and issues related to *test standardization and norming*. Our discussion includes examples from available assessments to illustrate how signed language test developers have sought to overcome these issues, including use of newer web-based technologies and initiatives to support tester training, including use of assessment findings to inform interventions with deaf signing children.

THE RESEARCH BASE ON SIGNED LANGUAGE ACQUISITION

Test development is influenced by what is known of language acquisition. Through knowledge of how different aspects of language develop and which areas take longer to master, test developers identify areas that an assessment should target. However, there continues to be far less research on signed language development in comparison with research on spoken languages (Woolfe et al., 2010). This means that the knowledge base for signed language acquisition is less well established and that gaps remain. One example of the limited knowledge available on signed languages is the lack of vocabulary frequency lists. Such lists document the size and content of children's lexicons at different stages (e.g., 1,000, 2,000, 5,000 words, and data on age of acquisition of different words are of great value, particularly when selecting items for vocabulary assessments. Frequency lists (e.g., Bååth, 2010; Cobb, 1998) are widely available for spoken languages but rare in signed languages, although there have been recent efforts to establish such norms for British Sign Language (Vinson et al., 2008) and for American Sign

Language (ASL) (Caselli et al., 2017). There are also only a few studies that have investigated the acquisition of grammatical features in native signers, all of which have focused on BSL. Most of these studies are based on children older than 3 years (e.g., Herman & Roy, 2006; Morgan, 2006).

Although research continues to grow in the field of signed language acquisition, most studies have been based on the acquisition of ASL (e.g., Mayberry & Squires, 2006), which has the longest history of signed language research. Although there are parallels between different signed languages in some areas (e.g., vocabulary and narrative development; Chen Pichler, 2012), findings from ASL cannot automatically be generalized to another signed language. For example, with phonological development, different signed languages have different phonological systems (Johnston & Schembri, 2007), just like different spoken languages, therefore developmental patterns will vary according to the particular phonology (e.g., handshapes used in the language). More research is needed into different aspects of acquisition and in different signed languages to direct test developers to which features of signed language to assess.

Studies of signed language acquisition that are available are usually based on native signers—that is, children in deaf families—who as mentioned above, represent only 5–10% of the deaf population (Mitchell & Karchmer, 2004). Studies therefore include small numbers of participants, ranging from single case studies to groups of up to 30 participants (see Haug, 2011, for an overview of studies and sample sizes), in contrast to studies of hearing children, where samples are much larger. In view of the wide variations in development observed in typically developing hearing children acquiring spoken languages (e.g., Foster-Cohen, 2014), caution must be taken when interpreting studies on small samples. Indeed, there is potentially more variation in deaf children's signed language development compared to hearing children's spoken language development due to delayed exposure to signed language and limited access to fluent signers. As there are relatively few studies that investigate signed language development in deaf children, it is important to carry out further studies to investigate the extent of variability in signed languages in a range of areas and to collect more data on typical signed language development.

KNOWLEDGE AND SKILLS OF TEST DEVELOPERS AND ADMINISTRATORS

As with development of any test, test developers must be familiar with the principles of assessment, such as item generation, reliability, validity, and so forth. In addition, to test signed language development, a high degree of fluency in the language and linguistic knowledge is vital. Knowledge of how signed language acquisition compares to that of spoken language is necessary, along with skills in interacting flexibly with deaf children of different ages (Haug et al., 2018). For many of these areas, the involvement of deaf and native signed language users in the development of signed language assessment tools—and indeed in signed language research more broadly (Jones & Pullen, 1992; Ladd, 2003)—is of central importance. Hearing non-native signers generally have limited signed language fluency and lack the insights and cultural knowledge possessed by deaf and especially native signers. These are crucial in determining whether tests items are culturally or linguistically appropriate for the target group. Given the lack of available research, as mentioned earlier, native signers with knowledge of child development can bring valuable insights into typical signed language acquisition and to the analysis of signed language samples that may be otherwise missed by hearing researchers.

Deaf skilled or native signers play a significant role in administering signed language tests to ensure test stimuli are delivered in a natural, child-oriented register and that signed language samples are representative of the child's potential. Deaf children are skilled at modifying their language when encountering signers who lack fluency, hence use of non-native signers can negatively affect the validity of a language sample collected. Although the involvement of fluent signers during the development and administration of signed language assessments is of paramount importance, very few fluent signers have the necessary training or qualifications to carry out such assessments. This calls for a multidisciplinary approach where qualified and nonqualified test administrators work together to provide a holistic approach to assessing deaf children's signed language skills. For example, speech and language therapists working with deaf children have the requisite training to carry out language assessments and to interpret test scores in order to create targeted interventions, but they may not have sufficient signed language skills to carry out assessments themselves. In such situations, working collaboratively with fluent signers can ensure valid test administration, and, in addition, the assessment team can work together to identify areas of strengths and weaknesses (Hoskin, 2017).

With any research, during the early stages of test development, considerable time and access to child participants is needed. In the United Kingdom, deaf children are now far less likely to attend deaf schools or units and are increasingly educated in mainstream educational settings (78%; CRIDE, 2017). For researchers, this means that they are more difficult to locate. Deaf signers with strong links to the deaf community can be highly effective in communicating research aims to deaf families at events within the Deaf Community to facilitate the recruitment process. Thus, a key consideration when developing a measure of signed language acquisition is to include deaf and native signers as part of the test development team to contribute to the skill mix.

APPROPRIATE TEST METHODOLOGY

Manuals for tests of spoken language generally include guidelines for test administration, including a script that testers follow to ensure administration is standardized. Because there is no written form of signed language, this can affect the delivery of live assessments. Indeed, preliminary pilot work by Herman (1998b) identified inconsistencies in test administration because of precisely this problem. This issue was resolved by using pre-recorded test stimuli, which served to standardize test administration and reduce pressure on testers when administering the BSL Receptive Skills Test (BSL RST; Herman et al., 1999) and subsequent adaptations of this test (Enns et al., 2016; Herman et al., 2016). Later work on signed language assessment has adopted a similar pre-recorded format and gone further, delivering tests via the web (e.g., the American Sign Language Assessment Instrument; Hoffmeister et al., 2014; the BSL Vocabulary Test; Mann & Marshall, 2012).

The development of targets and valid distractor items is a challenge when developing a test in any language. For a receptive test of signed language, attention must be paid to different features when compared with a spoken language. For example, selection of items for a receptive measure must not only take account of the linguistic features of signs, but also *sign iconicity*, which is where form is often closely related to meaning in visually motivated signs, as in the BSL signs for TREE and BALL (Perniss et al., 2010). Other signs (e.g., DRINK, SMOKE) are visually motivated by actions and also highly iconic. These types of signs and others, such as signs indicated by pointing to body parts, may render the target too easy to identify or the distractors too easy to eliminate. A further aspect is the amount of *mouthing* (where English words are visible on the mouth) that accompanies the sign since this may make the item more or less easy to speechread (lipread). The BSL RST (Herman et al., 1999) involves children viewing signed sentences and selecting the one from a choice of pictures that best matches the signed content. During the development of the test, some limited trialing with hearing child participants who had no prior knowledge of sign was carried out to identify and eliminate items that were easy to guess because of either sign iconicity or speechreadability.

Development of measures to assess signed production raises further difficulties. One of these is the need for tester skill in language analysis; another is the lack of a quick and accessible method of transcribing signed language, even with test administrators who are fluent in signed language. For these reasons, relatively few tests of signed production exist. One of them, the BSL Production Test (Herman et al., 2004), is based on a narrative recall task. Children are asked to retell a story viewed on video to a deaf signer who (the child thinks) does not know the story. Children's stories are video-recorded for later analysis. The authors used coding of children's signed utterances to eliminate the need for transcription. Testers undergo a period of training, and their coding reliability is checked before they can be registered to use the test (Herman et al., 2004). These are some of the ways that test developers have attempted to overcome the specific challenges presented when assessing a visuo-gestural language.

DEVELOPING TEST NORMS

When standardizing tests, an essential factor to consider is sample size. It is generally accepted that norms for tests of spoken languages should be based on large numbers of native users. For example, Fenson et al. (2000) collected data from 1,130 children for the Toddler Form and 569 children for the Infant Form of the MacArthur Communicative Development Inventory (CDI), a parent checklist designed to document language development in hearing children from 8 to 36 months. Such large samples of native language users are usually not available for researchers of sign languages. For example, to compare, the CDI was adapted for use with BSL signers and only 29 native signers were recruited (Woolfe et al., 2010). This is partly because of the prevalence of deafness in the general population, which is at 1:1000 births (Fortnum et al., 2001), but also because of the small number of native signers (Mitchell & Karchmer, 2004).

One way of increasing sample size is to include deaf and hearing children from signing families since both grow up to be native signers. However, it cannot be assumed that deaf and hearing children of deaf parents, even if they received the same amount of exposure to sign language, are truly equivalent in terms of language acquisition. Herman and Roy (2000) noted that hearing children in deaf families are likely to be bilingual from an early age, whereas deaf children are more likely to grow up monolingual with sign until they start school. Although no significant differences were found in a study comparing deaf and hearing native signers' performance on a test measuring comprehension of BSL morphosyntax (Herman & Woll, 1998), differences have been observed at earlier stages of development. For example, Gayner (2007) reported differences in the onset of first signs when comparing the developmental trajectories of deaf and hearing native signers. This highlights the need, at least initially, to establish monolingual norms in signed language as a basis for measuring deaf children's progress in language development.

However, for the majority of deaf children with hearing parents, their first exposure to signed language is typically late (the age of exposure varies according to age of diagnosis) because parents usually do not know a signed language and therefore need to learn it themselves first before using it to communicate with their child. Furthermore, sign fluency levels of hearing parents—and indeed of professionals working with deaf children—vary considerably (Woolfe et al., 2010). Hearing families are less likely to use signed language beyond direct interactions with the deaf child; consequently, the deaf child misses out on opportunities for incidental language learning (Lu et al., 2016). If deaf children experience delayed and/or limited exposure to signed language, it impacts the successful mastery of language (Lu et al., 2016; Mayberry, 2007). Research has shown that comprehension skills of deaf children with hearing parents tend to be lower and their morphological skills vary more widely compared to native signers (Kyle, 1990; Mayberry, 2007; Newport, 1990).

Test developers need to be aware of these differences within the deaf population when developing and standardizing measures for use with deaf children. In the development of the first standardized test of any signed language, Herman and colleagues (1999) used native signers to pilot the format of the BSL RST, develop test items, and derive an order of difficulty. However, children from hearing families on bilingual and total communication (a combination of speech with signs; usually signs and spoken words are produced simultaneously in the order of the majority spoken language in a given country) programs were included at a later stage to standardize the measure. Ideally, one should collect data from different subgroups of signing children, both for comparison of test performance, but also because ultimately the wider deaf population consists of such subgroups. From a statistical perspective it is rarely possible to develop separate norms for these different groups since numbers are already small.

Collecting repeated datasets on the same group of children is one way of doing this. Anderson and Reilly (2002) used such an approach when developing the ASL version of the CDI, which was based entirely on data collected from native signers. Of the 69 deaf native signers recruited, 34 were tested longitudinally, yielding 110 datasets. Woolfe et al. (2010) adopted a similar approach in their adaptation of the CDI to BSL. Their sample represented approximately 30% of the estimated number of deaf children born to deaf parents in the United Kingdom within the designated age range (8–36 months). Although small, Woolfe and colleagues argued that their sample represented a much larger proportion of the potential population than is found in any other test standardizations (Woolfe et al., 2010). The approach of collecting repeated data from the same sample has also been used with other signed languages (e.g., Sign Language of the Netherlands; Hermans et al., 2010).

The use of new technologies is rapidly expanding the range of available test formats in sign, for use with both child and adult learners, and offers new opportunities to those involved in the assessment of signed languages (Herman et al., 2020). For example, the BSL RST, originally developed as a video-based test, has now been adapted to a web-based format (Haug et al., 2014; Herman et al., 2016). This has allowed new data to be collected via the internet to update test norms (Herman & Curtin, 2017). These approaches present potential solutions to the challenge of updating test norms on a diminishing population of signed language users.

FUTURE DIRECTIONS

This chapter has presented challenges that face researchers when developing assessments of signed language acquisition for use with deaf children. Despite these difficulties, a number of assessments for different signed languages are now available and used by professionals working in schools to monitor deaf children's language acquisition in sign. A multidisciplinary approach to assessment is necessary, involving the key contribution of fluent or native signers, to ensure an accurate evaluation of deaf children's signed language abilities.

Signed language assessments are also valuable for research that includes signing deaf children. Importantly, the availability of assessments has contributed to our understanding of atypical patterns of signed language development, including the identification of developmental language disorder in signing deaf children (Mason et al., 2010; Quinto-Pozos et al., 2011).

Future developments in signed language assessment will see the increased use of web-based technologies (Herman et al., 2020), offering new possibilities for test formats and opportunities to collect normative data via the internet (Herman & Curtin, 2017, also see Chapters 12.1–12.3 in this volume on new technologies).

However, although much progress has been made over the past 20 years, there is still a long way to go. More assessments are needed to investigate diverse areas of language and for groups of children for whom no assessments are currently available. This includes assessments of higher-level language skills that are important to literacy and learning in older children and assessments appropriate for deaf children with additional needs.

Signed language assessments are only beneficial if the people who administer them do so accurately and are able to understand and make use of assessment findings. A major issue to date has been the lack of fluent and/or native signers, known in the United Kingdom as *Deaf*

Language Specialists (DLSs), working with signing deaf children and the limited and variable training that exists for them. This is compounded by the lack of sign fluency and Deaf cultural awareness in many hearing professionals (Hoskin, 2017, also see Chapter 3.2 in this volume). DLSss' roles include working in multidisciplinary teams with a specific focus on assessing signed language acquisition and supporting the development of children's sign language skills. In the United Kingdom, some DLSs and hearing colleagues receive training in assessment by attending the training course that accompanies the BSL Production Test (Herman et al., 2004). Such courses are important in promoting the development of knowledge, skills, and teamwork in the area of sign language assessment, but more is needed.

A new initiative, "Developing Online Training for Deaf Language Specialists" (*DOTDeaf* https://researchcentres.city.ac.uk/language-and-communication-science/developing-online-training-for-deaf-language-specialists-dotdeaf) based at City, University of London is taking the concept of training in signed language assessment further. Involving teams from the United Kingdom, Spain, Portugal, and Brazil, *DOTDeaf* is creating a range of online modules available in different signed languages aimed at Deaf and hearing staff working in this area. Modules will focus on signed language acquisition and its application to understanding assessment results, approaches to assessment, intervention planning and delivery, and development of a shared vocabulary for Deaf and hearing colleagues. The training developed through *DOTDeaf* seeks to share best practice between different national contexts and improve the skills of professionals, to the benefit of deaf children (also see Chapters 11.1–11.3 in this volume on assessment literacy).

REFERENCES

Anderson, D., & Reilly, J. (2002). The MacArthur communicative development inventory: normative data for American Sign Language. *Journal of Deaf Studies and Deaf Education*, 7(2), 83–106.

Bååth, R. (2010). ChildFreq: An online tool to explore word frequencies in child language. *LUCS Minor*, 16. http://childfreq.sumsar.net/

Botting, N., Jones, A., Marshall, C., Denmark, T., Atkinson, J., & Morgan, G. (2017). Nonverbal executive function is mediated by language: A study of deaf and hearing children. *Child Development*, *88*(5), 1689–1700. https://doi.org/10.1111/cdev.12659

Bouvet, D. (1990). *The path to language: Toward bilingual education for deaf children*. Multilingual Matters Ltd.

British Deaf Association. (2019). www.bda.org.uk

Caselli, N. K., Sehyr, Z. S., Cohen-Goldberg, A. M., & Emmorey, K. (2017). ASL-LEX: A lexical database of American Sign Language. *Behavior Research Methods*, *49*(2), 784–801. https://doi.org/10.3758/s13428-016-0742-0

Chen Pichler, D. (2012). Chapter 29: Language acquisition. In R. Pfau, B. Woll and M. Steinbach (Eds.), *Handbook of Linguistics and Communication Science: Sign Language*. Berlin: de Gruyter.

Cobb, T. (1998). Why and how to use frequency lists to learn words. https://lextutor.ca/research/

Consortium for Research into Deaf Education (CRIDE). (2017). *UK Wide Summary*. https://www.batod.org.uk/wp-content/uploads/2018/02/CRIDEUK2017.pdf

Enns, C. Haug, T., Herman, R., Hoffmeister, R., Mann, W., & McQuarrie, L. (2016). Exploring signed language assessment tools in Europe and North America. In M. Marschark, V. Lampropoulou, & E. K. Skordilis (Eds.), *Diversity in deaf education* (pp. 171–218). Oxford University Press. https://doi.org/10.1093/acprof:oso/9780190493073.003.0007

Fenson, L., Bates, E., Dale, P., Goodman, J., Reznick, S., & Thal, D. (2000). Measuring variability in early child language: Don't shoot the messenger. Comment on Feldman et al. *Child Development, 71*, 323–328.

Fortnum, H. M., Summerfield, A. Q., Marshall, D. H., Davis, A. C., & Bamford, J. M. (2001). Prevalence of permanent childhood hearing impairment in the United Kingdom and implications for universal neonatal hearing screening: questionnaire based ascertainment study. *BMJ* (Clinical research ed.), *323*(7312), 536–540. https://doi.org/10.1136/bmj.323.7312.536

Foster-Cohen, S. H. (2014). *An introduction to child language development*. Routledge.

Gayner, L. (2007). *Language development in deaf and hearing native signers. Unpublished dissertation*. University College London.

Haug, T. (2011). *Adaptation and evaluation of a German Sign Language test: A computer-based receptive skills test for deaf children ages 4–8 years old*. Hamburg University Press. https://doi.org/10.15460/HUP.111

Haug, T., Herman, R., & Woll, B. (2014). Constructing an Online Test Framework, Using the Example of a Sign Language Receptive Skills Test. *Deafness & Education International*. doi: http://dx.doi.org/10.1179/1557069X14Y.0000000035

Haug, T., Mann, W., Boers-Visker, E., Contreras, J., Enns, C., Herman, R., & Rowley, K. (2018). *Guidelines for sign language test development, evaluation, and use*. Unpublished document. http://www.signlang-assessment.info/

Herman, R. (1998b). Issues in designing an assessment of British Sign Language development. *Proceedings of the Conference of the Royal College of Speech & Language Therapists*, 332–337.

Herman, R., & Curtin, M. (2017). *British Sign Language receptive skills: How much has changed in 18 years?* Paper presented at the Annual Conference of the Royal College of Speech & Language Therapists, Glasgow.

Herman, R., Grove, N., Haug, T., Mann, W., & Prinz, P. (2020). The assessment of signed languages. In G. Morgan (Ed.), *Understanding deafness, language and cognitive development: Essays in honour of Bencie Woll* (pp. 53–72). John Benjamins Publishing. https://doi.org/10.1075/tilar.25.04her

Herman, R., Grove, N., Holmes, S., Morgan, G., Sutherland, H., & Woll, B. (2004). *Assessing BSL Development: Production Test (Narrative Skills)*. City University Publication.

Herman, R., & Woll, B. (1998). *Design and standardization of an assessment of British Sign Language Development for use with deaf children: Final report, 1998.* Manuscript. Department of Language & Communication Science, City University London, UK.
Herman, R., Holmes, S., & Woll, B. (1999). *Assessing BSL Development: Receptive Skills Test.* Forest Books (out of print).
Herman, R., Rowley, K., & Woll, B. (2016). *Assessing BSL Development: Receptive Skills Test.* www.dcalportal.org
Herman, R., & Roy, P. (2006). Evidence from the Extended Use of the BSL Receptive Skills Test. *Deafness & Education International, 8*(1), 33–47.
Herman, R., & Woll, B. (1998). Design and Standardisation of an Assessment of British Sign Language Development for use with Young Deaf Children: Final Report to North Thames RHA.
Hermans, D., Knoors, H., & Verhoeven, L. (2010). Assessment of Sign Language Development: The Case of Deaf Children in the Netherlands. *The Journal of Deaf Studies and Deaf Education, 15*(2), 107–119, https://doi.org/10.1093/deafed/enp030
Hoffmeister, R. J., Caldwell-Harris, C. L., Henner, J., Benedict, R., Fish, S., Rosenburg, P., Conlin-Luippold, F., & Novogrodsky, R. (2014). *The American Sign Language Assessment Instrument (ASLAI): Progress report and preliminary findings.* Working paper: Center for the Study of Communication and the Deaf.
Hoskin, J. (2017). *Language therapy in British Sign Language: A study exploring the use of therapeutic strategies and resources by Deaf adults working with young people who have language learning difficulties in British Sign Language (BSL).* Unpublished PhD Dissertation, University College London, UK.
Humphries, T., Kushalnagar, P., Mathur, G., Napoli, D. J., Rathmann, C., & Smith, S. (2014). Bilingualism: A pearl to overcome certain perils of cochlear implants, *Journal of Medical Speech-Language Pathology*, 21(2), 107–125. https://www.ncbi.nlm.nih.gov/pmc/articles/PMC4237221/pdf/nihms589649.pdf
Irwing, P., Booth, T., & Hughes, D. J. (2018) (Eds.). *The Wiley handbook of psychometric testing: A multidisciplinary approach to survey, scale and test development.* Wiley, Chichester, UK.
Johnston, T., & Schembri, A. (2007). *Australian Sign Language: An introduction to sign language linguistics.* Cambridge University Press.
Jones, L., & Pullen, G. (1992). Cultural Differences: Deaf and Hearing Researchers Working Together. *Disability, Handicap and Society, 7*(2), 189–196.
Ladd, P. (2003). *Understanding Deaf Culture.* Clevedon: Multilingual Matters.
Lu, J., Jones, A., & Morgan, G. (2016). The impact of input quality on early sign development in native and non-native language learners. *Journal of Child Language, 43*(3), 537–552. https://doi.org/10.1017/S0305000915000835
Mahshie, S. M. (1995). *Educating deaf children bilingually.* Gallaudet University Press.
Mann, W., & Marshall, C. R. (2012). Investigating deaf children's vocabulary knowledge in British Sign Language. *Language Learning, 62*(4), 1024–1051. https://doi.org/10.1111/j.1467-9922.2011.00670.x
Mason, K., Rowley, K., Marshall, C. R., Atkinson, J. R., Herman, R., Woll, B., & Morgan, G. (2010). Identifying specific language impairment in deaf children acquiring British Sign Language: Implications for theory and practice. *British*

Journal of Developmental Psychology, 28(1), 33–49. https://doi.org/10.1348/026151009X484190
Mayberry, R. (2007). When timing is everything: Age of first-language acquisition effects on second-language learning. *Applied Psycholinguistics, 28*, 537–549.
Mayberry, R., Giudice, A., & Lieberman, A. (2010). Reading achievement in relation to phonological coding and awareness in deaf readers: A meta-analysis. *Journal of Deaf Studies and Deaf Education, 16*(2), 164–188. https://doi.org/10.1093/deafed/e$1$2
Mayberry, R, L., & Squires, B. (2006). Sign language acquisition. In E. Lieven & Keith Brown (Eds.), *Language acquisition: Vol. 11. Encyclopedia of language and linguistics* (2nd ed., pp. 291–295). Oxford: Elsevier.
Mitchell, R., & Karchmer, M. (2004). Chasing the mythical ten percent: Parental hearing status of deaf and hard of hearing students in the United States. *Sign Language Studies, 4*(2), 138–163. https://doi.org/10.1353/sls.2004.0005
Morgan, G. (2006). 'Children are just lingual': The development of phonology in British Sign Language (BSL). *Lingua, 116*(10), 1507–1523. doi:10.1016/j.lingua.2005.07.010
Newport, E. L. (1990). Maturational constraints on language learning. *Cognitive Science, 14*(1), 11–28.
Perniss, P., Thompson, R., & Vigliocco, G. (2010). Iconicity as a general property of language: Evidence from spoken and signed languages. *Frontiers in Psychology, 1*. https://doi.org/10.3389/fpsyg.2010.00227
Pickersgill, M. (1998). Bilingualism, current policy and practice. In S. Gregory, P. Knight, W. McCracken, S. Powers, & L. Watson (Eds.), *Issues in deaf education* (88–97). Fulton Publishers.
Quinto-Pozos, D., Forber-Pratt, A., & Singleton, J. (2011). Do developmental communication disorders exist in the signed modality? Reporting on the experience of language professionals and educators from schools for the deaf. *Language, Speech and Hearing Services in Schools, 42*, 423–443. https://doi.org/10.1044/0161-1461
Strong, M., & Stuckless, R. (1995). A review of bilingual/bicultural programs for deaf children in North America. *American Annals of the Deaf, 140*(2), 83–94. https://doi.org/10.1353/aad.2012.0860
Vinson, D. P., Cormier, K., Denmark, T., Schembri, A., & Vigliocco, G. (2008). The British sign language (BSL) norms for age of acquisition, familiarity and iconicity. *Behavior Research Methods, 40*, 1079–1087.
Woolfe, T., Herman, R., Roy, P., & Woll, B. (2010). Early vocabulary development in deaf native signers: A British Sign Language adaptation of the Communicative Development Inventories. *Journal of Child Psychology and Psychiatry, 51*(3), 322–331. https://doi.org/10.1111/j.1469-7610.2009.02151.x
Yoshinaga-Itano, C., Baca, R. L., & Sedey, A. L. (2010). Describing the trajectory of language development in the presence of severe to profound hearing loss: A closer look at children with cochlear implants versus hearing aids. *Otology & Neurotology, 31*(8), 1268–1274. https://doi.org/10.1097/MAO.0b013e3181f1ce07

1.3

Discussion of Issues Related to Spoken and Signed Language Test Design for L1 Children

Shula Chiat, Rosalind Herman, Katherine Rowley, and Penny Roy

In this discussion of our paired chapters, we highlight the common issues and challenges in spoken and signed language assessment as well as the differences. We consider how experience with spoken language assessment may inform test development in signed language, but also how awareness of issues in signed language assessment may increase awareness of similar issues that are easily overlooked in spoken language assessment—for example, the range of communication contexts and partners that children regularly encounter—and stimulate critical reflection on the use of language tests in general.

HOW SPOKEN LANGUAGE ASSESSMENT HAS INFORMED SIGNED LANGUAGE TEST DEVELOPMENT

As Herman and Rowley point out in Chapter 1.2, a wide variety of tests are available for assessing spoken language, with a particular abundance of English language tests standardized in the United States and/or United Kingdom. As discussed by Roy and Chiat (Chapter 1.1), some of these tests provide comprehensive assessment of receptive and expressive language using a variety of tasks to target many aspects of language, while others target specific aspects such as vocabulary, morphosyntax/grammar, discourse/narrative, and pragmatic language. Where tests are rigorously developed and standardized, as outlined by Roy and Chiat (see Chapters 8.1–8.3 in this volume on test validation), they allow for systematic comparison of an individual child to determine their level of performance and identify difficulties and needs in the area tested. The rich materials available clearly put the assessment of spoken English at a great advantage relative to most spoken languages and any signed languages, but these benefits are not without

Shula Chiat, Rosalind Herman, Katherine Rowley, and Penny Roy, *Discussion of Issues related to Spoken and Signed Language Test Design for L1 Children* In: *The Handbook of Language Assessment Across Modalities*. Edited by: Tobias Haug, Wolfgang Mann, and Ute Knoch, Oxford University Press. © Oxford University Press 2022. DOI: 10.1093/oso/9780190885052.003.0004 caveats that bear on the development of signed language assessments, as discussed by Herman and Rowley.

The sheer range of available spoken language assessments and their value to testers have undoubtedly informed the signed language tests that have been developed to date. In part, this is because spoken and signed languages share many parallels, in terms of both linguistic structure and broad patterns of the acquisition process, in addition to the fact that signed language test developers may be grounded in and draw from assessments of spoken language. This does not mean that unique aspects of signed language acquisition are less important. For example, the development of turn-taking, a key precursor to the acquisition of any language, is particularly significant in the acquisition of signed languages since failure to attend visually to a visually transmitted language means that input is missed. Yet because hearing parents do not naturally share their deaf child's visual perspective, the process of turn-taking in the visual modality often fails to be mastered (Harris & Mohay, 1997; Swisher, 1992). Despite the importance of turn-taking skills, and although not solely the domain of a standardized test, to date no agreed approach to assessment exists.

HOW SIGNED LANGUAGE TEST DEVELOPMENT MAY INFORM SPOKEN LANGUAGE ASSESSMENT

When assessing spoken language development, most testers have a high degree of fluency in the language and are also likely to have received professional training in conducting language assessments and interpreting test scores. As Herman and Rowley point out in Chapter 1.2, the same cannot be assumed for assessors of signed language, where one or the other of these may be absent. Hearing staff are likely to lack signed language fluency, and Deaf staff rarely have access to relevant training on language assessment (Hoskin, 2017), therefore collaborative practice within a team that shares the requisite skills is necessary and recommended. One advantage of this is that, done well, it encourages a focus not only on a single assessment session, but also on a child's broader communication skills with different communication partners, both hearing and deaf. This approach is equally good practice when assessing spoken language development, especially for children with multilingual input. As such it serves as a useful reminder of the need to consider the range of communication contexts in which hearing children typically find themselves and their corresponding contribution to a child's language development.

Variability in tester skill has determined the format of many available tests of signed language, such that prerecorded test stimuli are frequently used because of the need to standardize test administration. In comparison, tests of spoken language are generally considered to be reliable when presented live. The development of signed language assessments has benefited from advances in technology, which permit tests to be administered and scored via desktop, laptop, or tablet devices. These formats convey advantages not only of standardizing test administration but also scoring procedures and, in addition, allow testing to be completed more independently by children and, in some cases, enable groups of children to be tested at the same time. Although not led specifically by developments in signed language assessments, similar moves to computerize tests of spoken language are under way. However, there is a difference between converting a test from hard copy to computerized or web-based format and developing a test for initial use in digital format. For example, the digital construction of the BSL Vocabulary Test (Mann & Marshall, 2012) enables automated selection of appropriate stimuli based on a child's earlier test responses in order to provide a detailed profile of different aspects of their vocabulary knowledge. This would be extremely demanding for the tester in a live assessment session because each child's journey through the assessment is uniquely based on their previous performance. The majority of tests of spoken language development have been designed for live presentation, hence do not capitalize on the digital format in the same way.

ADDRESSING CHALLENGES IN BOTH SPOKEN AND SIGNED LANGUAGE ASSESSMENT

As pointed out earlier, rigorous assessment relies on comparison to relevant peers. Ideally, comparison would be with children who share similar language experience, assuming a relatively homogeneous population. But what about a child who has had significantly less exposure to the test language than all or most children in the standardization sample? Herman and Rowley (Chapter 1.2) highlight the limited research on the acquisition of signed language compared with spoken language and the challenges in identifying which deaf children and how many to include when standardizing an assessment of signed language development. However, it is important to acknowledge that the first two decades of research on English language acquisition focused largely on middle-class monolingual children. A turning point in child language research was a book by Hart and Risley (1995) that opened researchers' eyes to the wide disparity in vocabulary experienced by children from more or less advantaged socioeconomic backgrounds and the corresponding disparity in their language development. These differences have since been confirmed and extended with a plethora of research on socioeconomic factors in language development (see Roy & Chiat, 2013, for a review). Likewise, there is increasing awareness of multilingualism and issues involved in assessing children exposed to different languages (see Chapters 6.1–6.3 in this volume on assessing multilingual children) and with variable and sometimes unknown levels of exposure to the language of testing. This is an issue that is equally relevant when assessing children's signed language acquisition, where exposure is typically from hearing adults who lack fluency in signed language.

In requiring that the standardization sample is socioeconomically and geographically representative of the target population, standardization of tests goes some way to address the potential impact of differences in experience on children's scores. However, with reference to tests of spoken language development, the resulting norms are an aggregation of the groups within the sample, and this must be taken into account when considering reports that a third to half of children in low socioeconomic groups meet criteria for moderate to severe impairment on standardized tests of receptive and expressive language (Roy & Chiat, 2013). This raises the possibility that children be assessed in relation to performance in their own community rather than the aggregated performance norms of the population, which would require different norms to be provided for different subgroups. But what would be the purpose of such standardization? What information would it provide about these children's language development and knowledge? And how would subgroup norms help in assessing children in multilingual populations who have disparate language experience (i.e., populations that cannot be classified into substantial subgroups sharing similar language experience)?

Considerations of standardization sample size present a major challenge in the field of deafness where the population of signing deaf children is small and heterogeneous; therefore, developing norms for subgroups is even more problematic. Increasingly, the dwindling population of deaf signing children in the United Kingdom and elsewhere in recent years falls into two distinct subgroups: children in deaf families who typically have no additional difficulties and benefit from early and fluent language exposure, and children in hearing families, among whom those with additional difficulties are heavily represented, who receive later and less fluent input and who subsequently fail to achieve age-equivalent language skills (Herman & Curtin, 2017). To address the issue of small population size, it has become accepted that developers of signed language assessments generally include much smaller numbers when developing test norms and also look at alternative ways of increasing sample size, such as collecting longitudinal data from the same small group of children. It should be pointed out that both of these approaches bring risks because small numbers are more likely to contain greater variability, and anomalies in a small dataset are potentially amplified by the inclusion of repeated measures.

In the case of spoken language, dilemmas arising from different profiles of subgroups of the population have led to a useful distinction between language proficiency and language ability (Gathercole et al., 2016) and differentiation of tests to assess these. Standardized tests of receptive and expressive language provide a useful indication of the child's language knowledge and proficiency and, importantly, their readiness to meet the language demands of the classroom. If children score within or above the normal range, they should not have problems. However, test developers need to caution test users about the interpretation of scores that are below the normal range because tests do not reveal whether children's performance is low due to limited language experience or whether it is low due to a language disorder (also see Chapters 3.1–3.3 of this volume on dynamic assessment). These different sources of difficulty have different implications for the support that children need, but teasing them apart is no easy matter, particularly when assessing children who use signed language. For these children, careful consideration must be given to the timing, quality, and quantity of language exposure, and decisions about language disorder must be determined based on these factors and from comparisons with children who have similar language experiences.

Although far from solving the problem of variability in input, in the field of spoken language assessment there is increasing interest in assessments that require limited if any exposure to a particular language and can therefore help to distinguish language *abilities* from language *knowledge and proficiency*. The Early Sociocognitive Battery discussed by Roy and Chiat in Chapter 1.1 is an example of such an assessment, targeting sociocognitive skills that are known to underpin the development of social communication and language and to be impaired in some children with delayed and disordered language. Skills in phonological processing and memory are also prerequisites for language development that can to some extent be tested independently of language experience by using nonword repetition tasks which require the child to repeat a phonological form they have never heard before. We would expect standardized tests using such tasks to be valid regardless of language experience, whether socioeconomic, geographical, or cultural. Evidence on the Early Sociocognitive Battery (Roy et al., 2019) has shown this to be the case (Roy & Chiat, 2019), and most though not all research on nonword repetition has found that performance is independent of socioeconomic and language background and is indicative of language abilities (see Chiat & Polišenská, 2016). A test of non-sign repetition has been developed to target similar skills in British Sign Language (Mann & Marshall, 2010), although for different purposes, and future research is needed to indicate whether performance on this type of measure is equally predictive of later language skills.

Another example is *novel word-learning*: novel word-learning tasks target crucial language-learning skills (the ability to link a new phonological form to a meaning and retain this over time) and have been a focus of dynamic assessments aimed at children from different backgrounds using spoken (Peña et al., 2001) and signed languages (Mann et al., 2014) (also see Chapters 3.1–3.3 in this volume). However, while word-learning tasks can be standardized, for a number of reasons they do not lend themselves to standardization. The process of introducing children to new words and testing their understanding and production of the new words is difficult to systematize and is necessarily spread over time; the number of items tested is therefore limited, and, particularly where prompts are given (as in dynamic assessment) and partially correct responses are credited, devising systematic and reliable criteria for scoring is challenging. This illustrates the tensions of test development that can arise between the selection of optimally informative targets (e.g., word-learning, and turn-taking) and selection of psychometrically optimal methods (with precisely specified targets, responses, and scoring to ensure reliability of scores and allow rigorous comparison with peers). Nonetheless, given the importance of word-learning abilities for language acquisition, it is worth addressing the challenges of standardizing word-learning tests in future in order to realize their potential as universally valid assessments of key skills.

CONCLUSIONS ON SPOKEN AND SIGNED LANGUAGE ASSESSMENT

Looking across test development issues in spoken and signed languages reveals some areas that are comparable in both types of language and others that contrast. Inevitably, since tests of spoken language were developed before the first tests of signed language, they have been influential in directing the focus and approach adopted by those developing tests of signed language. However, the more recent development of signed language tests during a period of rapid technological growth has ensured that they maximize the potential of the digital medium, whereas computerized tests of spoken language development are likely to be a direct adaptation of the original "hardcopy" test.

Directions for the future in the field of spoken and signed language assessment include tests of skills that underpin language and avoid language exposure limitations to better distinguish language proficiency and knowledge. More tests of signed languages are needed, including tests that extend to older children for whom no measures currently exist. Finally, developers of signed language measures should consider areas unique to signed communication that are important for language development as the focus for future assessments.

REFERENCES

Chiat, S., & Polišenská, K. (2016). A framework for crosslinguistic nonword repetition tests: Effects of bilingualism and socioeconomic status on children's performance. *Journal of Speech, Language, and Hearing Research, 59*(5), 1179–1189. https://doi.org/10.1044/2016_JSLHR-L-15-0293

Gathercole, V. C. M., Kennedy, I., & Thomas, E. M. (2016). Socioeconomic level and bilinguals' performance on language and cognitive measures. *Bilingualism: Language and Cognition, 19*(5), 1057–1078. https://doi.org/10.1017/S1366728915000504

Harris, M., & Mohay, H. (1997). Learning to look in the right place: A comparison of attentional behavior in deaf children with deaf and hearing mothers. *Journal of Deaf Studies and Deaf Education, 2*(2), 95–103. https://doi.org/10.1093/oxfordjournals.deafed.a014316

Hart, B., & Risley, T. R. (1995). *Meaningful differences in the everyday experience of young American children*. Brookes.

Herman, R., & Curtin, M. (2017). *The BSL Receptive Skills Test: How much has changed in 18 years?* Paper presented at the National Conference of the Royal College of Speech & Language Therapists, Glasgow.

Hoskin, J. (2017). *Language therapy in British Sign Language: A study exploring the use of therapeutic strategies and resources by Deaf adults working with young people who have language learning difficulties in British Sign Language (BSL).* Unpublished dissertation, University College London.

Mann, W., & Marshall, C. (2010). Building an assessment use argument for sign language: The BSL Nonsense Sign Repetition Test. *International Journal of Bilingual Education and Bilingualism, 13*(2), 243–258. https://doi.org/10.1080/13670050903474127

Mann, W., & Marshall, C. (2012). Investigating deaf children's vocabulary knowledge. *Language Learning, 62*(4), 1024–1051. doi: 10.1111/j.1467-9922.2011.00670.x

Mann, W., Peña, E. D., & Morgan, G. (2014). Exploring the use of dynamic language assessment with deaf children, who use American Sign Language: Two case studies. *Journal of Communication Disorders, 52*, 16–30. https://doi.org/10.1016/j.jcomdis.2014.05.002

Peña, E., Iglesias, A., & Lidz, C. S. (2001). Reducing test bias through dynamic assessment of children's word learning ability. *American Journal of Speech-Language Pathology, 10*(2), 138–152. https://doi.org/10.1044/1058-0360(2001/014)

Roy, P., & Chiat, S. (2013). Teasing apart disadvantage from disorder: The case of poor language. In Marshall, C. (Ed.), *Current issues in developmental disorders* (pp. 125–150). Routledge.

Roy, P., & Chiat, S. (2019). The Early Sociocognitive Battery: A clinical tool for early identification of children at risk for social communication difficulties and ASD? *International Journal of Language and Communication Disorders, 54*(5), 794–805. https://doi.org/10.1111/1460-6984.12477

Roy, P., Chiat, S., & Warwick, J. (2019). *Early Sociocognitive Battery*. Hogrefe.

Swisher, M. V. (1992). The role of parents in developing visual turn-taking in their young deaf children. *American Annals of the Deaf, 137*(2), 92–100. https://doi.org/10.1353/aad.2012.1086

Topic 2

Score Use and Interpretation of First Language Assessments for L1 Children

2.1

Score Use and Interpretation of First Spoken Language Assessments

Bernard Camilleri

Assessments of a hearing child's first language (L1) abilities are usually carried out by a speech and language therapist/pathologist in the context of a concern being raised about the child's language, either by a parent, teacher, or other relevant person in the child's environment. In this context, several elements are involved in collecting information to reach decisions regarding the child's eligibility for services as well as about clinical management more broadly (Roseberry-McKibbin, 2007). The use of "standardized," "norm-referenced" language assessments, where a child's score is compared to the mean and range of scores obtained by a standardization (normative) sample of children, is but one of these elements. Also, these assessments can only be adopted when they have been developed using a sample of children with a linguistic and social-cultural context that approximates the child's own (Friberg, 2010). For example, assessments developed in the United States cannot be used in the United Kingdom or Australia without adaptations and fresh normative data, which reflects the responses and therefore the norms that are specific to children within those contexts. A case in point is the UK fifth edition of the Clinical Evaluation of Linguistic Fundamentals (CELF-5 UK; Wiig et al., 2013), which was originally developed in the United States but subsequently adapted and renormed for UK populations. A separate version of the CELF, with different test items (i.e., not simply translated) was developed specifically for the Hispanic population in the United States using normative data from speakers of Spanish as an L1 in the United States. It goes without saying that standardized assessments for one L1 cannot simply be translated for a child with a different L1 (American Speech-Language-Hearing Association [ASHA], 2019). While the use of suitable standardized assessments is not always possible, in English-speaking countries and in other contexts where a range of standardized and locally normed assessments are indeed available, clinicians have

Bernard Camilleri, *Score Use and Interpretation of First Spoken Language Assessments* In: *The Handbook of Language Assessment Across Modalities*. Edited by: Tobias Haug, Wolfgang Mann, and Ute Knoch, Oxford University Press.
 DOI: 10.1093/oso/9780190885052.003.0005

tended to put a lot of emphasis on these measures when making clinical decisions (Friberg, 2010).

The use of standardized assessments of language mirrors that of the traditional use of IQ tests in the field of educational psychology, which is the context in which norm-referenced assessments of cognitive functioning or "intelligence" were originally developed (Gould, 1997). As pointed out by Gould (1997), intelligence or other cognitive functions, such as language, are not "things" that can be measured as one might measure a square or a rectangle, and therefore choice of assessment and interpretation of scores on these assessments need to be carried out with some caution. Any scores derived from a standardized assessment will need to be interpreted on the basis of a range of factors to do with the assessment's properties, the child, and the questions that the professional seeks to address (Friberg, 2010). This chapter discusses key issues that need to be considered when scoring and interpreting standardized assessments of L1. The evolving role of standardized assessments in the context of working with children with L1 difficulties will also be addressed (see also Chapter 5.1). First, however, factors that influence the choice of standardized assessment will be addressed. Scores derived from an assessment and subsequent interpretations are only useful if the right assessment has been chosen in the first place.

CHOOSING AN ASSESSMENT

While there are elements shared in common across standardized assessments, there are also aspects that will be unique to each individual test. As Friberg (2010) points out, each commercially available, standardized language assessment comes with an examiner's manual that enables the user to explore the features that pertain to the specific test and to make an informed decision as to whether it will help address the appropriate questions. The manual will also provide information regarding the assessment's reliability and validity and other important statistical characteristics, such as standard error of measurement (SEM), internal consistency, test-retest reliability, and concurrent validity (Wiig, 2001).

One other common element is that the manual will prescribe procedures for carrying out the assessment. This should ensure that each individual's performance, and therefore their score on the assessment, is not affected by extraneous variables such as tester bias or variations in presentation of materials. A precise description of how the procedure needs to be carried out is one of the crucial criteria identified by Friberg (2010) when choosing a standardized assessment. Any difference in how the assessment is carried out compared to its use with the standardization sample (the group of children used to establish normative data) renders the scores and subsequent interpretation invalid

(Friberg, 2010). Friberg (2010) also specifies that the assessment should include information on the purpose of the test. This is important because some assessments might be designed to identify the presence or absence of a language disorder, while others may be used to determine severity or a recognized disorder or to help specify goals for intervention. The latter are likely to be assessments that address one aspect of language specifically and in some detail (e.g., assessments of expressive grammatical skills or narrative skills).

Assessments that cover various aspects of language are used to determine the absence or presence of a language disorder as well as to identify areas of relative strength and weakness across language areas. Even when an assessment aims to cover language skills broadly, the underlying theoretical constructs may vary. So, for example, the CELF-5 (Wiig et al., 2013) looks at linguistic skills as well as the interface between linguistic skills and auditory memory, retrieval, and recall. Other assessments will focus more exclusively on linguistic aspects to do with understanding and expression of semantics and syntax, such as the New Reynell Developmental Scales (Edwards et al., 2011). When interpreting the results of an assessment, the clinician needs to have chosen an assessment that matches the clinician's purposes and questions (Friberg, 2010).

One of the most important elements to consider when choosing an assessment is that the standardization sample should be clearly specified and of sufficient size to be representative when comparing the individual child's score to the normative data. Friberg (2010) specified a standardization sample of at least 100 children per age subgroup as being a requisite for valid conclusions to be reached from test scores. Perhaps even more critical is the description of the geographical, socioeconomic, and linguistic status of the children included in the standardization sample. A child's scores on a language assessment and any resulting interpretations are only valid if the child's linguistic, geographical, and socioeconomic status is represented within the test itself (Friberg, 2010). Another crucial factor in interpreting assessment results is whether children with identified language disorders were included in the standardization sample. Where children with language impairments have been included in the sample, the assessments have been found to be less accurate for the purpose of identification of children with language disorders (Peña et al., 2006). These assessments are more suitable for determining the severity of difficulty as opposed to identifying a difficulty.

SCORING AND INTERPRETING STANDARDIZED ASSESSMENTS

Standardized, norm-referenced assessments fundamentally enable test administrators to answer this question: "How does the individual compare to the average and range in the standardization population on given tasks?." Assessment manuals need to provide the data to allow the assessor to make this comparison. When a child carries out tasks on a standardized assessment they achieve a score, which typically is the tally of correct responses to items on the test. With some assessments, this unconverted or "raw" score can be compared against data (in the manual) regarding the means and ranges of scores for the child's relevant age group.

With most standardized assessments, however, the unconverted or "raw" score is not used directly to compare the child's performance with the standardization sample. Rather, the child's raw score is converted to a *standard score* using tabulated information in the handbook. One of the advantages of converting raw scores to standard scores is that the mean as well as the standard deviation (a figure which specifies the distribution of scores) for standard scores are stable across age groups as well as across different subtests of a given standardized assessment. For example, the manual might specify that the mean score is 100 and the standard deviation is 15 (this is the case with many standardized assessments, including IQ tests and assessments of language) across the age range for the assessment (see Figure 2.1.1).

If a child were assessed at two points in time (e.g., at age 4 years and 5 years), they would achieve different raw scores (naturally, higher at

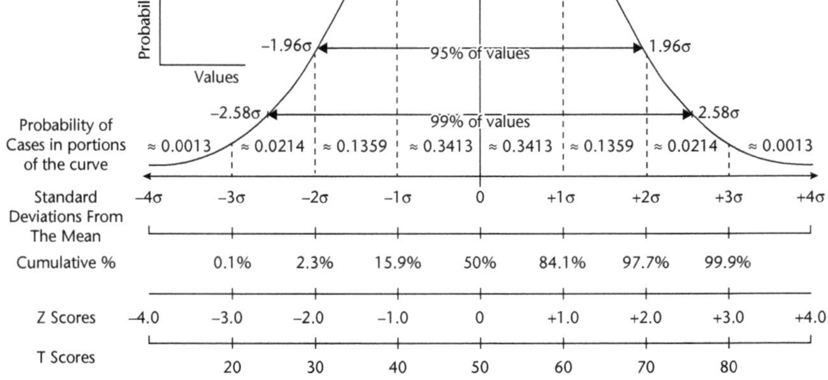

Figure 2.1.1 Standard scores and their percentile equivalents on a normal distribution with a mean of 100 and a standard deviation of 15.

age 5). However, if at both points in time, their raw scores were found to be equivalent to a standard score of 100, one could conclude that the child was functioning at a perfectly average or typical level for his or her age on both occasions.

An important point to make is that standardized assessments of L1 (as of other cognitive domains) are based on the assumption that language skills follow a normal distribution (as in Figure 2.1.1), with predictable proportions of children achieving scores at set intervals (standard deviations) from the mean. A detailed discussion of normal distributions and the assumptions on which they are based is beyond the scope of this chapter. However, it is worth mentioning here that, with any normal distribution, 68% of the population will achieve a score within one standard deviation from the mean and 95% of the population will achieve a score within two standard deviations of the mean, distributed equally either side of the mean. These scores are also usually accessed by using tabulated data within the assessment manual and/or can be represented visually, as in Figure 2.1.1.

A *percentile* score translates the standard score to a measure which informs the assessor of how many children out of 100 would achieve a score that is lower or higher than the child being assessed. With a mean of 100 and a standard deviation of 15, the assessment manual would indicate that a child achieving a standard score of 85 would equate to the 16th percentile (as can be seen in Figure 2.1.1). Out of 100 children, 15 would achieve a lower score, while 84 would achieve a higher score. A child achieving a standard score of 70 (exactly two standard deviations below the mean) would be on the second percentile—with only 1 out of 100 children achieving a lower score. Standard or percentile score can be compared across different subtests of an assessment or indeed across different assessments, allowing for an estimate of a child's relative areas of strength and weakness.

The *age equivalent score* is an estimate of the age at which the raw score achieved would equate to an average score for that age. For example, a 5-year-old might achieve a raw score which equates to a standard score of 85 (percentile score of 16). However, the same raw score would be equivalent to a standard score of 100 for a younger child—for example a 4-year-old. In this case, the raw score for the 5-year-old child would therefore equate to an age-equivalent score of 4 years. As pointed out by some authors of standardized assessment themselves (e.g., Wiig et al., 2013), age equivalent scores need to be used with caution, partly because the conclusion that the child is performing like a typically developing younger child might be erroneously reached. The quantitative score could easily mask the fact that the child's performance in the test was qualitatively very different from that of a younger "average" child in terms of which elements of the test are completed correctly and which are not. This, of course, raises the point that every performance on a standardized assessment can be qualitatively analyzed for these different patterns, particularly as a child may demonstrate patterns of strength and weakness across different items or elements of the test. If the emphasis is on purely quantitative interpretation of numerical scores, this can be easily overlooked.

INTERPRETATION: CAN YOU TRUST THOSE SCORES?

An important consideration in interpreting the standard score obtained by a child relates to the reliability of the assessment and specifically to the *standard error of measurement* (SEM) of the assessment. Every standardized assessment has a built-in element of error, which means that a specific score may be an over- or underrepresentation of the child's skills. An error of measurement is the difference between a person's hypothetical true score and the actual score obtained when an assessment is carried out. Many assessments will use (or convert) the SEM figures to a 90% or 95% confidence interval range. This provides information on the range within which a child's true score is likely to be with a given score on a single administration of the test. So, if a child obtained a standardized score of 85, with a 90% confidence interval range of (for example) plus or minus 6, the score of 85 cannot be guaranteed to be correct. However, we can be 90% certain that the child's true score falls within the range of 79–91. If we could hypothetically give this child the same test 100 times without any learning effects, then 90 times the child would obtain a score between 79 and 91. In both research and clinical contexts, standardized scores or percentile scores are often adopted without mention of confidence intervals, but rather are reported as children's "true" scores. Wiig (2001) cautions against the use of exact scores for diagnostic purposes, putting forward the 90% confidence range as being the more appropriate scores on which to base decisions. The built-in margin of error could be considered one of the limitations of a standardized assessment. Perhaps a greater limitation arises from the lack of awareness of the implications of this when interpreting scores without considering confidence intervals.

RECENT DEVELOPMENTS IN THE INTERPRETATION OF STANDARDIZED ASSESSMENTS: DIAGNOSTIC CRITERIA VERSUS DIAGNOSTIC TOOLS

A recent multinational and multidisciplinary consensus study (CATALISE) by Bishop and colleagues (2016) set out to bring together expert researchers and practitioners across different English-speaking countries in the field of child language toward reaching agreement on several key aspects to do with the identification and classification of language impairments in children. Assessment of children's L1 was not the only focus of this study, but the use and interpretation of different assessments generally and of standardized assessments in particular constituted a recurrent theme.

The first key consensus statement reached by Bishop et al. (2016) reinforces the point made at the start of this chapter, as well as by several others (e.g., ASHA, 2019; Friberg, 2010; Wiig, 2001), which is that multiple sources of information should be combined in assessing a child's language. These should include gathering information from relevant caregivers and professionals and direct observations within naturalistic setting, as well as scoring and interpreting performance scores on norm-referenced assessments. They emphasize that standardized assessments are particularly useful at highlighting relative strengths or weaknesses in specific components of language, including areas that might otherwise go unnoticed—for example, difficulties with understanding the L1. They also highlight the point that there is no clear cutoff between what should be considered a low score within the normal range and a score that clearly indicates an impairment, but rather that children falling on the extreme lower end of the scale will require intervention because they are unlikely to "catch up" with their peers (Bishop et al., 2016). Simultaneously, children achieving low scores closer to the mean may still be clinically considered as requiring intervention and may continue to experience longer term difficulties into adolescence (Spaulding et al., 2006, 2012; Tomblin, 2008). The extent to which a child's language difficulty affects performance within their social and educational context needs to be considered alongside a child's performance on standardized assessments.

Another consensus statement that specifically relates to standardized assessments is that these should be used in a staged way, such that an initial assessment would assess a range of skills to include both receptive (understanding language) and expressive (speaking) elements. This would indicate the broad nature and severity of any existing difficulty. The CELF-5 is one such assessment (Wiig et al., 2013). Wiig (2001) cautions against interpreting the results of individual subtests of such broad assessments for diagnostic purpose, but rather advocates for the use of the composite score, which combines both receptive and expressive elements. The exception would be a situation where there was a marked discrepancy between receptive and expressive skills or where the 90% confidence intervals for receptive and expressive scores did not overlap—indicating a markedly greater difficulty in either aspect of language. The use of a broad assessment of language for initial diagnostic purposes could be followed by more specific evaluations as necessary. For example, a test of a child's expressive syntactic skills or of narrative skills could be adopted if this was an area that required further investigation. This is where the choice of standardized assessments needs to be carefully considered (Friberg, 2010), as discussed in the previous section. Specific components of language could also be assessed alongside an intervention, using a range of information-gathering tools not restricted to norm-referenced assessments. Aspects of language that are difficult to assess with norm-referenced tests, such as pragmatic skills, are likely to be evaluated alongside an intervention by adopting a range of means. These can include formal (but not norm-referenced) assessments that provide the clinician with a framework for making clinical decisions. Checklists, such as the Children's Communication Checklist (Norbury et al., 2004) or the Language Use Inventory for Young Children (O'Neill, 2007), are completed by or with caregivers and other relevant people and are perhaps the most useful approach to identifying children with pragmatic difficulties that have a functional impact on children's lives (Bishop et al., 2016). The CELF-5 (Wiig et al., 2013) contains a Pragmatic Activities Checklist (PAC) for this purpose. With these formal (but not norm-referenced) assessments, a specified pattern of responses is indicative of a diagnosis of pragmatic language difficulty. They can also constitute a source of qualitative information about the individual child's profile of difficulties in this area of language.

The most controversial aspect addressed by the consensus study (Bishop et al., 2016) was whether the diagnosis of a language disorder should be reserved to cases where there is a mismatch between language abilities and nonverbal abilities as measured by performance scores on standardized language assessments and nonverbal IQ tests, respectively (see Chapters 5.1–5.3 for a detailed discussion). The overall conclusion was that, while there may be occasions where researchers may wish to adopt exclusionary criteria and look at children with "pure" or "specific" language impairments, in clinical settings this is not appropriate (Bishop et al., 2016). The view that a child with language difficulties but average (or above average) nonverbal ability would be one eligible for intervention is based on the implicit belief that the discrepancy between verbal and nonverbal ability represents a gap that needs to be bridged, whereas a profile of difficulty across both verbal and nonverbal skills does not warrant intervention (Bishop et al., 2006). This argument has been shown to be invalid on several grounds, starting with criticisms of the measures themselves and the fact that discrepancy scores are too unstable to constitute a reliable basis of classification (Cole et al., 1995). As Bishop et al. (2016) argue, the key question—certainly in clinical practice—should always be whether a child is functionally affected by a language difficulty within their daily lives and whether they would benefit from intervention. Neither of these two questions is influenced by nonverbal IQ. The International Classification of Disease (ICD 11; WHO, 2019), which is currently available in "release" version online, omits both the explicit need for a discrepancy between language and nonverbal ability and the specification of cutoff points on standardized

L1 assessment while adopting terminology which mirrors that adopted by the CATALISE project (Bishop et al., 2016).

With regards to assessment, the Royal College of Speech and Language Therapists (RCSLT; the professional body for the profession in the United Kingdom) reiterate several points made by Bishop et al. (2016), but also explicitly state that assessment of nonverbal IQ by an educational psychologist is not required in order to reach a diagnosis of developmental language disorder (DLD) (Royal College SLT, 2020). It is worth noting that this does not imply that educational psychologists or other professionals should not be involved when assessing children's L1 abilities. In fact, the more inclusive criteria for DLD (compared to "specific" language difficulties) only serve to increase the heterogeneity of children requiring both assessment and intervention. The best provision can only be determined with input from different disciplines. Bishop et al. (2016) as well as the RCSLT (2017) and the American Speech-Language-Hearing Association (ASHA, 2019) highlight the need for assessments other than standardized ones. They make specific mention of dynamic assessment (also see Chapters 3.1–3.3) as a promising option, particularly when working with children from diverse cultural and linguistic backgrounds (Camilleri & Botting, 2013; Camilleri & Law, 2014).

The part that norm-referenced assessment has to play in both clinical and research contexts is evolving. This is not to say that these assessments cannot or should not play a role in the identification and diagnosis of children with language disorders, but rather that it is a more complex undertaking than simply specifying cutoff scores on a mixture of norm-referenced language and nonverbal measures. Rather than being used as diagnostic criteria, standardized assessments constitute a diagnostic tool that should be combined with other sources of information, enabling the speech and language therapist to make informed management decisions.

CONCLUSION AND FUTURE DIRECTIONS

Therapists' use of standardized assessments as baseline assessments of language, as aspects of diagnostic assessment as well as to measure progress, will undoubtedly continue. It is important to recall that, for diagnostic purposes, rather than using the actual score obtained by the child, the range of scores within the 90% confidence interval should be adopted (Wiig, 2001). The child's true language ability is likely to be reflected in that range of scores, not in the exact standard score.

The use of standardized assessments to measure progress reflects an implicit belief: that there will be a measurable change from the baseline assessment to the later (post-intervention) assessment. This is certainly achievable for some children but may not be for others. Bishop

(2017) makes the point that evaluations of progress based solely on language tests as outcome measures may underestimate the benefits of intervention. Standardized test(s) may not be sensitive enough to measure the changes that have been achieved, and an intervention may well have addressed aspects that are not measurable by these tests. Conversely, one misconception may be that intervention should address specific items that are found to be deficient on a child's performance on a test (Wiig, 2001). This would actually invalidate the use of the assessment to monitor progress without actually helping the child in addressing the real underlying deficits (Wiig, 2001). Bishop (2017) suggests that outcome measures should include measures of quality of life and functional change, including family functioning, social integration, and self-esteem. Dynamic assessments (see also Chapters 3.1–3.3) may also be more appropriate measures of progress when standardized assessments are not sufficiently sensitive to change (Glaspey & Stoel-Gammon, 2007).

The reduced reliance on cutoff scores and the increased emphasis on a range of sources of information means that the question of whether language abilities are stable cognitive abilities that can be used to classify children in a "once and for always" manner becomes a moot point. The change in emphasis also fits more comfortably within a sociocultural view of language which underlies speech and language interventions. The underlying principle is that positive changes to a child's language experience will lead to growth that would not otherwise have happened, but also that a child can function better within an environment that more flexibly adapts to his or her needs (Bishop, 2017).

Researchers in the field now have important choices to make. The need to specify clearly the participants within a given study remains. This is essential if findings from a study are to be applicable to other children whose profile matches that of the participants. The extent to which cutoff points on standardized assessments are used as selection criteria may vary—and should depend on the questions being addressed and the populations involved. Researchers are likely to continue to adopt combinations of cutoffs on language assessments as well as on nonverbal IQ measures. However, rather than using them only as inclusion/exclusion criteria, they can be also be used alongside other variables to define different groups of children with L1 difficulties. So, for example, studies could explicitly compare response to intervention for children with DLD with and without concomitant low nonverbal IQ.

The issue that scores derived from norm-referenced assessments, whether of language or of nonverbal IQ, are not necessarily accurate measurements of a child's skills is an important consideration for researchers when making decisions on participants' inclusion in a research study. It is also important for clinicians making decisions on eligibility for intervention or on other aspects of clinical management. The possibility of using other measures that look at aspects that are not easily evaluated by standardized assessments also needs to be considered in both research and clinical contexts. The latest developments in the field have repositioned the use and interpretation of standardized assessments without reneging their role.

REFERENCES

American Speech-Language-Hearing Association (ASHA). (2019). *Spoken language disorders*. https://www.asha.org/Practice-Portal/Clinical-Topics/Spoken-Language-Disorders/

Bishop, D. V. M. (2017). Why is it so hard to reach agreement on terminology? The case of developmental language disorder (DLD). *International Journal of Language and Communication Disorders, 52*(6), 671–680. https://doi.org/10.1111/1460-6984.12335

Bishop, D. V. M., Snowling, M. J., Thompson, P. A., Greenhalgh, T., & CATALISE consortium (2016). CATALISE: A multinational and multidisciplinary Delphi consensus study. Identifying language impairments in children. *Plos One, 11*(7), 1–26. https://doi.org/10.1371/journal.pone.0158753

Camilleri, B., & Botting, N. (2013). Beyond static assessment of children's receptive vocabulary: The dynamic assessment of word learning (DAWL). *International Journal of Language and Communication Disorders, 48*(5), 565–581. https://doi.org/10.1111/1460-6984.12033

Camilleri, B., & Law, J. (2014). Dynamic assessment of word learning skills of pre-school children with primary language impairment. *International Journal of Speech and Language Pathology, 16*(5), 507–516. https://doi.org/10.3109/17549507.2013.847497

Cole, K. N., Schwartz, I. S., Notari, A. R., Dale, P. S., & Mills, P. E. (1995). Examination of the stability of two methods of defining specific language impairment. *Applied Psycholinguistics, 16*, 103–123.

Edwards, S., Letts, C., & Sinka, I. (2011). *The new Reynell Developmental Language Scales*. GL Assessment Limited.

Friberg, J. C. (2010). Considerations for test selection: How do validity and reliability impact diagnostic decisions? *Child Language Teaching and Therapy, 26*(1), 77–92. https://doi.org/10.1177/0265659009349972

Gould, S. J. (1997). *The mismeasure of man*. Reinehart.

Glaspey, A. M., & Stoel-Gammon, C. (2007). A dynamic approach to phonological assessment. *Advances in Speech and Language Pathology, 9*(4), 286–296. https://doi.org/10.1080/14417040701435418

Norbury, C. F., Nash, M., Bishop, D. V. M., & Baird, G. (2004). Using parental checklists to identify diagnostic groups in children with communication impairment: A validation of the Children's Communication Checklist–2. *International Journal of Language and Communication Disorders, 39*(3), 345–364. https://doi.org/10.1080/13682820410001654883

O'Neil, D. K. (2007). The language use inventory for young children: A parent-report measure of pragmatic language development for 18- to 47-month-old children. *Journal of Speech Language and Hearing Research, 50*(1), 214–228. https://doi.org/10.1044/1092-4388(2007/017)

Peña, E. D., Spaulding, T. J., & Plante, E. (2006). The composition of normative groups and diagnostic decision- making: Shooting ourselves in the foot. *American Journal of Speech–Language Pathology, 15*(3), 247–254. https://doi.org/10.1044/1058-0360(2006/023)

Roseberry-McKibbin, C. (2007). *Language disorders in children: A multicultural and case perspective.* Allyn and Bacon.

RCSLT (2020). RCSLT briefing paper on Language Disorder with a specific focus on Developmental Language Disorder. https://www.rcslt.org/wp-content/uploads/media/docs/Covid/language-disorder-briefing-paper-with-edit.pdf?la=en&hash=98B6A1E60824DEE9D52CCDFFACCE5EE6D67749D9

Spaulding, T. J., Plante, E., & Farinella, K. A. (2006). Eligibility criteria for language impairment: Is the low end of normal always appropriate? *Language, Speech, and Hearing Services in Schools, 37*(1), 61–72. https://doi.org/10.1044/0161-1461(2006/007)

Spaulding, T. J., Swartwout Szulga, M., Figueroa, C. (2012). Using norm-referenced tests to determine severity of language impairment in children: Disconnect between U.S. policy makers and test developers. *Language, Speech, and Hearing Services in Schools, 43*(2), 176–190. https://doi.org/10.1044/0161-1461(2011/10-0103)

Tomblin, J. B. (2008). Validating diagnostic standards for SLI using adolescent outcomes. In C. F. Norbury, J. B. Tomblin, & D. V. M. Bishop (Eds.), *Understanding developmental language disorders* (pp. 93–114). Routledge.

Wiig, E. H. (2001). Multi-perspective, clinical-educational assessments of language disorder. In A. S. Kaufman & N. L. Kaufman (Eds.), *Specific learning disabilities and difficulties in children and adolescents* (pp. 247–278). Cambridge University Press.

Wiig, E. H., Semel, E., & Secord, W. A. (2013). *Clinical Evaluation of Language Fundamentals–Fifth Edition (CELF-5).* NCS Pearson.

World Health Organization. (2019). *The ICD-11 for mortality and morbidity statistics.* WHO. https://icd.who.int/browse11/l-m/en

2.2

Score Use and Interpretation of First Signed Language Assessments

Charlotte Enns and Patrick Boudreault

BACKGROUND

In the past, the assessment of signed language abilities in deaf children was generally considered unnecessary because it did not seem to relate to children's educational programming and ~~because~~ teachers were not aware of the bilingual connection between signed language and spoken/written language development. So assessments were either not done at all or done through informal measures (Hoffmeister et al., 2013). As educational programming during the 1980s shifted to incorporate a cultural perspective of Deaf people, greater emphasis was placed on assessing and monitoring the development of children's signed language skills. At that time, formal assessments typically consisted of adapting existing spoken language tests to be administered in signed language; for example, the Peabody Picture Vocabulary Test-III (Dunn & Dunn, 1997) and the Test of Early Reading Ability-Deaf/Hard of Hearing (Reid et al., 1991) both had signed language (Signed English) versions. However, the results of these translated assessments were not accurate and often did not focus on vocabulary with a similar level of difficulty or appropriate structures of signed languages (Hoffmeister et al., 2013). For these reasons, there has been increased international research interest over the past two decades in tests specifically developed and designed to assess signed languages using tasks and materials (video, pictures, spatial arrangements) that fit with the visual learning needs of deaf children. Some examples of these newly developed tests include the BSL Receptive Skills Test (Herman et al., 1999), the American Sign Language (ASL) Assessment Instrument (Hoffmeister et al., 2014), and the BSL Vocabulary Test (Mann & Marshall, 2012).

The issues of interpreting signed language test scores cannot be fully understood without an overview of the complexities involved in identifying and defining the L1 of deaf signers. Among children born deaf, fewer than 8% come from families with at least one deaf parent (Mitchell & Karchmer, 2004) and have the opportunity to acquire signed

Charlotte Enns and Patrick Boudreault, *Score Use and Interpretation of First Signed Language Assessments* In: *The Handbook of Language Assessment Across Modalities.* Edited by: Tobias Haug, Wolfgang Mann, and Ute Knoch, Oxford University Press. © Oxford University Press 2022. DOI: 10.1093/oso/9780190885052.003.0006 language naturally. The situation is quite different for the other 92% of deaf children, where preschool language experiences vary significantly due to access to and availability of services and parental choices. Understanding the language acquisition context for deaf children can provide insight into the complexity of accurately assessing signed language development. The diversity of language acquisition experiences among deaf signers emphasizes the potential pitfalls of signed language assessment with this population of L1 users and the impact of interpreting test results.

PURPOSE OF ASSESSMENT

The purpose of administering a signed language assessment to deaf children can vary and can include both educational and research objectives (Enns & Herman, 2011). First, one purpose for assessment is to establish a baseline for language intervention or therapy, school programming, or research investigation. With a baseline measure, the educator or researcher can monitor progression through language development milestones and identify any language strengths and difficulties (see Chapter 2.1). Second, a key educational purpose of assessment is to guide instruction (Stiggins, 2002). This can be accomplished through both formal and informal measures. Although some formal, standardized tests can provide useful information for program planning or determining appropriate educational and linguistic goals, they are often more effective in determining the current level of functioning or to monitor progress. Third, assessment is used for accountability purposes in educational settings. Assessment results are typically required for formal reporting purposes to parents and administrators of deaf programs and schools so that they can be aware of language functioning and progress. Formal scores and normed results can help the education system provide appropriate support for deaf L1 users' learning needs.

Given that assessments serve various purposes, it is crucial for test administrators to clarify the purpose of the assessment beforehand so that the appropriate test is selected (see Chapter 2.1). It is also crucial to consider that several different tests might be needed to provide a complete picture of a child's signed language abilities. For example, if a child with limited exposure to signed language is entering a new educational program where instruction is provided via signed language, administering a signed language vocabulary test to monitor the child's acquisition of new signs would be appropriate. Here, the purpose of assessment becomes to monitor progress following exposure to new programming. If the purpose of assessment is to access additional educational supports for a deaf child, then administering a formal, standardized signed language measure might be most appropriate. The assessment would then demonstrate if the child is significantly delayed in comparison to the norms, and including this information in a report for funding might convince the authorities to provide the needed supports.

TEST ADMINISTRATION PROCEDURES

The administration of signed language assessments requires consistent procedures to prevent scoring errors or misinterpretation of the results (Zucker, 2004). Formal training or experience in administering tests in general and specific tests is critical to valid and reliable scoring. Such training can be a challenge given that there is no profession specifically focused on signed language assessment akin to how speech therapists/pathologists assess spoken language. Some professionals working with deaf children, such as psychologists, educational specialists, and speech-language pathologists, may have general knowledge of test administration but usually lack experience in administering signed language tests due to gaps in their training or limited signed language fluency. However, there is a shifting trend for Deaf ASL specialists to administer such tests. ASL specialists are typically teachers, fluent in signed language, who have formally or informally developed their knowledge of signed language linguistics, acquisition, and assessment. Again, due to the lack of professional preparation in this area, anyone administering signed language assessments often learns the process through hands-on practice.

Appropriate test administration is important, particularly for standardized assessments where it is essential that testing is conducted the same way for each child so that scores can be accurately compared with the norms. In this context the use of video-recorded instructions or test materials can facilitate consistency in administering signed language assessments (Haug & Mann, 2008). If the instructions, elicitation prompts, and scoring guidelines are only available to examiners in written form, then a transcription system must be used to outline the expected signed responses for scorers and examiners. Although there are some basic linguistic conventions, including spoken language "glosses" (translated words) that represent signs in writing, the lack of a standardized system frequently leads to significant variation in how the information is conveyed in signed language. The interpretation of signed forms linked to glosses also depends on the examiner's linguistic knowledge. Assessments should include a printed or video appendix of the complete signed language forms, at either the lexical or sentence level.

The examiner's signed language proficiency can influence assessment results and scoring. Deaf children will naturally modify their signing in the presence of a nonfluent signer, such as signing slower, using shorter sentences, and incorporating less space and complex morphological structure; as a result the administrator misses the opportunity to see children produce complex grammatical structures (Lucas & Valli, 1992; Quinto-Pozos & Adam, 2013), leading to the possibility of a skewed score. If the examiner is unable to use direct communication, the presence of a signed language interpreter can also influence test results, especially if the interpreter is not familiar with the test's goals and inadvertently modifies standardized instructions or the child's responses (Higgens et al., 2016; Roger & Code, 2011). Even among educational interpreters trained in a wide range of topics related to signed language, the phenomenon of *contact language* (modifying signing to follow spoken language patterns) will persist. Each administrator and examiner involved with the testing process should be fully cognizant of all the possible circumstances to ensure a fair, appropriate process. Please refer to Chapter 1.2 for more details on considerations for test administration.

INTERPRETATION AND APPLICATION OF TEST SCORES

The interpretation and application of signed language assessment results among deaf children is multifaceted, and the scores can have implications for children's educational, clinical, vocational, and social achievements. Ideally, assessment information helps to identify the child's needs and provides guidance in meeting those needs, whether through educational programming, therapy/remediation, or enhancing social interaction at school or at home. Even if the results of assessment suggest the child is functioning below average, the results should be used to build on relative strengths and fill the gaps in the child's development.

A considerable challenge for signed language assessments is determining how to establish norms given the diversity of the Deaf population and their language and educational experiences (Enns & Herman, 2011; Herman, 1998; Johnston, 2004). To establish a baseline of typical language acquisition, the collection of the normed data should be based on children who have had full access to signed language from birth (e.g., deaf children of deaf parents), or before the age of 3 years (Morford & Mayberry, 2000; Singleton & Newport, 2004). Using specific norms helps maintain high expectations for deaf children's language benchmarks and more accurately reflects the impact of signed language deprivation during the preschool years (Enns & Herman, 2011). Furthermore, a key factor in determining inclusion criteria for normative samples is cognitive abilities, which are closely linked to language skills. Cognitive abilities of deaf children are best assessed with measures of nonverbal IQ in order to reduce the impact of language differences and cultural bias (Fraine & McDade, 2009). Examiners should be aware of the approach to normative sampling implemented in the signed language tests they administer so they can make accurate comparisons and interpretations of the scores for each tested child. The interpretation of the scores should be enhanced by other non-normative observations to conduct a holistic assessment of signed language proficiency.

Representative Scores

For most signed language assessments, the results are reflected in a numerical score. In formal, standardized assessments, this score is typically compared to the normative sample to determine whether the result falls within the mean, usually plus or minus one standard deviation, and either above or below the range. Percentile ranking is also another common scoring system used to compare a child's performance to the normative group.

An accurate interpretation of the test-taker's functioning first involves an assessment of whether the score is representative of the child's abilities. This includes consideration of questions such as: Was the test administered accurately? Was the child fatigued or distracted? Did the child understand the test task? Was the child's score influenced by cultural bias, visual acuity, or some other factors not specific to language skills? Each of these factors may invalidate the test results and render the scores useless.

If the examiner judges the score to be representative of the child's abilities, then the next consideration is how well the normative group represents the child. The primary consideration for signed language assessments is usually the age of acquisition/exposure to the signed language, but other factors, such as nonverbal intelligence (IQ), presence of disabilities (learning, cognitive, behavioral), and home language, must also be considered when interpreting and reporting scores. All factors and considerations should be reported to provide an appropriate context for how accurately the child's score reflects his or her abilities and is comparable to the norms.

Diagnostic Information

A primary purpose of language assessment is to determine children's areas of strength and need and/or to identify gaps in their exposure and learning (i.e., provide diagnostic information). Due to the limited number of tests available for signed language assessment, deaf children's overall language abilities are often incorrectly based on the results of only one test. Simply assessing a child's vocabulary in a signed language does not provide information about that child's knowledge of grammar or discourse structures in that language. In fact, several tests (ASL Phonological Awareness Test [McQuarrie et al., 2012] or BSL/ASL/DGS Receptive Skills Tests [Herman et al., 1999; Enns et al.,

2013; Haug, 2011]) require a pre-test of the vocabulary used in the test to ensure that the child has acquired these signs and the test specifically measures the phonological and grammatical structures included in the assessment. Similarly, if one assesses a child's receptive signed language abilities, it does not always follow that they have a similar level of skills in expressive use of the language. Determining the child's performance across different measures can more clearly pinpoint the areas where they excel or have gaps. Consequently, a compilation of various signed language tests can facilitate the identification of unique language acquisition patterns and determine how these patterns fit with other developmental, cognitive, and learning difficulties.

The pattern of errors within tests must also be considered when interpreting test results. Test interpretation does not end once the score is standardized and placed within the broad normative categories (below, average, above, or other rankings). In many cases, the mean and standard deviations of these categories may not categorize test takers' true abilities accurately. For example, a specific pattern of errors within the total test score was observed during the administration of the ASL Receptive Skills Test (Enns et. al., 2013) when a child obtained an overall average score but incorrectly responded to all the items involving negation, even those acquired by most children at early ages. With further analysis, it was discovered that school personnel had observed this child to have autistic tendencies, including difficulties with nonverbal cues. The test results reinforced the previous observations, since negation in ASL is usually marked by headshakes and facial expressions. With this information, the child was then referred for further diagnostic assessment so that appropriate educational supports could be provided. A similar observation was noted in the administration of the BSL Vocabulary Test, where an unusual response pattern in one student diagnosed with autism spectrum disorder was revealed even though there was no significant effect of this additional disability on vocabulary performance (Mann et al., 2013). This type of careful analysis is particularly important for signed language assessments because it builds on the limited information available regarding the linguistic patterns that occur in deaf children with developmental differences and disabilities.

Nature of Test Tasks and Scoring Procedures

The nature and difficulty of test tasks should also be recognized to accurately interpret test results. With many signed language assessments, as is the case with spoken language assessments, cognitive and linguistic skills are required to complete the test tasks (Gatherole et al., 2004). A basic receptive language task like watching a signed sentence and selecting the correct picture from a choice of four involves the cognitive skills of memory, matching, and visual discrimination. Other more complex language assessment tasks, such as story retelling, require higher-level cognitive processing as well as more experiences with the world, depending on the story topic. Formal assessments often consist of tasks that provide only a single opportunity to determine the child's performance. This is a particular concern with formal assessments of signed languages; most do not have alternate versions of the same level, so immediate retesting is not possible, and longitudinal follow-up may emerge as a challenge as children become more familiar with the test tasks/items with every retesting.

A checklist assessment approach addresses this by allowing for scoring across different environments (home, school, clinic) and providing multiple opportunities for the child to demonstrate language abilities compared to normed tests. However, contrary to this breadth of assessment, checklists are also open to more variable interpretation. Some computer-based tests are scored automatically, which reduces the possibilities for tallying errors and subjective interpretation. Signed language assessments that require analysis of expressive language samples are particularly open to a variety of interpretations. For example, in a story retelling task there is often a typical classifier handshape that the child is expected to use when referring to a particular object (e.g., INDEX for person), but there may be other acceptable alternatives (e.g., V for legs). If all the correct possibilities are not known or agreed upon by different scorers, the children's scores will vary. The use of a scoring rubric or answer sheet may facilitate scoring consistency, but the analysis of language samples raises the issue of interrater reliability and the process of training consistency among raters. (The regulation and proficiency of raters is further discussed in Chapter 9.2 "Scoring Issues.")

A thorough understanding of what the test tasks entail also allows the examiner to modify the standardized administration of the test to gain additional information about the child's linguistic skills. In such cases, applying the standardized score would not be appropriate, but the insight gained may make the effort to adapt or modify the instrument worthwhile. For example, the standardized administration of an assessment often imposes a time limit for completing each item. If the test administration protocol is modified to extend (or remove) the time limit, and then the child is able to respond to the items accurately, this may indicate that the child has acquired the linguistic concepts but is delayed or developing differently in terms of cognitive processing skills. Although comparing the score to the norms may not be possible, key insights regarding the child's language and cognitive level of functioning can be gained. Future testing might then use the child's previous score for comparison to determine a measure of growth and development. Another example of an alternative to standardized testing methods that has been applied to signed language is dynamic assessment (Mann et al., 2014; also see Chapters 3.1–3.3). Through the process of mediated learning experiences guided by initial assessment results, instructors gain a better understanding of children's strategies and learning potential. The results have implications for teaching and more effective planning for future educational programming.

Reporting Test Scores

Whether the purpose of testing is to establish a baseline, monitor progress, or determine developmental delays or difficulties, reporting of test scores (numerically) should also include a full description of the testing context and meaningful interpretation of the results. With formal assessments, the emphasis may shift to the specific scores and whether results fall within or outside of the normal range. Formal assessments are often required for educational funding applications, where the significance of the child's delay or disorder determines the amount of funding provided or level of access to special services (such as an Individual Education Plan [IEP] in the United States as mandated by the Individuals with Disabilities Education Act [IDEA]). Identifying children's needs can then place them in educational environments (i.e., signing environment) that more appropriately meet their needs. Similarly, if students experience a beneficial change in educational placement or programming, their progress can be validated through increases in formal test scores.

Through the process of sharing signed language assessment reports with parents, the parents can gain a better understanding of their child's learning needs. For this reason, it is important that reports are written and explained in a way that parents can understand them. In some cases, sharing results directly with the child may also be appropriate and can support the development of self-advocacy skills. It is imperative to obtain parental support in making changes to children's educational programming. Formal signed language assessment reports are beneficial in showing parents the differences between conversational language skills, which they see in everyday interactions with their child, and the academic language skills needed for school success. A similar process is also needed for classroom teachers. A key purpose of assessment is to guide instruction. Sharing the results of testing with teachers can inform them about the connections between signed language abilities and the concepts they teach in their classrooms. In particular, the links between signed language and written language literacy must be emphasized in the classroom to maximize the reading and writing potential of deaf students.

A particular concern in the area of signed language assessments with children is that a child's level of functioning should not be determined by the results of one particular test. It is important to consider individual test scores within the context of various informal and formal language assessments that evaluate different components of language (receptive, expressive, phonology, vocabulary, grammar, pragmatics).

Yet the difficulty with signed language assessment is that too few tests have been developed to assess all components of signed languages (Singleton & Supalla, 2011). It may be necessary to combine holistic assessment (classroom/home observation, checklists, informal language tasks) and dynamic assessment (including mediated learning experiences) with normative scores to provide a more complete picture of the results. Professionals must look beyond the numerical score of signed language assessments with children to gain a deeper interpretation. This can be accomplished by considering how the child's abilities are represented, the pattern of errors, the nature and difficulty of test tasks, the characteristics of both the test-taker and test administrator, and the purpose and place for reporting results.

FUTURE DIRECTIONS

For ongoing development in the area of L1 signed language assessment, a larger norming data pool is needed to support the understanding of "normal" signed language development. Although this may not be possible in all signed languages, particularly those in smaller countries with limited users (including dialects within a signed language), a larger database of key signed languages has the potential for cross-linguistic application. More research focused on assessing deaf children and collecting language acquisition data will help test developers establish appropriate norms. These developmental standards will, in turn, ensure that families and educators have age-appropriate expectations for deaf children's signed language development.

A better understanding of signed language acquisition and norms, not only for researchers but also practitioners, will also facilitate more effective training for test administration, scoring, and interpretation. Since there are currently no formal professional or training requirements for administering signed language assessments (see Chapters 11.1–11.3), individuals with varying experience and knowledge are currently conducting the tests and interpreting the results with varied outcomes. There is a need to establish standardized credentials as well as procedures for individuals to achieve these skills to ensure accurate and consistent assessment of signed language abilities.

Currently, signed language assessments are primarily available only in the areas of vocabulary (both receptive and expressive), receptive grammar (morphology and syntax), narrative (expressive grammar and narrative structure), and some aspects of sign phonology. Additional formal and commercially available measures in the areas of signed language phonology, expressive morphology/syntax, and discourse or pragmatic abilities are still needed to strengthen the links between language and literacy development. Tests to measure these various aspects of signed languages are needed to better diagnose any potential language development issues. Signed language abilities contribute to a child's overall literacy and academic learning. Through the process of determining strengths and weaknesses in children's signing skills, more effective instruction can be implemented to help deaf children reach their full potential.

Additional research is also needed to develop tests in a variety of different signed languages. Most of the current tests have been developed for BSL or ASL, with some adaptations of these tests created in other signed languages throughout Europe.

In summary, the future needs for improving the interpretation of signed language assessment scores for children requires (1) more data on typical signed language acquisition (to inform norms and enhance examiner understanding), (2) standardized credentialing for administering and interpreting signed language tests, (3) a greater variety of assessments measuring a variety of signed language components to provide accurate and thorough diagnostic information, and (4) assessments available in all signed languages around the world. The ongoing research related to signed language acquisition is an excellent foundation for further development of much needed effective and appropriate tools to assess children's signed language development with an efficient and reliable process for score interpretation.

REFERENCES

Dunn, L. M., & Dunn, D. M. (1997). *Peabody picture vocabulary test* (3rd ed.). American Guidance Services.

Enns, C., & Herman, R. (2011). Adapting the Assessing British Sign Language Development Receptive Skills Test into American Sign Language. *Journal of Deaf Studies and Deaf Education, 16*(3), 362–374. https://doi.org/10.1093/deafed/enr004

Enns, C., Zimmer, K., Boudreault, P., Rabu, S., & Broszeit, C. (2013). *American Sign Language: Receptive Skills Test*. Northern Signs Research, Inc.

Fraine, N., & McDade, R. (2009). Reducing bias in psychometric assessment of culturally and linguistically diverse students from refugee backgrounds in Australian schools: A process approach. *Australian Psychologist, 44*(1), 16–26. https://doi.org/10.1080/00050060802582026

Gatherole, S. E., Pickering, S. J., Ambridge, B., & Wearing, H. (2004). The structure of working memory from 4–15 years of age. *Developmental Psychology, 40*(2), 177–190. https://doi.org/10.1037/0012-1649.40.2.177

Haug, T. (2011). Approaching sign language test construction: Adaptation of the German Sign Language receptive skills test. *Journal of Deaf Studies and Deaf Education, 16*(3), 343–361. https://doi.org/10.1093/deafed/enq062

Haug, T., & Mann, W. (2008). Adapting tests of sign language assessment for other sign languages: A review of linguistic, cultural, and psychometric problems. *Journal of Deaf Studies and Deaf Education, 13*(1), 138–147. https://doi.org/10.1093/deafed/enm027

Herman, R. (1998). Issue in designing an assessment of British Sign Language development. *Proceedings of the Conference of the Royal College of Speech & Language Therapists* (pp. 332–337). Liverpool, UK.

Herman, R., Holmes, S., & Woll, B. (1999). *Assessing BSL development: Receptive Skills Test*. Forest Bookshop.

Higgens, J. A., Famularo, L., Cawthon, S. W., Kurz, C. A., Reis, J. E., & Moers, L. M. (2016). Development of American Sign Language guidelines for K–12 academic assessments. *Journal of Deaf Studies and Deaf Education, 21*(4), 383–392. https://doi.org/10.1093/deafed/enw051

Hoffmeister, R. J., Caldwell-Harris, C. L., Henner, J., Benedict, R., Fish, S., Rosenburg, P., Conlin-Luippold, F., & Novogrodsky, R. (2014). *The American Sign Language Assessment Instrument (ASLAI): Progress report and preliminary findings*. Working paper. Center for the Study of Communication and the Deaf.

Hoffmeister, R. J., Kuntze, M., & Fish, S. A. (2013). Assessing American Sign Language. In A. J. Kunnan (Ed.), *The companion to language assessment* (pp. 1731–1741). Wiley. https://doi.org/10.1002/9781118411360.wbcla088

Johnston, T. (2004). The assessment and achievement of proficiency in a native sign language within a sign bilingual program: The pilot Auslan receptive skills test. *Deafness and Education International, 6*(2), 57–81. https://doi.org/10.1179/146431504790560582

Lucas, C., & Valli, C. (1992). *Language contact in the American deaf community*. Academic Press.

Mann, W., & Marshall, C. (2012). Investigating deaf children's vocabulary knowledge in British Sign Language. *Language Learning, 62*(4), 1024–1051. https://doi.org/10.1111/j.1467-9922.2011.00670.x

Mann, W., Pena, E., & Morgan, G. (2014). Exploring the use of dynamic language assessment with deaf children, who use American Sign Language: Two case studies. *Journal of Communication Disorders, 52*, 16–30. https://doi.org/10.1016/j.jcomdis.2014.05.002

Mann, W., Roy, P., & Marshall, C. (2013). A look at the other 90 percent: Investigating British Sign Language vocabulary knowledge in deaf children from different language learning backgrounds. *Deafness & Education International, 15*(2), 91–116. https://doi.org/10.1179/1557069X12Y.0000000017

McQuarrie, L., Abbott, M., & Spady, S. (January, 2012). American Sign Language phonological awareness: Test development and design. *Proceedings of the 10th Annual Hawaii International Conference on Education* (pp. 142–158), Honolulu, Hawaii.

Mitchell, R., & Karchmer, M. (2004). Chasing the mythical ten percent: Parental hearing status of deaf and hard of hearing students in the United States. *Sign Language Studies, 4*(2), 138–163. https://doi.org/10.1353/sls.2004.0005

Morford, J. P., & Mayberry, R. I. (2000). A reexamination of "early exposure" and its implications for language acquisition by eye. In C. Chamberlain, J. P. Morford, & R. I. Mayberry (Eds.), *Language acquisition by Eye* (pp. 110–127). Lawrence Erlbaum Associates.

Quinto-Pozos, D., & Adam, R. (2013). Sign language contact. In R. Bayley, R. Cameron, & C. Lucas (Eds.), *The Oxford handbook of sociolinguistics* (pp. 379–401). Oxford University Press.

Reid, D. K., Hammill, D., Wiltshire, S., & Hresko, W. (1991). *Test of Early Reading Ability Deaf or Hard of Hearing (TERADHH)*. ProEd.

Roger, P., & Code, C. (2011). Lost in translation? Issues of content validity in interpreter-mediated aphasia assessments. *International Journal of Speech-Language Pathology, 13*(1), 61–73. https://doi.org/10.3109/17549507.2011.549241

Singleton, J. L., & Newport, E. L. (2004). When learners surpass their models: The acquisition of American Sign Language from inconsistent input. *Cognitive Psychology, 49*(4), 370–407. https://doi.org/10.1016/j.cogpsych.2004.05.001

Singleton, J. L., & Supalla, S. (2011). Assessing children's proficiency in natural signed languages. In N. Peter, M. Marschark & P. E. Spencer (eds.), *The Oxford Handbook of Deaf Studies, Language and Education, Volume 1, 2nd Edition* (pp. 306–321). Oxford University Press.

Stiggins, R. J. (2002). Assessment crisis: The absence of assessment for learning. *Phi Delta Kappan, 83*(10), 758–765. https://doi.org/10.1177/003172170208301010

Zucker, S. (2004). *Assessment report: Administration practices for standardized assessment*. Pearson Education.

2.3

Discussion of Issues Related to Score Use and Interpretation of First Spoken and Signed Language Assessments

Patrick Boudreault, Bernard Camilleri, and Charlotte Enns

ASPECTS OF SIGNED LANGUAGE ASSESSMENT THAT ARE APPLICABLE TO SPOKEN LANGUAGE ASSESSMENT

It might seem reasonable to assume that the use and interpretation of standardized assessments of language would share much in common across signed and spoken mediums. Insofar as the use of standardized assessment involves the comparison of an individual's performance to normative data, this is true. It is also the case that the normative data are intended to capture the mean and range of "typical development" for the language in question. So, a standardized assessment of spoken English language (or other spoken languages) will collect data from native, monolingual speakers, thus establishing what is the range of receptive and/or expressive abilities of children across different ages. Similarly, normative data for standardized assessments of signed language are established by collecting data from native signing deaf children. Where the difference arises is the way in which the normative data relate to the target populations and the individuals within those populations who are being assessed. While standardized assessments of spoken language are normed on and predominantly intended for use with native speakers of that language, standardized assessments of signed language are intrinsically designed for use with a heterogenous group of children, of whom only a minority have the opportunity of learning signed language as their native language. This can be seen as a possible source of "error" when using assessments of signed language, but perhaps a different interpretation can be adopted—one

Patrick Boudreault, Bernard Camilleri, and Charlotte Enns, *Discussion of Issues Related to Score Use and Interpretation of First Spoken and Signed Language Assessments* In: *The Handbook of Language Assessment Across Modalities.* Edited by: Tobias Haug, Wolfgang Mann, and Ute Knoch, Oxford University Press. © Oxford University Press 2022.
DOI: 10.1093/oso/9780190885052.003.0007

which enables standardized assessments to be used productively with a wider range of children.

When a spoken language assessment is used, it can only be used correctly with children who have a similar experience of (and exposure to) language as the children in the normative data. This is one of the key points identified by Friberg (2010). In other words, monolingual native speakers of the language in question (e.g., English) are assessed with assessments that have been normed with monolingual English speakers. This enables a "fair" comparison between the child's language skills and the normative data. Unless norms have been established for children learning a language (e.g., English) alongside an additional language (as is the case with the Clinical Evaluation of Language Fundamentals [CELF] developed for use with the Hispanic population in the United States; also see Chapter 6.1), a standardized assessment cannot be used to accurately measure bilingual children's language, for example. When choosing to use a standardized assessment with a child, the underlying assumption is that the child has had broadly similar opportunities to learn English (or the spoken language being assessed), and, therefore, any differences between the child's performance and expected norms is uncovering a difference in a (relatively) stable underlying characteristic.

The approach of using standardized assessments of signed language is rather different. As discussed in Chapter 2.2, the normative data for signed language assessments tend to be based on children who have accessed signed language from birth or from very early in life, in general before 2 or 3 years of age. This sets an adequately high benchmark of typical native signed language development but does not preclude the use of these assessments with children who have had limited exposure to the signed language in question. On the contrary, using native signers as a baseline is seen as an opportunity to measure the impact of signed language deprivation (Enns & Herman, 2011) and consequently identify the need for educational and other measures to be put in place. While the use of standardized signed language assessments means it can be hard to differentiate between test-takers' difficulties due to language deprivation and difficulties due to language disorders or impairments (see also Chapters 5.1–5.3), it also means that all signing children can be assessed. Of course, it is crucial that the interpretation of the assessment incorporates a wider range of sources of information—most importantly an evaluation of the child's language history and their exposure to signed language.

The same principles can equally be applied when using standardized assessment of a spoken language with children who have different exposure to the language in question, typically alongside exposure to another language. In an increasingly diverse society, many standardized tests of English (or of the majority language) are being used with children for whom the majority language is not their first or their only language. Recent research (Floccia et al., 2018) has been exploring the possibility of developing experience-adjusted norms for standardized assessments for spoken language users. This involves combining information about the relative exposure to the different languages as well as the characteristics of the different languages in making judgments about the child's observed proficiency in either the majority language or both languages. The perfect solution may still be a long way ahead, but, in the meantime, standardized assessments can be used to quantify as well as to provide qualitative information about the diversity of children's spoken language skills in the context of different exposure to the language in question. The crucial point in doing so will be to ensure that any scores are *not* interpreted as measures of a stable characteristic, but as measures of current performance—open to considerable change if and when exposure changes.

ASPECTS OF SPOKEN LANGUAGE ASSESSMENT THAT ARE APPLICABLE TO SIGNED LANGUAGE ASSESSMENT

In the two chapters regarding assessment for spoken and signed languages (Chapters 2.1 and 2.2), discussion took place on how signed language could benefit from best practices observed in spoken language assessment and what challenges exist in implementing such best practices. Three critical aspects need to be considered when interpreting results from spoken language assessments effectively.

First, spoken language assessments have a long history of normed, standardized tests being validated based on psychometrics, and the professionals (such as speech-language pathologists, psychologists, or other language specialists) trained in using these measures are familiar with implementing the procedures and interpreting scores. This is often not the case with professionals administering signed language assessment; therefore, additional preparation or certification needs to be part of the training of signed language specialists so they can accurately administer, interpret, diagnose, and apply the results and implement effective interventions with deaf children.

Second, historically, and even today, the number of tests available for assessing signed language has been very limited. This has created a crucial gap in signed language assessment and analysis. To address the problem, professionals, such as speech-language pathologists or teachers of the deaf and/or hard of hearing (D/HH), tended to translate available assessment materials from spoken language and rely on results that were the not necessarily valid for an informal interpretation of the score. However, this practice is not typically used with spoken language assessment since translating an assessment can lead to inaccurate data and uncertainty in interpreting the scores. Consequently, such unsound practice, especially with a different language modality of visuo-spatial language grammar, often results in misdiagnoses, with potentially grave consequences. To avoid this requires the development of norm-referenced assessments for signed languages, including linguistic variations if applicable, in order to allow the attainment of the best possible interpretation of the results.

Third, there is a need to identify and diagnose a language disability in a deaf child to enable effective and successful intervention just as it is the case for hearing children using spoken language. For this reason, it is important for a test developer to understand how norms are established and then to define possible developmental language disorder (DLD) among native signing deaf children (see also Chapter 5.2) versus the non-native and delayed language acquisition population. Identifying a possible language disability among native signers is complex for two reasons: the small sample size and unknown types of language disability emerging within this population. Also, intervention is less likely to be effective when the interpretation of the results is vague or uncertain due to lack of professional training among experts and limited access to tests developed specifically for research. An assessment may be helpful with identifying a global language delay (i.e., typically determined as a score of two standard deviations below the mean) in a deaf test-taker, but not the atypical patterns of a specific linguistic feature. For instance, in a case study of a deaf native signing child with unusual language behavior, a diagnosis of DLD was determined through an array of assessment tools ranging from normed and research-based tests to informal measures (Quinto-Pozos et al., 2017). Using various tests along with the expertise of a Deaf specialist can be an alternative strategy to address this conundrum, although not yet widely discussed. Therefore, a thoughtful consideration of the cultural and linguistic differences between the assessor and the deaf child must take place before determining the likelihood of a language disability.

SUGGESTIONS FROM SIGNED LANGUAGE TO ADVANCE KEY ISSUES IN SPOKEN LANGUAGE ASSESSMENT

The reliance on normative data presents an interesting difference between the fields of signed language assessment and spoken language assessment, specifically when related to children. Determining "normal" language acquisition in deaf children who use signed languages remains one of the key challenges due to children's inconsistent access to language, which often results in language deprivation. The need to determine what deaf children are capable of when provided with early and rich exposure to language is a key prerequisite for accurate assessment. On the other hand, there is concern from the spoken language perspective that an overreliance on norms, through the use of standardized tests, may result in an inaccurate representation of children's individual differences. Whereas the field of signed languages is still working toward establishing norms, colleagues focusing on assessing spoken languages may have perhaps defined their norms too narrowly. For this reason, spoken language assessment could benefit from strategies used in signed language assessment by expanding the use of informal observation, performance (nonverbal) IQ, and analysis of error patterns, as described next.

Informal Observation

Prior to the availability of the first standardized tests in the late 1990s, naturalistic observations have been a critical part of the assessment of deaf children, specifically when it comes to determining their linguistic mastery. Integrating naturalistic approaches with selected normed scores from particular tests to evaluate and determine language functioning can also be useful for spoken language. This will allow cross-validation between norm-based (formal) results and naturalistic observations (informal). Historically with deaf students, such informal assessments were often carried out by professionals who were not native or fluent in signed language or not even part of the assessed child's ethnocultural experience. This results in a liability to misdiagnosing the results or making unwarranted assumptions about children's language proficiency. In order for professionals to accurately implement and interpret informal observations beyond normed scores, whether in signed or spoken language, they must be fluent in the target language and also have a cultural understanding of their tested population. Examiners' linguistic proficiency and cultural competency can be more easily overlooked when interpreting language abilities solely based on a normed test score as reference.

Performance IQ

In signed language assessment, performance IQ (nonverbal), not verbal IQ, is recommended to determine whether or not cognitive ability is interfering with the acquisition of language. This nonlinguistic assessment helps the signed language professionals to rule out potential cognitive issues that may be present in deaf children who are below 2 standard deviations from the mean. The preliminary results from the IQ measure can act as an indicator that standardized language test results need to be looked at with great caution and may require further interpretation. Performance IQ is a powerful and reliable alternative to verbal IQ assessment, specifically when used with deaf children, because it measures the cognitive abilities they constantly have access to in their visual surroundings, including deductive reasoning, visuospatial skills, and independent problem-solving. Including this test for hearing children as a baseline or gatekeeper could be useful in cases where there is suspicion of a language impairment.

Analysis of Error Patterns

It is possible for children to obtain a "normal" or "average" overall score on a language test but still demonstrate significant difficulties with a particular linguistic structure. For example, a child may present with overall average narrative abilities but problems with producing pronouns accurately. Looking beyond the overall score can reveal potential errors that are primarily related to particular linguistic features. Further assessment specific to these areas can then help to determine the language needs that may be contributing to a child's social or academic difficulties. Future directions in spoken language assessment can focus on using modified assessments within standardized measures to explore and determine specific areas of difficulty and seek strategies for remediation.

SUGGESTIONS FROM SPOKEN LANGUAGE TO ADVANCE KEY ISSUES IN SIGNED LANGUAGE ASSESSMENT

The use of standardized assessments in signed language presents some unique challenges that are not typically paralleled in the field of assessing hearing children's spoken language. One such challenge is linked to the considerable variation in signed language proficiency by the assessor. Other challenges experienced in signed language assessment are more common for the field of spoken language assessment. As highlighted in Chapters 2.1 and 2.2, choosing the right assessment to address the clinical question at hand (e.g., whether a difficulty is present versus elaborating which aspects of expressive syntax are causing difficulty) is one such common challenge. An assessment that is designed to diagnose a language disorder or disability in a native signer needs to measure a wide range of skills that are both receptive and expressive. As identified by the authors of Chapter 2.2, such assessments are lacking in the field of signed languages. Both the breadth (number) and the depth (different kinds) of signed language assessments need to be enhanced, but it is only natural that this will take time as our understanding of signed language development grows.

One particular challenge identified by Boudreault and Enns (Chapter 2.2) is the difficulty in establishing normative data. As they pointed out, normative data tend to be based on native signers. While this has some advantage (as discussed earlier), it also means that there is currently no objective way to measure the language skills of those children who were exposed to signed language at a later stage (e.g., after enrolling in a program that uses signed language as the means of communication and instruction). In essence, this challenge is very similar to the one faced by assessors of spoken language when that language is the dominant societal language but not the home language (as is the case for many bilingual children in the United Kingdom and the United States).

The necessity to develop norms that take into account non-native signers is particularly acute because this subgroup constitutes the vast majority of deaf signers who are not born to parents who are deaf signers themselves. While the author of Chapter 2.1 agrees with his colleagues from signed language that norms based on native signers can be useful, it is also true that other norms that take exposure into account, such as deaf children with hearing parents or late learners, would be particularly useful. It may be possible to identify further subgroups of non-native signers that have sufficiently similar exposure to signed language that would enable separate norms to be established. This approach has its flaws, particularly regarding the potential variability of the sample and the lowering of expectations, but it has been used with some success where the exposure to spoken language (e.g., English and Spanish) is sufficiently similar within a group of speakers (but different from other groups), as is the case with Hispanic children in the United States (Semel et al., 2006). While this model may or may not be applicable to non-native signers, it would seem to be an area that needs addressing as a priority in the field of signed language assessment.

FUTURE DIRECTIONS

It is important to keep in mind that all standardized assessments, whether developed to measure spoken languages or signed languages, have a margin of error. Even when the child being assessed matches the normative data (typically based on native language learners), a 90% confidence interval should be applied to account for factors influencing performance (e.g., distraction, attention, chance) whenever the assessment manual provides this information. Where this information is not provided in the assessment manual, it is still important to bear in mind that any assessment result will have a built-in margin of error. We propose, however, that instead of limiting the use of standardized assessments to categorize children, we broaden their purpose by using and interpreting them descriptively while at the same time acknowledging their limitations. Standardized assessments could be used with non-native spoken language learners, as is already the case with deaf children, but with the awareness that the results are descriptive of a child's current performance on specific tasks. This descriptive score is by no means indicative of the child's language abilities or potential in a broader sense and should not be used to reach diagnostic conclusions in terms of classifying the child as having a language disorder. A comparison to native learners (normative sample) could be used to justify additional input through intervention, therapy, home support, or educational placement. Most importantly, the limitations of the descriptive score must be understood and explicitly incorporated in reporting and interpreting results whether in the field of signed language assessment or spoken language assessment.

As previously mentioned, the norms for standardized assessments of signed languages have usually been generated based on children with deaf parents or those with early exposure to signed language even though they are not representative of the general population of deaf children. The rationale for basing a comparison group on a small minority of the population is to demonstrate the capabilities of deaf children when provided with full access to language. This comparison also serves to reveal the significant effects of language deprivation and advocate for early exposure to signed language for deaf children. Extending the application of standardized assessments for spoken language (based on monolingual children) in a similar way with bilingual hearing children could also serve to advocate for additional services (including language therapy, enhanced peer interaction, placement in a signing educational environment) rather than taking a "wait and see" approach (also see Chapters 6.1–6.3). The question of differentiating disorder from difference remains and is important for all children. This is even more of an issue for bilingual speakers and late signers, for whom low performance on a standardized assessment will almost certainly be affected by the relative lack of exposure, but may (or may not) also be due to a language learning deficit. For bilingual speakers, understanding the relative exposure to the two languages while comprehensively assessing children's skills in both languages can be helpful in distinguishing difference from disorder. Sometimes this is straightforward, as would be in the case of a child who is demonstrably highly proficient in their home language (with high exposure) but who has difficulties with the language used in school/society (with limited exposure). With many children, this distinction is much harder in practice. In the absence of clear distinctions between difference and disorder, but also in any situation where the child has difficulties using the language in their home/school settings (whether spoken or signed), every child should be given adequate support to achieve both social and educational competence in the language in question. This important area is addressed further in Chapters 5.1–5.3.

Another point of agreement between signed and spoken first language assessment is the importance of not relying on one measure to categorize a child's overall linguistic abilities. An appropriate balance of quantitative and qualitative information must be considered in determining an accurate assessment. In the case of signed languages, there are often limited formal measures available, so examiners should be cautious not to overrely on informal or measures translated from spoken language assessments while incorporating a range of sources of information. In contrast, the abundance of standardized assessments available for spoken languages should not be used as a reason for excluding informal observation or tasks when assessing children's spoken language abilities. Across both spoken and signed languages, professionals certainly need to gather information from those people in the home and school environment who know the child best.

Assessing a child's language is not like using a ruler to measure their height: there is no one definitive number or score that provides a representative result. The process of language assessment is complex and imprecise and therefore must include a critical discernment of both formal and informal measures, qualitative and quantitative evidence, and consideration of both the child's and the examiner's experience and learning context.

REFERENCES

Enns, C., & Herman, R. (2011). Adapting the assessing British Sign Language development: Receptive Skills Test into American Sign Language. *Journal of Deaf Studies and Deaf Education*, *16*(3), 362–374. https://doi.org/10.1093/deafed/enr004

Floccia, C., Sambrook, T. D., Delle Luche, C., Kwok, R., Goslin, J., White, L., Cattani, A., Sullivan, E., Abbot-Smith, K., Krott, A., Mills, D., Rowland, C., Gervain, J., & Plunkett, K. (2018). Vocabulary of 2-year-old learning English and an additional language: Norms and effects of linguistic distance. *Monographs of the Society for Research in Child Development*, *83*(1), 7–80. https://doi.org/10.1111/mono.12348

Friberg, J. C. (2010). Considerations for test selection: How do validity and reliability impact diagnostic decisions? *Child Language Teaching and Therapy*, *26*(1), 77–92. https://doi.org/10.1177/0265659009349972

Quinto-Pozos, D., Singleton, J., & Hauser, P. (2017). A case of specific language impairment in a deaf signer of American Sign Language. *Journal of Deaf Studies and Deaf Education*, *22*(2), 204–218. https://doi.org/10.1093/deafed/enw074

Semel, E., Wiig, E. H., & Secord, W. A. (2006). *Clinical Evaluation of Linguistic Fundamentals 4th edition (CELF4) Spanish*. Psychorp.

Topic 3

Dynamic Assessment of Language Learning in L1 Children

3.1

Dynamic Assessment of Learners of a Spoken Language

Natalie Hasson

Dynamic assessment (DA) relates to a model in which the ability of an individual to learn is evaluated, rather than the achievement of the individual in learning to date. This model allows for a small amount of teaching or intervention to be carried out *within* an assessment to determine how well the individual responds to teaching and to enable future intervention to be planned accordingly. The concepts originate within the assessment of intelligence, in the fields of educational and cognitive psychology, and will be expanded further in this chapter.

The adaptation of DA to the assessment of spoken language is a recent and so far underresearched method. I believe that the construct of potential to learn lends itself well to the assessment of language. The *product*—namely the language that is known and used—is clearly distinguished from the *process* of learning. It is therefore both possible and useful to determine not only what language structures are known and used, but also what strategies for learning are used and are effective or which are weak and could benefit from intervention.

This chapter reviews the work that has been done on DA of spoken language, evaluates the usefulness of DA to supplement the shortcomings of standardized assessments, and considers future directions for research. I begin with a brief definition of DA.

WHAT IS DYNAMIC ASSESSMENT?

The term "dynamic assessment" is used interchangeably with other terms such as "interactive assessment" and "learning potential assessment." The most defining aspect is that active intervention by the examiner is incorporated into the test procedure, and the examinee's response to that intervention is measured (Haywood & Lidz, 2007). This broad definition encompasses all types of interventions within an assessment and a range of methods and materials for delivery of the intervention and evaluation of the learner's response to that intervention.

Natalie Hasson, *Dynamic Assessment of Learners of a Spoken Language* In: *The Handbook of Language Assessment Across Modalities*. Edited by: Tobias Haug, Wolfgang Mann, and Ute Knoch, Oxford University Press. © Oxford University Press 2022. DOI: 10.1093/oso/9780190885052.003.0008

Dynamic assessments are usually contrasted to "static," "standardized," or "normative" assessments, although some researchers have devised dynamic tests that are standardized and psychometrically validated (Hessels et al., 2008). The more useful contrast to a dynamic assessment is a *static* test that looks at an individual's independent performance on a given task at a given point in time.

DA is rooted in Vygotsky's sociocultural theory, with the influence of others in the environment being a key part of shaping learning. The assessment is based on one of Vygotsky's key constructs: namely, the *zone of proximal development* (ZPD) (Vygotsky, 1986). It aims to measure how much more a child can achieve with support from an adult or more experienced peer compared to what he can manage independently. Vygotsky used the notion of ZPD in the context of devising appropriate instruction for children, rather than as assessment for any other purpose. (Vygotsky, 1986). He described establishing differing ZPD in two children with the same measured "intelligence age." One of these children was able to achieve tasks several years above his measured age when strategies were mediated to him by a teacher. The other child could only manage tasks up to 1 year above his age. The difference is described as the first child having a substantially greater ZPD than the other. This difference means that some individuals will grasp what is being taught easily and progress toward managing it on their own, while others will not be able to succeed even with facilitation. DA is focused on this measurement of the ZPD: it looks at the level one can reach with intervention and the nature of the assistance required to achieve that maximal level.

The concepts of DA were first presented by Andre Ray in the 1930s, but only formally operationalized by Reuven Feuerstein in the 1970s (Feuerstein et al., 1979). Since then, usage has largely been geared to the assessment of broad concepts of intelligence, and the adaptation to assessment of language skills is more recent, starting around 1990 (see Peña & Iglesias, 1992).

DYNAMIC ASSESSMENT TO ADDRESS THE SHORTCOMINGS OF STANDARDIZED TESTS

The assessment of spoken first language is largely the domain of speech and language therapists (SLTs), especially when competence or adequacy in these skills is questioned. Although static standardized tests are extensively used to assess language, there are some significant limitations to their use. Primarily, Dockrell (2001, p. 78) noted that measures of individual aspects of language are "inadequate at distinguishing between children with typical development and children with language impairments." At best, a battery of tests or a test comprising a number of subtests is needed to get a complete profile of an individual's skills;

so, for example, an assessment of vocabulary, use of grammatical items such as pronouns, morphological prefixes and suffixes, and sentence formulation would be useful. These tests still remain inconclusive when used alone, and clinical assessment is almost certainly needed to support diagnostic tests.

Second, the process of standardized assessment is to carry out the test in as fixed and consistent a way as possible. Instructions are scripted, and feedback is not permitted. Tests are therefore, of necessity, decontextualized, not naturalistic, and, as a result, lacking in ecological validity.

The standardization of normative tests is seldom inclusive of children with developmental or learning difficulties, children on the autistic spectrum, and children with attention deficits or hearing impairments. Furthermore, they are unsuitable for assessing children from diverse cultural and linguistic backgrounds due to content bias, linguistic bias, and difficulties with adopting normative data (Laing & Kamhi, 2003). As a result, large numbers of children requiring assessment cannot reliably be compared to the norms.

Finally, static tests do not set out to provide information on a child's readiness for intervention (Olswang et al., 1992), nor do they provide qualitative information regarding useful strategies and methods of intervention (Hasson & Joffe, 2007). In fact, the focus in the tests on identifying errors in a particular linguistic structure may lead therapists to address specific areas, rather than generalizable skills.

Clearly then, there is scope for the development and use of alternative and supplementary methods of assessment. DAs aim to fill some of these gaps.

THE USES OF DYNAMIC ASSESSMENT

What makes DA useful for the assessment of language is its focus on strategies that facilitate learning and the qualitative information that may be extracted from a DA procedure. Because there are no norms, there are no exclusions, and DAs are intended for use with a wide range of clinical populations, such as those with developmental language disorders (DLD; also see Chapters 5.1–5.3) or children with a range of educational needs, such as learning difficulties and attention deficits.

The use of extensive feedback and support for learners is consistent with the social interactionist theory upon which DA is based and which is intrinsic to language therapy. As SLTs, "our practice rests on at least an implicit belief that social interaction provides the context for and has the potential to effect developmental change" (Schneider & Watkins, 1996, p. 157). While this practice is reflected in therapy, it is not generally reflected in the assessment practices of SLTs or, indeed, educationalists.

As we will see, the intervention phase of a DA can take many forms. In different tests from Feuerstein's Learning Potential Assessment Device (LPAD) battery (Feuerstein et al., 2002), test-takers are offered multiple repetitions of stimuli, presentation in different modalities, reduction in the number of items presented, verbalization, and systematic trial and error as strategies for problem-solving to determine which may be useful. This information is extremely valuable for those setting out to facilitate improved language learning.

Feuerstein's fundamental method though, is intervention using a *mediated learning experience* (MLE) (Feuerstein et al., 2002; Haywood, 1993; Lidz, 1991). In the MLE, the mediator conveys explicitly to the learner what they are going to learn and why it is important or relevant, that she (the mediator) is going to help the learner to solve the problems, that she has confidence that the learner will achieve, and she elicits a reciprocal contribution from the learner. She then supports the learner to solve items himself by arranging easier items first so that he learns progressively, mediating the use of rules and strategies, and asking reflective questions. All of these techniques (and a great many more) comprise a specialist intervention in which mediators are specifically trained.

Mediated intervention sessions are usually embedded in a test-teach-retest paradigm, which is one of the key methodologies of DA. Other types of intervention are also employed in this way, with the performance at post-test assumed to be more representative of an individual's ability to learn and less influenced by prior experience and knowledge.

Another important component is the role of feedback. In a DA method termed "testing the limits," Carlson and Wiedl (1992) gave detailed feedback to the individual after his first attempt at a task item and monitored the improvement in performance on the next item. Carlson and Wiedl showed that the more detailed the feedback given, the better the gain on successive items. Feedback was explicit and included discussion with the learner about why he had responded as he did and what strategies might be useful.

DA is not, however, limited to qualitative evaluation. In an effort to research DA methods more empirically, researchers have adopted frameworks that can be scored, such as quantifying the amount or intensity of intervention that is required to bring about the problem-solving, a procedure known as "graduated prompts" (Campione & Brown, 1987). The graduated prompt score represents the number of cues provided to the learner to enable him or her to achieve a defined criterion. Individuals may be compared on the basis of the score they receive, to evaluate learning potential, and to determine service delivery decisions, such as who might receive direct intervention versus a waiting and review period. Similarly, an individual may be retested over a period of time and the graduated prompt score used to detect improvement—indeed, sometimes a small incremental improvement that would not be detected on a standardized test score. The prompts are predetermined and arranged in sequence from those that are most general and least supportive to those that are more specific in their guidance. The count of prompts reflects not only the number of cues needed by the learner, but also the intensity of facilitation. Graduated prompt methods do not usually contain pre-and post-tests and may be carried out in a single assessment session of no more than an hour.

EVIDENCE IN SUPPORT OF DYNAMIC ASSESSMENT OF LANGUAGE

Studies using a range of methods have addressed the learning of different aspects of the language system, for example phonological processing, vocabulary, grammar, and narrative. Many studies by educationalists have attempted to predict reading skills using DAs of phonological processing and word learning in order to plan early interventions (e.g., Swanson and Howard [2005], Bridges and Catts [2011], Gillam and Ford [2012]). Studies by SLTs have aimed to differentiate children with language disorders from those with English as an additional language (EAL or bilingual children) through dynamic assessments of vocabulary, word learning, expressive language, and narrative, as described here.

Dynamic Assessment of Vocabulary

Vocabulary learning, for instance, was investigated by Camilleri and Law (2007) in their DA of receptive vocabulary. This test procedure, which investigated "fast-mapping" skills, was developed to compare the performance of monolingual English-speaking preschoolers with children with EAL and of typically developing children with those referred to SLT services by nursery staff. Children were required to match new words to a referent and also retain the new word for receptive and expressive access. The pre-test, a static version of the British Picture Vocabulary Scale (BPVS, Dunn et al., 1997), was followed by an interactive phase which consisted of a picture-word matching game and expressive and receptive tasks that were scored.

It was found that the DA was able to differentiate between typically developing (TD) children and those referred to speech-language therapy services because the referred children obtained significantly lower scores on all of the DA measures than the TD children. Similarly, there was equal performance between monolingual children and children with EAL whose static scores on the BPVS differed. This suggests that the static test may not be suitable for children with EAL and risks overdiagnosing them as language impaired. At 6-month follow-up, it was seen that the BPVS scores at Time 1 (T1) were highly predictive of BPVS scores at T2, but only with regard to high-scoring children. The DA, however, added 20% of variance to the predictability of low-scoring children. The authors concluded that the DA of word learning may be utilized as an alternative or additional measure with children with EAL as well as monolingual children to provide a more valid measure of children's lexical abilities and that the DA of word learning could be used to distinguish between children who are likely to make progress from ones who are likely to have longer-lasting difficulties.

Similarly, Steele and Watkins (2010), investigating word learning from reading, noted that children with language learning disorders (LLD) and TD children were both expected to show improved word learning with more exposures to target words and with more context clues. Thirty children aged between 9 and 11 years were given four reading passages containing non-words and asked to say the words, define them, and give synonyms for the non-words using clues gleaned from the context. They found that, as expected, contextual clues were helpful to all of the children, although TD children demonstrated significantly more of a benefit. The prompting methodology made this difference clearer than was apparent from the static test. Children with LLD required more prompting to infer meanings than did TD children. Children may be taught to use context to determine meaning and may be taught skills of definition, but the amount of teaching required to achieve criteria varied between TD and LLD groups.

Dynamic Assessment of Morphology

Building on a DA of derivational morphology developed by Larsen and Nippold in 2007, Ram et al. (2013) constructed a graduated prompt method to determine if children can derive meanings of morphologically complex words from their component morphemes. For example, can a child derive the meaning of "beautify" given their knowledge of the morpheme "beauty" and their experience of the morpheme "-fy"? Ram et al. assessed a group of 30 grade 3 children, with a mean age of 9;1 years, and a further 31 grade 5 children to evaluate the developmental trend in the skills and the use of the cues in the prompt hierarchy. Children were first asked to give the meaning of a complex word. If they did not succeed in defining the word according to the given criteria, they were prompted through five increasingly directive cues until they were successful. They were then scored according to the number of prompts required for the 20 words in the test.

Results of the study showed a developmental trend, with older children requiring fewer prompts to succeed in the task. Grade 3 children were, however, able to determine meanings of complex words from parts with adult scaffolding. They were able to benefit from support, indicating that they were modifiable. Given the more supportive cue of sentence context, they were able to determine meanings with less need for adult support. The DA was thought to be useful to determine the strategies used by children in this task, one that is regularly met by secondary age children in curriculum learning.

Dynamic Assessment of Narrative

Studies of narrative have been variously used to distinguish children with DLDs (language impairment or LI) from both mono- and bilingual TD children. Miller, Gillam, and Peña (2006) first examined the classification ability of a DA of narrative ability in three subjects who were in first and second grade at school. The procedure made use of two parallel wordless story books which were used as pre- and post-tests. Two sessions of individualized mediational intervention were then carried out in the "teach" phase. After the second intervention session, the children were rated by examiners on criteria such as modifiability, receptiveness to intervention, and the ease with which examiners were able to elicit responses. All of the children performed better on the post-test after the two sessions of mediated intervention, but the TD children showed greater gains than those with LIs, suggesting that they were more able to benefit from the intervention on offer. This was borne out by the findings that pre-test measures of narrative alone did not accurately classify TD and LI children and that the best single predictor was the rating of modifiability carried out by the assessors after the intervention sessions. In other words, the DA assessed responsiveness of the individual to instruction, and it is this feature that best distinguishes children with language difficulties from their typically developing peers.

The DA of narrative procedure was subsequently modified and shortened by Petersen et al. (2017) with the intention of evaluating whether it could effectively be carried out in two 25-minute sessions, with real-time rating of modifiability. Participants in the study were 42 bilingual schoolchildren, aged between 6;4 and 9;6, 10 of whom met the criteria for LI. Two sessions were carried out, each with a pre-test narrative retell, a narrative teaching phase, and a post-test retell. The teaching phase comprised assessors moving through a set of four predetermined steps supporting retelling of a story. Story grammar components and causal subordinate clauses were targeted. Modifiability was rated by the examiner at the end of each teaching session, and the scoring of rating scales was further modified to include a single cutoff point at which the presence or absence of LI could be determined because the authors believed that this diagnostic capability increased the value of the test. Interrater reliability was monitored and maintained at a high level. The authors found that the procedure was able to achieve close to 100% classification accuracy between two groups of LI and TD young bilingual children.

The Petersen group study was motivated by the need to reduce the time taken for a DA to that which would be more clinically efficacious while preserving the demonstrated advantages of a DA of narrative.

Previous DAs of narrative have required time-consuming transcription of narratives in addition to 3 or 4 intervention sessions. While this was achieved, the identified next step in furthering clinical utility would be to determine the training required for clinicians to administer and score the narrative DA in real time. The authors note that research assistants were trained for only 30 minutes, which is still significantly longer than the time taken to learn scoring of a norm-referenced test. Nevertheless Petersen et al. are committed to increasing the use of DA by practicing clinicians.

Dynamic Assessment of Sentence Structure

Similar concerns regarding the need for training of clinicians and the time taken for a DA were explored by Hasson, Dodd, and Botting (2012) in the Dynamic Assessment of Sentence Structure (DASS). The sentence anagram procedure, in which the child was required to arrange a set of single words into two possible sentences, was presented as a "hybrid" of a graded prompt structure in which each level of prompting was delivered using techniques of mediated learning and individualized to the learner. Like the narrative study, this added quantified scoring that enabled comparison between test-takers to the qualitative clinical information elicited. The DASS procedure was shown to tease out the performance of a group of children aged 8–10 years with previously identified language disorders over a wide range of scores, whereas their scores on a standardized test had clustered around the lowest percentiles. The scoring of the graded prompts was shown to be transparent and reliable by interrater agreement with another examiner, but the need to train clinicians to administer and score the DASS is still a barrier to widespread use of the test. Nevertheless, the authors demonstrated that the information gained from the DA was useful to clinicians involved in the clinical management of the participants and that the participants benefited from the changes made to their intervention.

RELIABILITY AND VALIDITY OF DYNAMIC ASSESSMENT

Before moving on, it is worth noting that reliability and validity of a DA is difficult to establish for a number of reasons. One of these is that the intention of a DA is to induce change in the performance of the test-taker, and, as a result, re-test reliability is not possible. Furthermore, individualized mediational interventions result in nonstandard administration of the test and reduce the usefulness of interrater reliability. Construct validity has been demonstrated by partial but significant correlations between the findings of dynamic tests and comparable static measures. Little more than a partial correlation can be expected, as only the part of the DA that addresses language content overlaps with the targets of the static test. The remainder of the DA addresses the process of learning and learning potential that is not in common with a static test.

FEEDING BACK THE RESULTS OF A DYNAMIC ASSESSMENT

As more research into DA has been carried out in relation to assessment of "intelligence," it is from that context that research into the reporting of the results of a DA originates. Haywood and Lidz (2007), Deutsch and Reynolds (2000), Bosma and Resing (2010), and others have explored how a DA may be reported in a school report or incorporated into an Educational and Health Care Plan (EHCP). Primarily, because the procedure is largely unfamiliar to teachers, other educational psychologists (EPs), SLTs, and families, reports will always need to contain a description of the (dynamic) test, as well as the findings. This makes reports longer and more time-consuming to read, which is always a drawback because professionals are less inclined to read and retain the content of longer reports. Bosma and Resing (2010) found that the responses of teachers to the reports of a DA varied with age and experience, and they concluded that reports may also need to contain information about the theory of DA to give the readers some context for understanding the information. Deutsch and Reynolds (2000) also reiterated the need for clarity as the procedure contrasts significantly with the static test. Similarly, there is a need for expanded explanations to parents and caregivers whose experience of assessment is also most likely to be of static, content-based tests.

Freeman and Miller (2001) reported that, despite the unfamiliar content, reports of DA contained material that special educational needs (SEN) staff found particularly useful. The DA helped SEN teachers understand children's abilities and needs and how to alter these with intervention. Lauchlan and Elliott (1997), however, found that while the reports were well received by teachers of pupils with learning difficulties, they did not impact the work being done in the classrooms. Hasson (2011), also found that there was too much expectation placed on SLTs that they would be able to modify their intervention practices based on a brief report and information leaflet. It was recommended that videos of the DA be shown to the professionals involved in the care of the child.

It may indeed be useful for others to observe the dynamic testing, and Haywood and Lidz (2007) and Delclos, Burns, and Vye (1993) demonstrated benefits to observers of DA who gained more insight into the children in their care and made more optimistic predictions about what they may achieve.

All of these authors have commented that the findings of a DA can usefully be incorporated into a student's EHCP or equivalent. In doing so, it is important to specify the roles of the teacher, learning support assistants, and others in the multidisciplinary team in implementing goals, as the recommendations of the DA are domain-general and apply to general cognitive learning principles. This also applies to assessments of language, as the learning processes would best be supported throughout the learning environment and not limited to language therapy sessions.

LIMITATIONS OF DYNAMIC TESTING

As alluded to earlier, clinicians and educators must be trained to administer DAs. Training in DA and mediation for therapists and educationalists is difficult to find, although courses are offered in the United Kingdom and Europe by trainers of the Feuerstein Institute. There is no formal training specifically for SLTs. Researchers investigating DA or mediated teaching (Kok, 2011; Petersen et al., 2017; Shamir & Tzuriel, 2004) have trained assessors specifically for their research projects, with differing amounts of training:—30 minutes for Petersen's research assistants; 50 hours for teachers in the study by Kok, and seven sessions of unknown length for 8-year-old children as mediators in the study by Shamir and Tzuriel—but there is no consistent recommended training in mediation or for assessors in DA procedures.

Hasson (unpublished research) trained SLTs in the DASS procedure in sessions lasting approximately 90 minutes and including video examples. The project aimed to find out whether the SLTs would be able to score the DA reliably, use principles of mediation when carrying out the dynamic assessment of language, and would find the DA useful for planning management of children on their caseload. The SLTs were in fact found to use and score the procedure reliably, although they lacked confidence in their test administration and missed opportunities to probe the metacognitive awareness of the children. Hasson concluded that a more detailed training package was needed, and this was published in 2018 as the Dynamic Assessment of Language Learning.

The Dynamic Assessment of Language Learning (Hasson, 2018) focuses mainly on the DASS, but the greatest limitation to the spread of DA of language remains the paucity of other tools for DA of language. Methods and materials for DA of language are still in the experimental stages, and training therapists in DA would have little clinical application at this stage.

FUTURE DIRECTIONS

While it can be seen that DA has been used to good effect in the assessment of first language for both diagnostic differentiation and intervention purposes, there is still a long way to go to devise more DA instruments for the different parts of the language system and train clinicians in their use. Further research is needed to develop and trial assessment tools and evaluate their effectiveness for assessment of language. Nevertheless, I believe that disseminating information about DA and training clinicians and educators in the principles of DA will go some way toward decreasing the reliance on static tests and increasing the use of trial therapies and stimulability tests.

REFERENCES

Bosma, T., & Resing, W. (2010). Teacher's appraisal of dynamic assessment outcomes: Recommendations for weak mathematics performers. *Journal of Cognitive Education and Psychology*, *9*(2), 91–115. https://doi.org/10.1891/1945-8959.9.2.91

Bridges, M. S., & Catts, H. W. (2011). The use of a dynamic screening of phonological awareness to predict risk for reading disabilities in kindergarten children. *Journal of Learning Disabilities*, *44*(4) 330–338. https://doi.org/10.1177/0022219411407863

Camilleri, B., & Law, J. (2007). Assessing children referred to speech and language therapy: Static and dynamic assessment of receptive vocabulary. *International Journal of Speech-Language Pathology*, *9*(4), 312–322. https://doi.org/10.1080/14417040701624474

Campione, J. C., & Brown, A. L. (1987). Linking dynamic assessment with school achievement. In C. S. Lidz (Ed.), *Dynamic assessment: An interactional approach to evaluating learning potential* (pp. 82–115). Guilford Press.

Carlson, J. S., & Wiedl, K. H. (1992). Principles of dynamic assessment: The application of a specific model. *Learning and Individual Differences*, *4*(2), 153–166. https://doi.org/10.1016/1041-6080(92)90011-3

Delclos, V. R., Burns, M. S., & Vye, N. J. (1993). A comparison of teachers' responses to dynamic and traditional assessment reports. *Journal of Psychoeducational Assessment*, *11*(1), 46–55. https://doi.org/10.1177/073428299301100106

Deutsch, R., & Reynolds, Y. (2000). The use of dynamic assessment by educational psychologists in the UK. *Educational Psychology in Practice*, *16*(3), 311–331. https://doi.org/10.1080/713666083

Dockrell, J. E. (2001). Assessing language skills in preschool children. *Child Psychology and Psychiatry Review*, *6*(2), 74–84. https://doi.org/10.1017/S1360641701002532

Dunn, L. M., Dunn, L. M., Whetton, C., & Burley, J. (1997). *British Picture Vocabulary Scale 2nd edition (BPVS-II)*. NFER-Nelson.

Feuerstein, R., Rand, Y., & Hoffman, M. B. (1979). *The dynamic assessment of retarded performers: The learning potential assessment device, theory, instruments, and techniques*. University Park Press.

Feuerstein, R., Feuerstein, R. S., Falik, L. H., & Rand, Y. (2002). *The dynamic assessment of cognitive modifiability: The learning propensity assessment device: Theory, instruments and techniques*. ICELP Press.

Freeman, L., & Miller, A. (2001). Norm-referenced, criterion-referenced and dynamic assessment: What exactly is the point? *Educational Psychology in Practice*, *17*(1), 3–16. https://doi.org/10.1080/02667360120039942

Gillam, S. G., & Ford, M. B. (2012). Dynamic assessment of phonological awareness for children with speech sound disorders. *Child Language Teaching and Therapy, 28*(3), 297–308. https://doi.org/10.1177/0265659012448087

Hasson, N. (2011). Dynamic Assessment and Informed Intervention for Children with Language Impairment. (Unpublished Doctoral thesis) City University London. Online, http://openaccess.city.ac.uk/1119/

Hasson, N. (2018). *The dynamic assessment of language learning*. Routledge.

Hasson, N., & Joffe, V. (2007). The case for dynamic assessment in speech and language therapy. *Child Language Teaching and Therapy, 23*(1), 9–25. https://doi.org/10.1177/0265659007072142

Hasson, N., Dodd, B., & Botting, N. (2012). Dynamic Assessment of Sentence Structure (DASS): Design and evaluation of a novel procedure for assessment of syntax in children with language impairments. *International Journal of Speech Language and Communication Disorders, 47*(3), 285–299. https://doi.org/10.1111/j.1460-6984.2011.00108.x

Haywood, H. C. (1993). A mediational teaching style. *International Journal of Cognitive Education and Mediated Learning, 3*(1), 27–38.

Haywood, H. C., & Lidz, C. S. (2007). *Dynamic assessment in practice. Clinical and Educational Applications.* Cambridge University Press.

Hessels, M. G. P., Berger, J. L., & Bosson, M. (2008). Group assessment of learning potential of pupils in mainstream primary education and special education classes. *Journal of Cognitive Education and Psychology, 7*(1), 43–69. https://doi.org/10.1891/194589508787381971

Kok, S. Y. (2011). Developing children's cognitive functions and increasing learning effectiveness: An intervention using the Bright Start Cognitive Curriculum for young Children. Doctoral Thesis, Durham University. http://etheses.dur.ac.uk/625/

Laing, S. P., & Kamhi, A. (2003). Alternative assessment of language and literacy in culturally and linguistically diverse populations. *Language Speech and Hearing Services in Schools, 38*(3), 201–212. https://doi.org/10.1044/0161-1461(2003/005)

Larsen, J. A., & Nippold, M. A. (2007). Morphological analysis in school-age children: Dynamic assessment of a word learning strategy. *Language, Speech, and Hearing Services in Schools, 38*(3), 201–212. https://doi.org/10.1044/0161-1461(2007/021)

Lauchlan, F., & Elliott, J. (1997). Using dynamic assessment materials as a tool for providing cognitive intervention to children with complex learning difficulties. *Educational and Child Psychology, 14*(4), 137–148.

Lidz, C. S. (1991). *Practitioner's guide to dynamic assessment*. Guilford Press.

Miller, L., Gillam, R. B., & Peña, E. D. (2006). *Dynamic assessment and intervention: Improving children's narrative abilities*. Pro-Ed.

Olswang, L., Bain, B., & Johnson, G. (1992). Using dynamic assessment with children with language disorders. In S. Warren & J. Reichle (Eds.), *Causes and effects in communication and language intervention* (pp. 187–215). Paul H. Brookes.

Peña, E., & Iglesias, A. (1992). The application of dynamic methods to language assessment: A non-biased procedure. *The Journal of Special Education, 26*(3), 269–280. https://doi.org/10.1177/002246699202600304

Petersen, D. B., Chanthongthip, H., Ukrainetz, T., Spencer, T., & Steeve, R. (2017). Dynamic assessment of narratives: Efficient, accurate identification of language impairment in bilingual students. *Journal of Speech, Language, and Hearing Research*, 60(4), 983–998. https://doi.org/10.1044/2016_JSLHR-L-15-0426

Ram, G., Marinellie, S. A., Benigno, J., & McCarthy, J. (2013). Morphological analysis in context versus isolation: Use of a dynamic assessment task with school-age children. *Language, Speech, and Hearing Services in Schools, 44*(1), 32–47. https://doi.org/10.1044/0161-1461(2012/11-0023)

Schneider, P., & Watkins, R. V. (1996). Applying Vygotskian developmental theory to language intervention. *Language Speech and Hearing Services in Schools, 27*(2), 157–170. https://doi.org/10.1044/0161-1461.2702.157

Shamir, A., & Tzuriel, D. (2004). Children's mediational teaching style as a function of intervention for cross-age peer-mediation. *School Psychology International, 25*(1), 59–78. https://doi.org/10.1177/0143034304024782

Steele, S. C., & Watkins, R. V. (2010). Learning word meanings during reading by children with language learning disability and typically-developing peers. *Clinical Linguistics & Phonetics, 24*(7), 520–539. https://doi.org/10.3109/02699200903532474

Swanson, H. L., & Howard, C. B. (2005). Children with reading disabilities: Does dynamic assessment help in the classification? *Learning Disability Quarterly, 28*(1), 17–35. https://doi.org/10.2307/4126971

Vygotsky, L. S. (1986). *Thought and language*. MIT Press.

3.2

Dynamic Assessment of Learners of a Signed Language

Wolfgang Mann, Joanna Hoskin, and Hilary Dumbrill

RESEARCH ON DYNAMIC ASSESSMENT

There is limited literature on the use of dynamic assessment (DA) with signing children. One reason for this lack may be the status of signed language research in general, which, aside from American Sign Language (ASL), British Sign Language (BSL) and a few other signed languages, is rather underdeveloped (Mann & Haug, 2014, also see Chapter 1.2). Another reason might be the small population of deaf children who sign compared to those who are raised orally (only 5–10% of deaf children have deaf parents; see Mitchell & Karchmer, 2004). Most of the existing literature has been contributed by authors of this chapter. For instance, Mann, Peña, and Morgan (2014) were the first to apply DA to signed language by piloting a model of assessing lexical-semantic categorization skills with two deaf elementary students between 7 to 8 years of age who were native signers. Participants completed a set of pre-/post-vocabulary measures and received two 30-minute mediations (mediated learning experiences, MLE) in ASL between tests. Each session involved different activities focusing on the use of categorization, such as sorting objects of various shapes and sizes or matching animals, body parts, and/or clothes. Materials included cutouts, pictures, and video-recorded ASL signs. Both sessions were scripted, and scripts included the five mediation strategies by Lidz (1991): namely (1) intention to teach, (2) intention to meaning, (3) mediation of transcendence, (4) mediation of competence, and (5) mediation of transfer (for more detailed information, the reader is referred to Mann et al., 2014, 2015). Findings revealed differences between the children both with regard to their response to mediation as well as their abilities to make semantic categories. One child who had scored poorly on the pre-test also required more support in MLE compared to her peer who worked more independently during the session. Both children also showed differences in their ways of applying cognitive strategies (e.g., the

Wolfgang Mann, Joanna Hoskin, and Hilary Dumbrill, *Dynamic Assessment of Learners of a Signed Language* In: *The Handbook of Language Assessment Across Modalities.* Edited by: Tobias Haug, Wolfgang Mann, and Ute Knoch, Oxford University Press. © Oxford University Press 2022. DOI: 10.1093/oso/9780190885052.003.0009 willingness to accept alternative strategies and/or the ability to use multiple strategies). Observations made by the mediator during the sessions were compared with teacher ratings of students' language skills and found to be consistent.

In a follow-up study, Mann, Peña, and Morgan (2015) investigated semantic categorization in a larger group of deaf children signing at different levels in ASL. One aim of this study was to examine more closely the extent to which children's response to mediation and the effort required by the mediator, both together referred to as "child modifiability," can be used to differentiate signing deaf children based on their language skills. The study used the same intervention format and materials as described in Mann et al. (2014). Findings showed a considerable sensitivity of mediator ratings of modifiability to language learning ability (i.e., the combination of child responsivity, the ability to transfer new knowledge, and the amount of support provided by the examiner). In addition, the differences between strong and weak language learners were most apparent in the use of cognitive strategies during the learning sessions. These results are relevant for practice as they encourage clinicians to carefully profile and respond to the kinds of strategies that are measured during mediation, including the way the child responds to feedback or the child's ability to self-correct errors.

In a recent study, Hoskin (2017) along with four deaf practitioners, explored mediated learning practices and DA by working with deaf children who have language difficulties. As part of this study Hoskin developed a set of mediated learning screening tools for language therapy in BSL, some of which are similar to those used by Mann and colleagues. The study found that deaf practitioners need specific tools and resources, training, and supervision as well as guidelines for best practice to ensure that they, and hearing language professionals, are sufficiently equipped to use mediated learning strategies and identify and address deaf children's language learning difficulties in BSL.

WHAT MAKES DYNAMIC ASSESSMENT USEFUL FOR DEAF SIGNING CHILDREN FROM A CLINICIAN/PRACTITIONER'S VIEW?

Historically, deaf children who signed were part of the Deaf community and learned to sign from adults and peers who were fluent in the signed language of their community either at home or in schools for Deaf children (Sutton-Spence, 2010). As changes in identification of deafness, early intervention, and the increase in mainstream education have occurred, identification of "deaf, signing children" has become more complex (see Herman, 2015, for more detail). For instance, it is becoming increasingly recognized that some children who are part of the Deaf community may have language disorders (Herman et al., 2014; Mason et al., 2010; Quinto-Pozos, 2014). Similarly, it is recognized that children who are referred for cochlear implantation may present with a range of needs in addition to their deafness (Inscoe & Bones, 2016). In case of the latter. this can mean that exclusive use of a spoken language does not fully meet their needs in terms of reaching their potential for communication development. One challenge for practitioners working with deaf children is in identifying when interventions carried out in a signed language might be most appropriate for different groups of children including:

- Deaf children with language disorder whose parents engage with the Deaf community and who have good early access to language but still experience language difficulties (Hoskin, 2016; Pizer et al., 2013).
- Children who are deaf and in whom a language disorder associated with deafness in spoken English is suspected (Bishop et al., 2016a, 2016b)
- Children whose deafness is part of a more complex picture of health, learning, and/or social needs (Inscoe & Bones, 2016; Watson et al., 2008)

Although research has highlighted the needs of the first group (e.g., Herman et al., 2014; Mason et al., 2010), the needs of the next two groups in relation to language disorder can be more complex to understand. In their summary from the Delphi Consensus, where international experts shared their views on terminology to use for children who present with language disorders, Bishop and colleagues (2016a) point out that children may have "biomedical conditions in which language disorder occurs as part of a more complex pattern of impairments. This may indicate a specific intervention pathway. We recommend referring to 'language disorder associated with X, where X is the differentiating condition" (p. 7). In supplementary comments they identify differentiating conditions as autism spectrum disorder (ASD), brain injury, acquired epileptic aphasia in childhood, certain neurodegenerative conditions, genetic conditions such as Down syndrome, cerebral palsy, and/or oral language difficulties associated with sensorineural hearing loss. These are all cases where an association between a biomedical condition and language disorder is commonly seen. In such cases, the child requires support for the language problems, but the intervention pathway will also need to consider the distinctive features of that condition. It should be noted, however, that there is little research directly comparing language intervention approaches across conditions, so this inference is usually based on clinical judgment rather than research evidence. Furthermore, there are deaf children with delay in spoken language who have not had access to signed language due to parental preference for a spoken communication mode, conflicting ideologies of those supporting the child and family, concerns that to introduce sign will lessen the child's attention to and development of oral/aural skills, and/or lack of access to deaf role models who are native signers. Supporting these children may require an immediate change in language environment and then use of DA to monitor their response to such change. In this context, DA allows for flexibility and for priority to be given to first establishing a "working relationship" with the child. DA values co-working and co-creation, situations which can in themselves be healing for a child who has struggled to communicate and connect.

Understanding a child's language learning journey, the choices and preferences of parents (i.e., signed or spoken language), use of listening technology (hearing aid, cochlea implant), and so on, along with the services, support, and interventions that are accessible locally to a child, can make the assessment and intervention process quite complex. DA enables a wide remit in focusing not only on a deaf child's language skills but on their skills in different contexts. In several clinical examples, children's language difficulties have been reported to impact their ability to manage change in their environment, and ASD is suspected. However, when skilled deaf practitioners with fluent signed language engaged with them, their flexibility increased as language was modified to meet their language needs. In another clinical example, a young deaf person had access to fluent communication partners at home and in a clinical setting who were able to adapt their language to meet the needs of the child (rather than their signed language skills solely). His social-emotional difficulties were initially attributed to attention deficit hyperactivity disorder (ADHD). When his language difficulties were identified, explained to caregivers in both settings, and mediated language learning opportunities provided, the child's language learning and executive function skills increased and his hyperactivity and attention issues decreased (Hoskin, 2017). These anecdotes suggest two things: (1) that the difficulties experienced by the individuals being treated were linked to the skills or knowledge of different mediators or communication partners and (2) that the use of DA and mediated learning tools enabled change in the children's responses as well as the strategies used by their mediator/communication partner. By using this more holistic view, clinicians are less likely to focus on one small aspect of a child's language profile, which may be the case with conventional testing. In this context it is vital that they understand the child's access to key relationships and community, particularly with reference to the importance of these factors for mental health and cognitive development.

CHALLENGES OF ASSESSING DEAF CHILDREN WITH STANDARDIZED INSTRUMENTS

The appropriate assessment of signing deaf children's language is usually hindered by two elements: (1) variability in children's language input/environment and (2) a general shortage of appropriate, signed language assessments. Deaf children's environments and their early language experiences vary considerably, ranging from signing deaf parents to hearing parents who communicate exclusively through speech. Traditionally there have been few reliable and valid tests available to examine deaf children's signed language abilities, although this is slowly changing (for a review of existing instruments, see Enns et al., 2016). Deaf children tend to do poorly on standardized tests for spoken language in part because these tests have been developed for (and normed on) a different target population—namely, hearing children—and the language used is not as easily accessible to them.

An additional concern is the potential bias introduced when differences to the hearing population (or low performance) are interpreted as disorders. For instance, even the act of test-taking requires a child to have sufficient language to comprehend the test instructions, enough to know what she or he is supposed to do. Given the language delay many deaf, signing children experience, their familiarity with the content or wording of tests may be affected. Findings from a recent study on the effects of ASL as accommodation for deaf/hard of hearing (D/HH) test-takers of standardized math/reading assessments showed no significant differences between those who did and did not receive ASL accommodations (Cawthon et al., 2010). These findings suggest that mere translation of the instructions for tests designed for a hearing population is unlikely to address the underlying lack of experience with such language. Even when a signed language assessment has been specifically developed for deaf children who sign, some challenges remain, including the varying signing skills of the test administrator and the question of availability of test norms (also see Chapter 1.2).

Professionals conducting language assessments in a signed language are usually neither native signers (nor deaf), and many do not have a well-developed knowledge of the language (Mann & Prinz, 2006). As a result, these professionals may misinterpret signs they do not recognize as incorrect. This is particularly problematic on tests that assess productive skills. Test norms of a signed language assessment may not be equally appropriate for all test-takers, given the variability in deaf children's signed language experience. For instance, signed language tests that have been developed and normed on children with natural signed language input from birth may be less accurate in distinguishing children who began learning signed language (e.g., ASL) later or those using artificial signed systems representing spoken language (e.g., Sign-Supported English, Sign-Supported German, Signed-Exact English) from children with true language learning impairments. Here we propose that the mediated learning approach utilized in DA can complement existing measures and help to reduce effects of limited experience on performance. Of course, this requires signed language fluency by the mediator in order to be successful.

HOW DO WE DETERMINE THAT DYNAMIC ASSESSMENT IS APPROPRIATE FOR A PARTICULAR CHILD?

When children present with a complex language learning situation, their language and communication skills need to be considered along with their environmental communication context, the skills of their interactors, and the child's potential for change. This may require assessment over a period of time, which includes assessment of how a child approaches people and tasks and whether they have potential to change.

Changes in interaction and communication patterns employed with the child impact how a child engages and learns. DA makes it possible to observe and record the child's engagement using mediated learning session observation sheets (for examples, see Mann, 2018). This generates information to guide a clinician's decision about which future intervention strategies will be more (or less) helpful in supporting a specific child and/or provides information about the skills and strategies needed by adults and other children engaging with the child. Observations of the child's learning skills can also be linked to some of the work on deaf children's executive function (Botting et al., 2017), readiness to learn (Herman & Morgan, 2011), and the importance of a developmental approach that looks at where the child is now and what skills they could be expected to learn or use next (Herman et al., 2017). Using information about a child's response to mediated learning and their modifiability from DA may provide more information about the links between language and behavior (Stevenson et al., 2010) and how best to support that child's development.

More tools and resources are becoming available to support practitioners in gathering and reporting a child's language environment and communication partner access and needs. Groups of UK-based practitioners, for instance, are providing guidance for practitioners working with deaf children (Ackroyd et al., 2018; Swanwick et al., 2014). This may include information about the language skills and use of these skills by all staff and caregivers as well as those of parents, siblings, and friends. SmiLE therapy (Schamroth & Lawlor, 2015) is one intervention package that includes DA in the form of a test-teach-retest approach which involves the child in their own assessment. Including children in test-teach-test models of intervention by giving them the opportunity for "self-evaluation" can improve a child or young person's understanding of their own strengths and needs and support them in identifying goals that motivate them (Lauchlan & Carrigan, 2013).

HOW DO WE EVALUATE WHETHER DYNAMIC ASSESSMENT IS BENEFICIAL?

When using DA to identify and/or provide (mediated) learning strategies, it is important to consider whether this approach adds anything to current procedures. Does DA provide new or more detailed information? Are assessors able to use this (new) information to inform practitioners' understanding of the child's needs? Can this information and understanding inform clinicians' interventions and everyday interactions? Gathering the necessary information will require video and/or very detailed note-taking to highlight small but important changes. One way to make the collection of information during the assessment more manageable for assessors (i.e., clinicians) is by targeting specific factors; that is, learning principles that are particularly easy or difficult to modify during MLE and are agreed on by all involved prior to the assessment (Lauchlan & Carrigan, 2013). The information gathered on these factors can then be used to inform follow-up discussions about the child's learning style involving other practitioners and parents as well as the child him- or herself. This approach makes the process of assessment more manageable and the findings easier to communicate in a way that is understood by nonpractitioners. If the use of DA and MLE tools can support identification and use of more individualized intervention activities and procedures, the process will be of benefit to the child and those working to support that child's language learning. For the majority of children, both deaf and hearing, a language-rich environment is needed whereas, for some children with specific language learning needs, a language-modified environment is preferable. DA and MLE can help identify key aspects of how a language environment needs modification for a specific child.

WHO SHOULD BE INVOLVED IN DYNAMIC ASSESSMENT OF SIGNING DEAF CHILDREN?

One key feature of DA and MLE is the recognition of the role of the mediator in the process of assessment and the identification of the skills and strategies that the mediator may need to use to facilitate learning for a child or young person. Many deaf children are now educated within mainstream schools, supported by teaching assistants, communication support workers, and/or classroom assistants. This presents both challenges and opportunities when considering who is best suited to carry out DA and provide structured, mediated learning, whether spoken language–dominant mediators or signed language–dominant mediators.

On one hand, English/spoken language–dominant mediators have good access to training and information because as books and courses on language development are in English and the other dominant spoken languages of many countries. They can readily be provided with instruction on DA and MLE through information available online, in journal articles, and in books. As people who regularly work with deaf children on a daily basis, they already have insight into a child's learning processes and language use. Training and/or access to tools for MLE (e.g., checklists with learning principles, mediated learning observation forms) would support their work and potentially increase the sharing of information within the team of practitioners involved in a child's educational development. This process may be relatively smooth as, in most mainstream classes, the qualified teacher and support staff tend to be spoken language–dominant. However, although some English/spoken language–dominant mediators may be bilingual in signed language, many others are not. Some of the near-bilinguals may have acquired their "second" language (i.e., ASL or BSL) late as an adult. Consequently, their experience of typical child language development may be limited. For other mediators, their lack of signed language competency may impact a child's ability to use or learn language.

For signed language–dominant mediators, on the other hand, their experience of typical child language development is likely to be broader. They may have had more opportunity to develop skills in the natural process of language adaptation for communication with children. However, although their own language and language adaptations skills may be stronger, signed language–dominant mediators' access to training may not have been as straightforward or extensive because training is often delivered by spoken language–dominant qualified teachers without native BSL skills and/or through third-party interpreters. Training in DA and MLE could be useful for both groups of staff, with tailored input to maximize the skills and knowledge base of each group. The sharing of DA and MLE information with qualified teachers, parents, and the assessed child would be facilitated through such training. Coupled with the provision of materials to aid DA, the identification of the best support packages for a child would then be more structured and inclusive.

FUTURE DIRECTIONS FOR USING DYNAMIC ASSESSMENT WITH SIGNING DEAF CHILDREN

As demonstrated here, DA and mediated learning strategies support target development and outcomes that are meaningful for signing deaf children. Using the language that parents, teachers, or others use for desired behaviors enables children and those working with them to share goals within everyday activities. Supporting a child to understand how a language task will link to their everyday language use is an explicit activity for mediators using mediated learning strategies. Enabling a child to understand their goals and, where possible, co-produce them supports a child's ability to acknowledge and recognize change. This can be done in simple ways, and some examples of how we have shared information with a child are given later.

Child-friendly reports with pictures and words at the child's level have been used to ensure the child understands the test-teach-retest results from interventions. As well as highlighting change, reports are explicit about what behaviors the child used to help with the learning process (e.g., "You told your mum about what you did, so I knew you understood it"). Comparison between videos of initial sessions and later sessions can highlight changes in desired skills; sharing these videos using language appropriate for the child helps them **see** what they are doing rather than relying on "talking about talking," which means they are expressing metalinguistic awareness. This strategy was used with a boy and parent. Initial difficulties were identified during the assessment period, video clips of intervention provided examples of when he was able to show desired skills, and the mother was supported to praise desired behaviors rather than commenting when behaviors were not demonstrated. This enabled her to observe and comment on desired changes specifically related to "waiting," "taking a turn," "talking/signing about pictures," and "telling a story," thus reinforcing the boy's learning. Sharing "child-friendly" versions of goals and feedback helps parents and staff notice skills development and praise appropriately; using language the child relates to their skills because this language is used within structured mediated learning tasks. The use of DA and mediated learning strategies can be enhanced when a collaborative approach is taken by professionals working with children and their families. This collaborative approach is supported by ensuring that accessible training, with practical components, is available in the spoken and signed languages of team members and that shared discussion is facilitated to overcome any language competence issues within the team. When working with children who use sign, Deaf practitioners value and benefit from discussions in signed language. Although the spoken language–dominant team members find this challenges their skills, the benefits for shared understanding are immense (Hoskin, 2017).

Easy to use tools are required to enable practitioners to embed DA and MLE into their practice. Some tools used in research need adaptation to ensure they are easily accessible and quick to use in educational and therapeutic sessions. Some "static" signed language assessment tools are currently available online (see www.dcalportal.org) and automatically gather data about children's responses. Test developers need to be aware of the very stringent confidentiality rules related to children's information in health and education services and be able to reassure practitioners that tools do not breach these rules.

Practitioners need to share a language to discuss language. Developing shared spoken and signed terms for aspects of assessment, intervention, and children's language strengths and difficulties for professionals and families is a challenge. This has been highlighted for spoken language difficulties (Bishop et al., 2016b; Lindsey et al., 2012) and is even more of a challenge when spoken and signed language are involved (Hoskin, 2017). Ongoing supervision and case reflection are needed to support co-working within teams. Enabling a discussion of the process of DA and MLE ensures that team members can step away from specific discussion about individual children's needs in order to monitor and improve their skills and processes. Careful thought is needed within teams about how and when to share information with children and parents. This complex and time-consuming process, if done with careful consideration, can enable shared understanding and increased access to intervention in different communication environments (Enderby, 2012) and is thus time well-spent.

DA and MLE approaches have much to offer practitioners working with deaf children who sign. The individualized approach focuses on identifying and supporting a child's language learning in the best way for them through detailed assessment and observation.

REFERENCES

Ackroyd, V., Hayes, R., & Hoskin, J. (2018). The evolution of an innovation; the Communication Profile—Learning and Innovation go hand in hand. *International Journal on Mental Health and Deafness*, *4*(1), 37–48. https://www.ijmhd.org/index.php/ijmhd/article/view/48/27

Bishop, D. V. M., Snowling, M. J., Thompson, P. A., & Greenhalgh, T. (2016b). CATALISE: A multinational and multidisciplinary Delphi consensus study of problems with language development. Phase 2. Terminology. *Peer J Preprints*, 1–31. https://doi.org/10.7287/PEERJ.PREPRINTS.2484V1

Bishop, D. V. M., Snowling, M. J., Thompson, P. A., Greenhalgh, T., CATALISE consortium (2016a). CATALISE: A multinational and multidisciplinary Delphi consensus study. Identifying language impairments in children. *Plos One*, *11*(7), 1–26. https://doi.org/10.1371/journal.pone.0158753

Botting, N., Jones, A., Marshall, C., Denmark, T., Atkinson, J., & Morgan, G. (2017). Nonverbal executive function is mediated by language: A study of deaf and hearing children. *Child Development*, *88*(5), 1689–1700. https://doi.org/10.1111/cdev.12659

Cawthon, S. W., Winton, S. M., Garberoglio, C. L., & Gobble, M. E. (2010). The effects of American Sign Language as an assessment accommodation for students who are deaf or hard of hearing. *Journal of Deaf Studies and Deaf Education, 16*(2), 198–211. https://doi.org/10.1093/deafed/enq053

Enderby, P. (2012). How much therapy is enough? The impossible question! *International Journal of Speech-Language Pathology, 14*(5), 432–437. https://doi.org/10.3109/17549507.2012.686118

Enns, C., Haug, T., Herman, R., Hoffmeister, R., Mann, W., & McQuarrie, L. (2016). Exploring signed language assessment tools in Europe and North Europe. In M. Marschark, V. Lampropoulou, & E. K. Skordilis (Eds.), *Diversity in deaf education* (pp. 171–218). Oxford University Press.

Herman, R. (2015). Language assessment of deaf learners. In H. Knoors & M. Marschark (Eds.), *Educating deaf learners: Creating a global evidence base* (pp. 196–212). Oxford University Press.

Herman, R., & Morgan, G. (2011). Deafness, language and communication. In K. Hilari & N. Botting (Eds.), *The impact of communication disability across the lifespan* (pp. 101–121). J&R Press Ltd.

Herman, R., Rowley, K., Mason, K., & Morgan, G. (2014). Deficits in narrative abilities in child British Sign Language users with specific language impairment. *International Journal of Language & Communication Disorders/Royal College of Speech & Language Therapists, 49*(3), 343–353. https://doi.org/10.1111/1460-6984.12078

Herman, R., Roy, P., & Kyle, F. E. (2017). *Reading and dyslexia in deaf children.* Nuffield Foundation; City University London.

Hoskin, J. H. (2016, March). Deaf children have language difficulties too. *British Deaf News*, 30–32.

Hoskin, J. (2017). Supporting the language needs of deaf children in *Bulletin: Magazine of Royal College of Speech and Language Therapists* (June), 13–14.

Inscoe, J., & Bones, C. (2016). Additional difficulties associated with aetiologies of deafness: Outcomes from a parent questionnaire of 540 children using cochlear implants. *Cochlear Implants International, 171*(1), 21–30. https://doi.org/10.1179/1754762815Y.0000000017

Lauchlan, F., & Carrigan, D. (2013). *Improving learning through dynamic assessment: A practical classroom resource.* Jessica Kingsley Publishers.

Lidz, C. S. (1991). *Practitioners' guide to dynamic assessment.* New York: Guilford.

Lindsay, G., Dockrell, J., Law, J., & Roulstone, S. (2012). *The Better Communication Research Programme: Improving Provision for Children and Young People with Speech, Language and Communication Needs.* DFE-RR247-BCRP1, 1–38.

Mann, W. (2018). Measuring deaf learners' language progress in school. In M. Marschark & H. Knoors (Eds.), *Evidence-based practices in deaf education* (pp. 171–188). Oxford University Press.

Mann, W., & Haug, T. (2014). Mapping out guidelines for the development and use of sign language assessments: Some critical issues, comments and suggestions. In D. Quinto-Pozos (Ed.), *Multilingual aspects of signed language communication and disorder* (pp. 123–139). Multilingual Matters.

Mann, W., Peña, E. D., & Morgan, G. (2014). Exploring the use of dynamic language assessment with deaf children, who use American Sign Language: Two case studies. *Journal of Communication Disorders, 52*, 16–30. https://doi.org/10.1016/j.jcomdis.2014.05.002

Mann, W., Peña, E. D., & Morgan, G. (2015). Child modifiability as a predictor of language abilities in deaf children who use American Sign Language. *American Journal of Speech-Language Pathology, 24*(3), 374–385. https://doi.org/10.1044/2015_AJSLP-14-0072

Mann, W., & Prinz, P. M. (2006). An investigation of the need for sign language assessment in deaf education. *American Annals of the Deaf, 151*(3), 356–370. https://doi.org/10.1353/aad.2006.0036

Mason, K., Rowley, K., Marshall, C. R., Atkinson, J. R., Herman, R., Woll, B., & Morgan, G. (2010). Identifying specific language impairment in deaf children acquiring British Sign Language: Implications for theory and practice. *British Journal of Developmental Psychology, 28*(1), 33–49. https://doi.org/10.1348/026151009X484190

Mitchell, R. E., & Karchmer, M. (2004). Chasing the mythical ten percent: Parental hearing status of deaf and hard of hearing students in the United States. *Sign Language Studies, 4*(2), 138–163. https://doi.org/10.1353/sls.2004.0005

Pizer, G., Walters, K., & Meier, R. P. (2013). "We communicated that way for a reason": Language practices and language ideologies among hearing adults whose parents are deaf. *Journal of Deaf Studies and Deaf Education, 18*(1), 75–92. https://doi.org/10.1093/deafed/ens031

Quinto-Pozos, D. (2014). Considering communication disorders and differences in the signed language modality. In D. Quinto-Pozos (Ed.), *Multilingual aspects of signed language communication and disorder* (pp. 1–42). Multilingual Matters.

Schamroth, K., & Lawlor, E. (2015). *SmiLE therapy: Functional communication and social skills for deaf students and students with special needs*. Speechmark.

Stevenson, J., McCann, D., Watkin, P., Worsfold, S., & Kennedy, C. (2010). The relationship between language development and behaviour problems in children with hearing loss. *Journal of Child Psychology and Psychiatry, and Allied Disciplines, 51*(1), 77–83. https://doi.org/10.1111/j.1469-7610.2009.02124.x

Sutton-Spence, R. (2010). The role of sign language narratives in developing identity for deaf children. *Journal of Folklore Research, 47*(3), 265–305. https://doi.org/10.1353/jfr.2010.0014

Swanwick, R., Simpson, K., & Salter, J. (2014). Language planning in deaf education: Guidance for practitioners by practitioners. *The National Sensory Impairment Partnership*. Retrieved from https://deafed.leeds.ac.uk/language-planning/

Watson, L. M., Hardie, T., Archbold, S. M., & Wheeler, A. (2008). Parents' views on changing communication after cochlear implantation. *Journal of Deaf Studies and Deaf Education, 13*(1), 104–116. https://doi.org/10.1093/deafed/enm036

3.3

Discussion on Issues Related to the Use of Dynamic Assessment of Learners of a Spoken or Signed Language

Wolfgang Mann, Joanna Hoskin, Natalie Hasson, and Hilary Dumbrill

Following the presentation of key issues related to using dynamic assessment (DA) separately for signed and spoken language, we now turn to the discussion of particular key issues and possible implications for either field.

WHAT CAN DYNAMIC ASSESSMENT FOR SIGNED LANGUAGES LEARN FROM SPOKEN LANGUAGES?

A wider range of dynamic assessments. One aspect of spoken language assessment with great potential to inform new research in signed language is the number and detail of available approaches that test different parts of the language system. Whereas DA with signing children has been used exclusively for assessing vocabulary, approaches in spoken languages have also targeted morphology, phonology, sentence structure, and narrative discourse. This situation is comparable to the number and variety of available "static" assessment for signed language versus spoken language, leaving researchers, clinicians, and practitioners with limited resources that are appropriate for testing signing children. Undertaking studies that explore the potential of DA for use with this population may address current gaps in our knowledge about different aspects of sign and their development.

Use of graduated prompting. Another area of research on DA for spoken language that can inform the field of signed language assessment relates to the type of testing. So far, the available research for signed language has used mediated intervention sessions that were embedded in a test-teach-retest paradigm (Mann et al., 2014, 2015). Less

Wolfgang Mann, Joanna Hoskin, Natalie Hasson, and Hilary Dumbrill, *Discussion on Issues Related to the Use of Dynamic Assessment of Learners of a Spoken or Signed Language* In: *The Handbook of Language Assessment Across Modalities.* Edited by: Tobias Haug, Wolfgang Mann, and Ute Knoch, Oxford University Press. © Oxford University Press 2022. DOI: 10.1093/oso/9780190885052.003.0010 explored is the use of graduated prompting that enables the assessor to quantify the level of intervention required for successful problem-solving. Furthermore, this approach could help to address the lack of developmental norms within signed language research by establishing sequences for the development of skills in a way that is similar to the studies described in Chapter 3.1. If successful, this would enable assessors to determine which aspects of language to target for intervention, as well as the level of language the child is currently able to use. Environmental interventions with parents and other adults could then be more targeted and based on the language skills a child is able to use or has potential to develop. By providing a structure for guided prompting, including specific identification of helpful strategies, practitioners would be enabled to focus on the child's developing functional skills rather than age-related norms. For schools, which are often under pressure to demonstrate a student's progress, the score provided by graduated prompting might be useful to demonstrate ongoing incremental change and progress.

Feedback to stakeholders. A third area where signed language research could benefit from the experiences of colleagues in spoken language research relates to how information resulting from DA is reported to parents. Where some guidance for those giving feedback from DA for children using spoken language has already been produced, such guidelines would help clinicians and academic assessors of signing children with how to provide feedback to parents and educators.

Parents and caregivers could benefit from raised awareness and increased knowledge to improve their own skills in understanding DA and mediated learning experience (MLE) (see Deutsch & Reynolds, 2000, in Chapter 3.1), and educators might be facilitated to focus or draw on a child's area of strength rather than on their limitations. Researchers in DA of spoken language have drawn on the experience of educators working in the DA of cognitive skill, and the combined experience may be useful to inform researchers in signed language. This guidance on what information to provide is related to how we engage families in the process of DA, as highlighted in the next section.

WHAT CAN DYNAMIC ASSESSMENT FOR SPOKEN LANGUAGES LEARN FROM SIGNED LANGUAGES?

Involving stakeholders in setting goals. One area where the available research from signed language could help inform the use of DA for spoken language is the involvement of children and families in co-producing goals to guide assessment and intervention. While research on spoken language has focused on providing guidance and supporting professionals using DA in knowing how to share their experiences, colleagues in the field of signed language assessment have worked closely with families on co-producing goals, as described in the signed language chapter. The co-production of goals and strategies ensures that children and parents are engaged in the therapeutic process of change. This promotes the use of strategies on a daily basis, which increases the overall impact of any professional intervention (Royal College of Speech and Language Therapists, 2018; Enderby, 2012).

Shared interests and needs. Finally, we would like to point out a couple of aspects that are of equal relevance for both fields and which provide opportunities for increased interdisciplinary collaboration. One of these aspects is the need for (more) training for mediators. Due to the current lack of a consistent method of recommended training in mediation or other DA procedures in the United Kingdom, both signed language and spoken language assessment need the development of mediator training and accreditation. In the absence of formal training, one aspect that would be beneficial for practitioners in both fields is to develop shared training protocols for administering DA by means of mediated learning sessions as part of a test-teach-retest approach or in the form of graduated prompting. These shared protocols may also be able to support mediators using DA with children with needs additional to language learning.

Another aspect is the need to make DA reports and the language used in these reports more accessible to stakeholders, including parents, speech language therapists (SLT), teachers, teaching assistants (TA), and communication support workers (CSW). Work carried out in this area by Lauchlan and Carrigan (2013) has produced a set of valuable resources that could serve as a starting point. These include learning profiles, checklists of learning principles, and intervention strategies to support effective and/or cognitive learning.

Children who use both signed and spoken languages (e.g., hearing children in Deaf families and bilingual deaf children) may benefit greatly from future collaborative work. By sharing working models of DA, these children's language strengths and potential could be better understood by those around them, thus enabling them to develop a strong first language in a more timely manner while maintaining a focus on skills development for their additional language(s).

Despite the many benefits of DA for spoken and signed language users we have discussed in this set of chapters, there is still a lot of work to be done to achieve positive, high-quality, joint work around DA in a multidisciplinary team.

REFERENCES

Deutsch, R., & Reynolds, Y. (2000). The use of dynamic assessment by educational psychologists in the UK. *Educational Psychology in Practice, 16*(3), 311–331. https://doi.org/10.1080/713666083

Enderby, P. (2012). How much therapy is enough? The impossible question! *International Journal of Speech-Language Pathology*, *14*(5), 432–437. https://doi.org/10.3109/17549507.2012.686118

Lauchlan, F., & Carrigan, D. (2013). *Improving learning through dynamic assessment: A practical classroom resource*. Jessica Kingsley Publishers.

Mann, W., Peña, E. D., & Morgan, G. (2014). Exploring the use of dynamic language assessment with deaf children, who use American Sign Language: Two case studies. *Journal of Communication Disorders, 52*, 16–30. https://doi.org/10.1016/j.jcomdis.2014.05.002

Mann, W., Peña, E. D., & Morgan, G. (2015). Child modifiability as a predictor of language abilities in deaf children who use American Sign Language. *American Journal of Speech-Language Pathology*, *24*(3), 374–385. https://doi.org/10.1044/2015_AJSLP-14-0072

Royal College of Speech and Language Therapists (RCSLT). (2018). *Clinical Guidance: Bilingualism*. Royal College of Speech and Language Therapists. https://www.rcslt.org/members/clinical-guidance/bilingualism/bilingualism-guidance

Topic 4

Assessing Language Development in L1 Children with Autism Spectrum Disorder

4.1

Assessing Spoken Language Development in Children with Autism Spectrum Disorder

Amy Kissel Frisbie

When conducting an evaluation of spoken language, it is imperative to consider all aspects of communication. Expressive output of language cannot be assessed without an understanding of receptive abilities. When spoken (or "expressive") language impairments exist, it is crucial to determine if there are accompanying deficits in receptive language. Similarly, expressive language cannot be considered in isolation from the other communication domains of phonology, morphology, syntax, semantics, and pragmatics. Spoken language impairments often co-occur with other conditions, such as intellectual or developmental disabilities, attention deficit hyperactivity disorder (ADHD), autism spectrum disorder (ASD), or sensory impairments such as hearing loss. Youngsters with spoken language difficulties often present with impairments related to literacy and social communication as well.

As of 2018, it is estimated that 1 in 59 children have an ASD (CDC, 2018). When evaluating atypical language development in children with ASD, it is vital to consider the core deficits of ASD. Per the *Diagnostic and Statistical Manual of Mental Disorders* (DMS-5) ASD includes (1) "persistent deficits in social communication and social interaction across multiple contexts" and (2) "restricted, repetitive patterns of behavior, interests, or activities, as manifested by stereotypic or repetitive motor movements, adherence to routines, intense interests and/or unusual sensory presentations" (American Psychiatric Association [APA], 2013, p. 50).

Social communication and spoken language abilities are intimately related to one another because social communication skills are imperative for successful language expression in both verbal and written modalities. The core deficits in ASD related to social communication include many important areas for consideration. The American Speech Language and Hearing Association (ASHA) subdivides social communication into three areas: social interaction, social cognition,

Amy Kissel Frisbie, *Assessing Spoken Language Development in Children with Autism Spectrum Disorder* In: *The Handbook of Language Assessment Across Modalities.* Edited by: Tobias Haug, Wolfgang Mann, and Ute Knoch, Oxford University Press. © Oxford University Press 2022. DOI: 10.1093/oso/9780190885052.003.0011 and pragmatics (ASHA, 2005). *Social interaction* includes gender and cultural expectations around communication, while *social cognition* includes aspects of social interaction such as Theory of Mind (ToM), executive functioning, and joint attention. *Pragmatics* includes functional use of communication for various purposes (i.e., to ask a question versus to share information, etc.), speech prosody, use of gestures, facial expressions, and eye contact as well as the use of challenging behaviors as communication (e.g., elopement to avoid a non-preferred task, hitting to refuse). These aspects of social communication must be evaluated to develop an appropriate plan of care for any child with ASD.

When using the DSM-5 to diagnose ASD, levels of severity are given specifiers to describe an individual's level of support required to participate in daily activities. Social communication severity level 1 ("requiring support") suggests that without support, "deficits in social communication cause noticeable impairments," while Level 2 ("requiring substantial support") suggests that impairments are "apparent even with supports in place." Level 3 ("requiring very substantial support") is given when "severe deficits in verbal and nonverbal social communication skills cause severe impairments in functioning." The DSM-5 also allows for the clinicians to notate ASD "with or without accompanying language impairment" (APA, 2013, p. 52). According to Levy et al. (2010), 63.4% of children identified with ASD do have a co-occurring language disorder, making a thorough communication evaluation vitally important. In preparation for a comprehensive language evaluation, the speech language pathologist (SLP) should take advantage of the information often made available at the initial diagnosis of ASD, such as the level of support required and previous language assessments completed.

SPOKEN LANGUAGE EVALUATION COMPONENTS

Case History

Any assessment related to communication should include several components, according to universal best practice evaluation standards. An evaluation of spoken language should always start with a thorough case history. Important details such as birth, medical, and family history may be available in a medical record, but understanding the family's specific concerns and questions and learning about the child's home language environment (i.e., if they are exposed to a second language) and other aspects of communication can only be gathered through an ethnographic caregiver interview (Westby et al., 2003). Reaching out to other stakeholders can be helpful (e.g., teachers, relatives, pediatrician). Given the high incidence of hearing impairments in children with ASD, a hearing screening or evaluation must also be completed (preferably before the evaluation) to rule out any hearing loss that may be impacting spoken language. A previously passed newborn hearing screen is not adequate, and a current understanding of hearing abilities across frequencies is vital. As part of the evaluation, the SLP should complete a brief oral mechanism examination (i.e., dental occlusion; status of dentition; hard and soft palate integrity; function of the lips, jaw, tongue, and velum; placement of tongue at rest and during speech). It is important to collect family input regarding feeding, swallowing, and management of meal time expectations.

Finally, at a minimum, a brief exploration of literacy (or pre-literacy) skills must be included in a spoken language evaluation. While 5–10% of children with ASD are considered "hyperlexic" (i.e., able to decode words, but struggle to interpret what they read), phonology and phonetic decoding are often impaired in ASD, so children with ASD are at higher risk for having difficulty learning to read (Newman et al., 2006). There are various literacy assessments available as standardized test supplements. The Clinical Evaluation of Language Fundamentals 5 (CELF-5) (Wiig et al., 2013) and the Clinical Evaluation of Language Fundamentals Preschool 2 (CELF-P2) (Wigg et al., 2004) have a reading and writing supplement and a pre-literacy scale, respectively. The Comprehensive Test of Phonological Processing Second Edition (Wagner et al., 1999) can be used to evaluate phonological awareness and phonological memory. In a school setting, various standardized literacy measures are routinely given to all children and can be included as part of an evaluation of written communication skills.

Observations

Another important aspect of spoken evaluation is mindful observation by the evaluator. In a clinic setting, this step can start as soon as a child is greeted in the waiting room. Does he look at the SLP when his name is called? Does she verbally greet the examiner or check in visually with her parents? Does he show the SLP the toys and treasures he's brought along? Ogletree and colleagues (2002) also suggest observation of children and their caregivers engaged in typical play routines (i.e., "play like you might at home"). Consideration of a child's play skills is vital to a robust assessment and for driving intervention targets. Skills observed while watching the child play can be compared to various developmental checklists related to typical play development.

In a school setting, an SLP can observe a variety of natural interactions throughout the child's day: the SLP may observe that she uses long verbal utterances in class yet can't find a friend to play with at recess. Does an older child struggle to join a peer group during project-based learning, even though she is described as "the smartest kid in fifth grade" or as "talking all the time"? When these opportunities are not available, analog tasks can be simulated as part of a communication evaluation. One strategy described in the literature for older, verbal children with ASD is the "double interview" (Winner, 2002). The clinician first interviews the child, then provides them with an opportunity to interview the clinician. Do they respond to social bids? Do they ask the examiner questions or make comments to show they are listening? By using these strategies, the clinician has a better sense of which standardized assessment tools to use and what to target in therapy.

Dynamic Assessment

Emerging (or minimally verbal) communicators or those using behaviors as communication may require evaluation tools and strategies that break communication milestones down into even more foundational skills. These tools are often completed with caregivers, using parent or teacher interview, as part of an ongoing, dynamic assessment (DA). DA (also see Chapters 3.1–3.3) differs from standardized testing in that a child is first assessed, then targeted skills are directly taught and retested to determine next steps based on the assessment outcomes. The ASHA encourages the use of DA as "a method that seeks to identify an individual's skills as well as his or her learning potential. . . . Dynamic assessment is highly interactive and emphasizes the learning process over time . . . [and] it can be used in conjunction with standardized assessments" (ASHA, 2018a). Examples of these dynamic tools include:

- Communication Matrix (Rowland, 2004): to evaluate "anyone functioning at the early stages of communication or using forms of communication other than speaking or writing" (Communication Matrix, 2020).
- The Early Start Denver Model Curriculum Checklist for Young Children with Autism (Rogers & Dawson, 2010; formal use of this model requires certification): used with toddlers with ASD between 12 and 60 months of age to "define the child's most mature skills" in several domains.

Receptive Language Assessment Using Standardized Measures

Many standardized tests are available across all ages to measure receptive language abilities. One common mistake, however, is to correlate simple vocabulary knowledge with one's ability to understand natural communication. Tests that measure receptive vocabulary knowledge (such as the Peabody Picture Vocabulary Test, Fourth Edition [PPVT-4] by Dunn & Dunn, 2007) are fast and easy to administer, and they provide good information about the child's ability to store and recall names of items (and actions), but they should not be used in isolation. When combined with a verbal naming assessment, such as the Expressive Vocabulary Test, Second Edition (EVT-2) (Williams, 2007), even more information can be gained toward understanding the child's ability to encode and retrieve names for pictured items and say them.

It is important not to stop here, however, because evaluating receptive language abilities is far more complicated than evaluating one's knowledge of vocabulary alone. For children with ASD, vocabulary (or semantic) knowledge is often a strength, but evaluation in this area in isolation does not tell us enough about how the child is functionally comprehending the world (Walenski et al., 2007). Walenski points out that lexical (or word knowledge) and semantic memory are often "enhanced" in people diagnosed with ASD, while "episodic" (or personal narrative) memory abilities remain impaired. Sharing personal stories and participating in conversation requires much more than simply knowing the specific names of objects.

Some standardized assessments include subtests that evaluate the more demanding aspects of receptive and expressive language integration and higher-level thinking. The Clinical Evaluation of Language Fundamentals–Fifth Edition (CELF-5) (Wiig et al., 2013), for example, includes an Understanding Spoken Paragraphs subtest where the child is read a brief story (5–7 sentences) and asked to answer a series of questions. It breaks down the various types of questions asked into main idea, details, sequence, inference, prediction, and social context. A subtest such as this places more cognitive and memory demands on a child and comes closer to simulating a more natural set of demands related to understanding and interpreting language. Linguistic demands for both speaking and comprehending are quite high throughout the school years, and difficulty with these tasks will lead to significant academic struggle. Adding in the questions related to prediction and inferencing (i.e., "What do you think would happen if . . . ") gives the examiner more insight into the strengths of the test-taker and highlights areas of need.

Standardized assessment measures of receptive language, such as those listed here, may be used to evaluate the abilities of children with ASD. One must always consider, however, their cultural and linguistic appropriateness based on the specific child being evaluated. Generally, individual subtests are included on assessments to quantify various aspects of language comprehension. Examples may include subtests such as Word Classes, Sentence Structure, Following Directions (including concepts such as, sequencing, negation, passive voice, etc.), and Semantic Relationships. When evaluating children with ASD, it is imperative to consider the norming samples used in the specific test's development and make sure it is representative of the child and their diagnoses if you intend to report standard scores (Santhanam & Hewitt, 2015). Receptive language assessment tools for children common in the United States include:

- PPVT-4 (Dunn & Dunn, 2007)
- CELF-5(Wiig et al., 2013)
- CELF-Preschool-2 (Wiig et al., 2004)

- Preschool Language Scales, Fifth Edition (PLS-5) (Zimmerman et al., 2011)
- The Rossetti Infant-Toddler Language Scale (Rossetti, 2006)

Expressive Language Using Standardized Assessment

A thorough evaluation of spoken language must include examination of all domains of language and speech production including phonology, semantics, morphology, syntax, and pragmatics. Difficulty with the pragmatic (or "social") aspects of spoken language is often the core challenge for a child with ASD. *Phonology* refers to the sound system of a language, or the individual sounds or phonemes that make up any word in a specific language. *Syntax* and *morphology* refer to the structure of language and are often evaluated using a variety of standardized evaluation tools; often given as a *cloze procedure*, where the child finishes the clinician's utterance with a word or adds the appropriate tense marker to a targeted picture (i.e., verb + ed for past tense or verb + s for plural) in an expressive subtest. When a child demonstrates difficulty with syntax, his communication partners may struggle to understand the sequencing of his or her narratives or conversation related to the timing of events. Evaluation and differential diagnosis of the cause of these types of difficulties is imperative as it may suggest cognitive differences related to ordering and sequencing and/or difficulty related to speech production (or "speech articulation").

Standardized measures of spoken language include various subtests such as sentence combining, word ordering, relational vocabulary, sentence imitation, and supplemental subtests such as phonological and articulation screeners. Examples of tools common in the United States include:

- Test of Language Development-Primary: Fourth Edition (TOLD-P:4; Hammill & Newcomer, 2008)
- Test of Language Development-Intermediate: Fourth Edition (TOLD-I:4; Hammill & Newcomer, 2008)
- The WORD Test 3 Elementary (Bowers et al., 2014)
- EVT-2 (Williams, 2007)
- CELF-5 (Wiig et al., 2013)
- CELF-Preschool-2 (Wiig et al., 2004)
- PLS-5 (Zimmerman et al., 2011)
- The Rossetti Infant-Toddler Language Scale (Rossetti, 2006)

Language Sampling

In additional to the use of parent report tools and standardized measures, a comprehensive spoken language evaluation should also include a language sample taken for analysis. Language sampling should be of spontaneous output and can be collected in play, during conversation, or elicited in narration (storytelling or personal discourse). Various informal and analytical measures can be applied to a language sample to augment information gained in standardized testing. One framework to consider is *Brown's stages* (Brown, 1973). Brown outlined five stages of typical expressive language morphology and syntax development (in English) achieved between the first 12 and 46 months of life in typical language learners. Brown's stages also delineate the expected *mean length of utterance* (e.g., in Stage III, children aged 31–34 months use an average of 2.5–3.0 morphemes per utterance) in typical spoken language based on age. Comparing grammatical morphemes from a language sample to typical development can provide important information for intervention.

In children with ASD, a language sample will often reveal *echolalic speech* (repeating the spoken utterances of others, usually word for word). There is extensive research in the literature related to the use of echolalia in children with ASD. Immediate and delayed echolalia are often observed. *Immediate echolalia* is described as repeating something heard within two conversational turns of the original utterance, while *delayed echolalia* is produced more than two conversational turns later and is characterized by (1) higher linguistic complexity than the child has spontaneously or (2) reflects a learned (or memorized) verbal routine (Prizant & Rydell, 1984). Current understanding of echolalia in ASD has evolved and is now considered a good predictor of achieving some level of functional spoken language. Discussion of echolalia with familiar communication partners is imperative because some children use echoed phrases so skillfully that they can be mistaken for generative utterances (Prizant & Rydell, 1984). Determining if older children used echolalia in the past is also helpful information.

Speech Articulation Assessment

Any evaluation of spoken language must include an evaluation of the speech articulation abilities of the child. An experienced SLP can hear differences in speech (articulation) production by ear and may be able to identify specific treatment targets for remediation based on developmental expectations of consonants and vowels that are omitted or mispronounced. A standardized tool is sometimes required to qualify a child for intervention in a school or clinical setting, however. Standardized tests can assist in the identification of phonological processes (i.e., cluster reduction, stopping, fronting, etc.) based on developmental norms. In the special case of children with ASD, this aspect of evaluation is especially important. Tierney and colleagues (2015) conducted a recent study and found that speech disturbances often co-occur in children with ASD. They found that 63.6% of children diagnosed with ASD also have *childhood apraxia of speech* (CAS). CAS is defined by the ASHA Ad Hoc Committee's Position Statement on Apraxia of Speech in Children (2007) as "a neurological childhood (pediatric) speech sound disorder in which the precision and consistency of movements underlying speech are impaired in the absence of neuromuscular deficits (e.g., abnormal reflexes, abnormal tone). The core impairment in planning and/or programming spatiotemporal parameters of movement sequences results in errors in speech sound production and prosody." While there are some standardized tools for evaluating for CAS, the Ad Hoc committee has identified three observable traits to consider during an evaluation: "(a) inconsistent errors on consonants and vowels in repeated productions of syllables or words, (b) lengthened and disrupted coarticulatory transitions between sounds and syllables, and (c) inappropriate prosody, especially in the realization of lexical or phrasal stress."

When CAS is suspected, it is vital to also consider differences in the child's nonspeech oral-motor abilities (i.e., lip and tongue movements on demand/in imitation), voice, resonance, and the prosody of their speech. Prosodic features are clinically evaluated by listening for unusual rhythm, stress, or intonation of the child's connected speech utterances. Atypical prosody is common in children with ASD and is not predicted by a child's cognitive or linguistic abilities. In fact, Shriberg and colleagues (2001) found that verbal children with "high functioning" ASD differed from neurotypical children in their prosodic features of stress, resonance, and phrasing. Unusual prosody impacts social relationships and interactions with communication partners and should be targeted for intervention by a SLP. Examples of standardized tools to evaluate speech articulation and phonology include:

- Goldman-Fristoe Test of Articulation 3 (GFTA-3) (Goldman & Fristoe, 2015)
- Arizona Articulation and Phonology Scale, Fourth Edition (Fudala, 2017)
- HAPP-3 Hodson Assessment of Phonological Patterns (Third Edition) (Hodson, 2004)

AUGMENTATIVE AND ALTERNATIVE COMMUNICATION

When a severe speech sound disorder, such as CAS, is diagnosed, consideration related to the use of *augmentative and alternative communication* (AAC) systems should occur. Beukelman and Mirenda (2013) have developed a process (the Participation Model, p. 109) where feature matching is used to determine the best AAC system for a specific individual. In the Participation Model, AAC is advised when any unmet communication need is identified compared to same-age peers. Beukelman and Mirenda describe "unaided" AAC systems as those that require no additional supports (e.g., natural gestures or signing) and "aided" AAC systems as requiring something additional to the body. This may include the use of nonelectronic communication boards, speech-generating devices (SGDs), or other systems, such as the Picture Exchange Communication System (PECS) (Bondy & Frost, 1994).

In recent years, the use of SGDs has been made much more accessible to those with complex communication needs secondary to a diagnosis of ASD with the advent of personal, handheld technology, such as mobile telephones and tablets. Lower costs for this technology, combined with the availability of hundreds of apps developed specifically for communication, have prompted families to seek out these options for their children who are non- or minimally verbal. McNaughton and Light (2013) recently reminded clinicians, parents, and teachers that, despite the relatively easy access to new technologies, it remains imperative to determine the best AAC system for each individual based on their particular needs (i.e., physical access or auditory/visual limitations, receptive language abilities, etc.), rather than simply seeking the latest technology. SGDs can be helpful in both receptive and expressive language learning, as is well documented in both the ASD and AAC literature; this issue is beyond the scope of this chapter.

Social Communication Assessment

The final, and perhaps most important, aspect of spoken language evaluation in a child with ASD is that of their social communication abilities. By definition, any child diagnosed with ASD has impairments related to their social use of language. When impairments in social cognition are suspected, both formal and informal assessments should be used to evaluate the child's social communication skills (both spoken and gestural). There are a limited number of standardized tests available to assess social (pragmatic) language skills in children, and some of the above-mentioned comprehensive assessments include supplements to do so. The CELF include a Pragmatics Profile inventory (to be completed by a therapist, teacher, or caregiver) as well as a Pragmatic Activities Checklist that can be used to quantify observations related to verbal and nonverbal communication functions. These may include using and responding to greetings, turn-taking, asking and answering questions, sharing information, and showing social closeness. The CELF-5 Metalinguistics assessment (Wiig & Secord, 2014) can be used to evaluate the ability of children 9 years and older to make inferences, interpret conversation in a given context, understand multiple meanings, and understand figurative language.

Given the limited number of standardized tests related to social communication, a significant amount of information during evaluation is gathered using observation and by using informal measures. Skills observed can be compared to typical pragmatic milestones based on the child's age. Available reference tools such as the "Social Communication Benchmarks" document published by ASHA (2018b) are quite valuable. When considering the various aspects of social communication, this tool includes the three aforementioned categories: "social interaction," "social cognition," and "pragmatics."

One important element of "social cognition" includes abilities related to ToM. The literature is saturated with descriptions of how people with ASD struggle with ToM. Sussman (2006) describes ToM as "the ability to understand that other people's thoughts and feelings differ from our own . . . [T]heory of mind (ToM) impairment in autism describes a difficulty someone would have with perspective taking" (p. 70). One can imagine how difficulty with "perspective taking" can lead to significant social impairments for children and adolescents with ASD, especially when interacting with peers. Children with ASD often look much better when interacting with adults, as is frequently the case during standardized evaluations—another important reason for including peer observations. The final social communication category defined by ASHA (2018b) in the Benchmarks document is "pragmatics." This includes skills related to functional use of language for various purposes (e.g., to ask a question vs. to share information), speech prosody, use of spontaneous gestures, facial expressions, and eye contact and is vital to assess in this population.

FUTURE DIRECTIONS

As the incidence of ASD continues to rise, SLPs will continue to see more children with this diagnosis who require comprehensive evaluation of their spoken language and communication abilities. While several standardized diagnostic tools are available, the most important component of any assessment is a skilled and experienced diagnostician familiar with the core symptoms of ASD. While the primary purpose of assessment may be to determine a specific diagnosis, the most valuable outcome of a spoken language evaluation is the information gained to help drive intervention. Future directions must include the training of more clinicians able to identify and treat the needs of people with ASD, improved understanding of co-occurring diagnoses (e.g., sensory impairments such as hearing loss, chromosomal differences, and motor impairments), and ongoing, multidisciplinary teaming in both evaluation and intervention. The development of new evaluation tools must include norming samples that represent all aspects of culture and diversity, including those with ASD. So much has been learned about children and young adults with ASD, but much more work is needed.

REFERENCES

American Psychiatric Association (APA). (2013). *Diagnostic and statistical manual of mental disorders: DSM-5*. American Psychiatric Association.

American Speech-Language-Hearing Association (ASHA). (2005). *Evidence-based practice in communication disorders (Position statement)*. https://www.asha.org/policy

American Speech-Language-Hearing Association (ASHA). (2007). *Childhood apraxia of speech (Position Statement))*. https://www.asha.org/policy

American Speech-Language-Hearing Association (ASHA). (2018a). *Autism Spectrum Disorder: Assessment*. https://www.asha.org/Practice-Portal/Clinical-Topics/Autism

American Speech-Language-Hearing Association (ASHA). (2018b). *Social Communication Benchmarks*. https://www.asha.org/uploadedFiles/ASHA/Practice_Portal/Clinical_Topics/Social_Communication_Disorders_in_School-Age_Children/Social-Communication-Benchmarks.pdf

Beukelman, D. R., & Mirenda, P. (2013). *Augmentative and alternative communication: Supporting children and adults with complex communication needs*. Paul H. Brookes.

Bondy, A. S., & Frost, L. A. (1994). The Picture Exchange Communication System. *Focus on Autistic Behavior and Other Developmental Disabilities, 9*(3), 1–19. https://doi.org/10.1177/108835769400900301

Bowers, L., Huisingh, R., LoGiudice, C., & Orman, J. (2014). *The word test 3 elementary: Examiners manual*. LinguiSystems.

Brown, R. (1973). *A first language: The early stages*. George Allen & Unwin.

CDC. (2018). *Report: Examining the prevalence of autism among children in the United States*. https://www.psychiatryadvisor.com/autism-spectrum-disorders/cdc-prevalence-of-autism-in-us-children/article/764970/

Communication Matrix. (2020). *Assessment*. https://www.communicationmatrix.org/

Dunn, L. M., & Dunn, D. M. (2007). *PPVT-4: Peabody Picture Vocabulary Test*. Pearson.

Fudala, J. B. (2017). *Arizona articulation proficiency scale: Fourth Edition Manual*. Western Psychological Services.

Goldman, R., & Fristoe, M. (2015). *GFTA-3: Goldman Fristoe 3 test of articulation*. PsychCorp, an imprint of Pearson Clinical Assessment.

Hammill, D. D., & Newcomer, P. L. (2008). *Test of language development: Intermediate*. Pro-Ed.

Hodson, B. W (2004). *The Hodson Assessment of Phonological Patterns–Third Edition: (HAPP-3)*. Pro-Ed.

Levy, S. E., Giarelli, E., Lee, L., Schieve, L. A., Kirby, R. S., Cunniff, C., . . . Rice, C. E. (2010). Autism spectrum disorder and co-occurring developmental, psychiatric, and medical conditions among children in multiple populations of the United States. *Journal of Developmental & Behavioral Pediatrics, 31*(4), 267–275. https://doi.org/10.1097/dbp.0b013e3181d5d03b

McNaughton, D., & Light, J. (2013). The iPad and mobile technology revolution: Benefits and challenges for individuals who require augmentative and alternative communication. *Augmentative and Alternative Communication, 29*(2), 107–116. https://doi.org/10.3109/07434618.2013.784930

Newman, T. M., Macomber, D., Naples, A. J., Babitz, T., Volkmar, F., & Grigorenko, E. L. (2006). Hyperlexia in children with autism spectrum disorders. *Journal of Autism and Developmental Disorders, 37*(4), 760–774. https://doi.org/10.1007/s10803-006-0206-y

Ogletree, B. T., Pierce, K., Harn, W. E., & Fischer, M. A. (2002). Assessment of communication and language in classical autism: Issues and practices. *Assessment for Effective Intervention*, *27*(1–2), 61–71. https://doi.org/10.1177/073724770202700109

Prizant, B. M., & Rydell, P. J. (1984). Analysis of functions of delayed echolalia in autistic children. *Journal of Speech Language and Hearing Research*, *27*(2), 183–192. https://doi.org/10.1044/jshr.2702.183

Rogers, S. J., & Dawson, G. (2010). *Early Start Denver Model for young children with autism: Promoting language, learning, and engagement*. Guilford Press.

Rossetti, L. (2006). *The Rossetti Infant-Toddler Language Scale*. Super Duper Publications.

Rowland, C. (2004). *Communication matrix: A communication skill assessment*. Design to Learn.

Santhanam, S. P., & Hewitt, L. E. (2015). Evidence-based assessment and autism spectrum disorders: A scoping review. *Evidence-Based Communication Assessment and Intervention*, *9*(4), 140–181. https://doi.org/10.1080/17489539.2016.11$1$2

Shriberg, L. D., Paul, R., Mcsweeny, J. L., Klin, A., Cohen, D. J., & Volkmar, F. R. (2001). Speech and prosody characteristics of adolescents and adults with high-functioning autism and Asperger syndrome. *Journal of Speech Language and Hearing Research*, *44*(5), 1097–1115. https://doi.org/10.1044/1092-4388

Sussman, F. (2006). *TalkAbility: People skills for verbal children on the autism spectrum; a guide for parent*. Hanen Program.

Tierney, C., Mayes, S., Lohs, S. R., Black, A., Gisin, E., & Veglia, M. (2015). How valid is the Checklist for Autism Spectrum Disorder when a child has apraxia of speech? *Journal of Developmental & Behavioral Pediatrics*, *36*(8), 569–574. https://doi.org/10.1097/dbp.0000000000000189

Wagner, R. K., Torgesen, J. K., & Rashotte, C. A. (1999). *Comprehensive test of phonological processing (CTOPP)*. Pro-Ed.

Walenski, M., Mostofsky, S. H., Gidley-Larson, J. C., & Ullman, M. T. (2007). Brief report: Enhanced picture naming in autism. *Journal of Autism and Developmental Disorders*, *38*(7), 1395–1399. https://doi.org/10.1007/s10803-007-0513-y

Westby, C., Burda, A., & Mehta, Z. (2003). Asking the right questions in the right ways. *The ASHA Leader*, *8*(8), 4–17. doi:10.1044/leader.ftr3.08082003.4

Wiig, E., & Secord, W. (2014). *Clinical Evaluation of Language Fundamentals, Fifth Edition Metalinguistics (CELF-5 Metalinguistics)*. Pearson Assessments.

Wiig, E., Semel, E., & Secord, W. (2013). *Clinical Evaluation of Language Fundamentals–Fifth Edition (CELF-5)*. Pearson Assessments.

Wiig, E., Secord, W., & Semel, E. (2004). *Clinical Evaluation of Language Fundamentals—Preschool—Second Edition (CELF-P 2)*. Pearson Assessment.

Williams, K. T. (2007). *EVT-2: Expressive vocabulary test*. Pearson Assessments.

Winner, M. G. (2002). Assessment of social skills for students with Asperger syndrome and high-functioning autism. *Assessment for Effective Intervention*, 27(1–2), 73–80. https://doi.org/10.1177/073724770202700110

Zimmerman, I. L., Steiner, V. G., & Pond, R. E. (2011). *PLS-5 Preschool Language Scales: Fifth Edition*. NCS Pearson.

4.2

Assessing Signed Language Development in Deaf/ Signing Children with Autism Spectrum Disorder

Aaron Shield, Deborah Mood, Nicole Salamy, and Jonathan Henner

There are currently no instruments designed specifically for identifying autism spectrum disorder (ASD) in deaf and/or hard of hearing (D/HH) children who use a signed language. The standardized tool, the Autism Diagnostic Observation Schedule, Second Edition (ADOS-2; Lord et al., 2012), warns specifically against its use with D/HH children. Despite this, as of 2010, one in 59 D/HH American children had an ASD diagnosis (Szymanski et al., 2012). Clinicians who work with D/HH children are faced with specific challenges in identifying ASD. This chapter is an attempt to identify challenges facing clinicians who work with signing children and provide solutions whenever possible.

CHALLENGES OF ASSESSMENT WITH SIGNING CHILDREN

In this section, we discuss two specific considerations: (1) the wide variety of language experiences that D/HH children have and (2) norm differences between Deaf communities and hearing communities.

Heterogeneity of Language Experience

Although standard diagnostic tools exist for evaluating hearing children with ASD, applying this framework to D/HH children requires additional consideration (Szarkowski et al., 2014). First, although hearing children with ASD may have receptive and expressive language delays, language is readily accessible to them in the environment; that is, their parents are generally able to produce language input that they are capable of perceiving. By contrast, 90–95% of D/HH

Aaron Shield, Deborah Mood, Nicole Salamy, and Jonathan Henner, *Assessing Signed Language Development in Deaf/Signing Children with Autism Spectrum Disorder* In: *The Handbook of Language Assessment Across Modalities*. Edited by: Tobias Haug, Wolfgang Mann, and Ute Knoch, Oxford University Press.
DOI: 10.1093/oso/9780190885052.003.0012

children have hearing parents (Mitchell & Karchmer, 2004a), and only a small percentage of hearing parents of D/HH children eventually learn a signed language (~25%; Crowe et al., 2014; Gallaudet Research Institute, 2011; Mitchell & Karchmer, 2004b). Thus, even neurotypical D/HH children (i.e., those who do not have ASD) are at risk of *language deprivation*. Language deprivation occurs when children are not exposed adequately to a language that is fully accessible to them (i.e., a signed language; Hall et al., 2017). A lack of adequate language exposure can affect not just language but also related cognitive skills, such as Theory of Mind (ToM). Although D/HH children of Deaf adults typically demonstrate ToM skills similar to their hearing peers, ToM is often delayed among D/HH children who lack adequate language exposure (Schick et al., 2007). Since children with ASD also often present with ToM deficits (Baron-Cohen et al., 1985), it is essential that clinicians be aware of the consequences of inadequate language exposure and be able to differentiate such a trajectory from that of children with ASD.

Signing D/HH students' exposure to sign in educational settings is likely to be variable as well. It may include exposure to a natural signed language such as American Sign Language (ASL), but most D/HH children receive language modeling through a signed language interpreter (who may or may not be qualified to interpret in an educational environment; Schick et al., 1999); a combination of spoken and signed language (in which the signed language is often degraded in quality; Wilbur & Petersen, 1998); an artificial manual communication system such as Signing Exact English, which follows English syntax and was invented for the purpose of increasing deaf children's English literacy (Hoffmeister, 1996); or a combination of these (Gallaudet Research Institute, 2011). The quantity and quality of language children have been exposed to should be considered when identifying symptoms of ASD. For example, D/HH children whose hearing family members communicate through gestures may develop their own "home signs," which may appear to be idiosyncratic to an outside observer. These signs must be distinguished from true idiosyncratic signs that could be symptomatic of ASD (i.e., unconventional signs that a child persists in using despite exposure to formal signs from the signed language lexicon). Furthermore, children with language deprivation may present with symptoms that mimic symptoms of ASD (e.g., repetitive behaviors in response to communication frustration, reduced conversational ability). Careful clinical evaluation guided by an understanding of the developmental impact of both ASD and language deprivation is warranted.

Different Norms of Behavior

Assessment of ASD necessitates an evaluation of whether children appear to be following the unwritten rules of their community that are, as such, culturally bound and culturally specific (Matson et al., 2011; Norbury & Sparks, 2013). Therefore, an appropriate language assessment must take into consideration the individual's culture(s), including Deaf culture. Most language assessment tools used commonly in the English-speaking world were developed primarily based on an understanding of white, hearing English speakers (Annamma et al., 2013). Therefore, a reliance on these tools alone would fail to take into consideration the cultural norms of the Deaf community, such as attention-getting behaviors such as taps and hand waves (Baker, 1977; Lieberman, 2015), shifts in visual attention between objects and people (Lieberman et al., 2014; Spencer, 2000), and strategies for joining conversations (Lieberman, 2015) and holding the floor during conversation (Coates & Sutton-Spence, 2001).

The visual-gestural modality of sign itself also has important consequences for the language of children with ASD. Here we address specific areas of signed languages that differ from spoken languages and how they could be affected by ASD.

WHICH AREAS OF SIGN ARE AFFECTED BY AUTISM SPECTRUM DISORDER?

One of the primary challenges in assessing language in signing D/HH children with ASD is that a number of social skills that play a primary role in the production and comprehension of signed languages are often affected. Here we delineate these skills and postulate the ways in which they may affect the acquisition of sign.

Visual Referencing and Joint Attention

D/HH children engage in episodes of joint attention with their caregivers from the first years of life (Lieberman et al., 2014). Unlike hearing children, however, D/HH children must shift their visual attention from a visual object to a visual linguistic symbol, whereas hearing children may simultaneously gaze at a visual object while hearing an auditory linguistic symbol. Thus, for children with ASD, the sign-learning task may be more difficult if the ability to engage in joint attention (and thus to gaze-shift) is compromised. Such impairment may lead to decreased opportunities for sign learning, resulting in language delay or disorder. This is even more likely for D/HH children of hearing parents who spend less time than Deaf parents engaged in episodes of sustained joint attention with their children, produce fewer words in such episodes, and are less responsive to their toddler's attention focus (Gale & Schick, 2009; Spencer & Meadow-Orlans, 1996). Early intervention in appropriate learning environments is key to addressing challenges with joint attention.

Perspective-Taking and Imitation

Children with ASD have well-documented deficits in ToM, the ability to impute mental states to others (Baron-Cohen et al., 1985). Similarly, D/HH children who are not exposed to a signed language are also at risk for delayed ToM (Schick et al., 2007). Shield, Pyers, Martin, and Tager-Flusberg (2016) found that native-sign–exposed deaf children with ASD also showed impaired ToM relative to a control group of neurotypical native-sign–exposed deaf children. Thus, D/HH children with ASD are at particular risk for delayed ToM development, even if they are exposed to sign from birth, but especially if they are not exposed to sign.

Visual perspective-taking (the ability to take the visual perspective of others) is a skill related to ToM. Some studies have found evidence of visual perspective-taking deficits in ASD (e.g., Hamilton et al., 2009) while others have not (e.g., Reed & Peterson, 1990). To date, only one study has examined the visual perspective-taking abilities of D/HH children with ASD (Shield et al., 2016), finding impairments in this ability relative to neurotypical deaf children. These visual perspective-taking abilities are of particular interest when discussing signing D/HH children because the ability to take another person's visual perspective is crucial for understanding a signed language. For example, the space in front of signers is used to depict spatial layouts (e.g., for giving directions), setting up referential loci, and establishing linguistic agreement between referents. These depictions require addressees to engage in perspective-taking and mental rotation in order to correctly comprehend the signed utterance. There is some evidence that D/HH children with ASD may not engage in perspective-taking as neurotypical signing children do, resulting in errors in sign formation (i.e., palm orientation reversals; Shield & Meier, 2012). Clinicians assessing D/HH children for ASD should be aware that D/HH children with ASD may reverse the orientation of their palm while signing, thus producing signs that appear to look "backward" (e.g., fingerspelling or using signs to spell out a word with the palm oriented toward the self rather than toward the addressee). Despite the fact that this phenomenon has also been documented in studies of gesture imitation by hearing individuals with ASD (e.g., Ohta, 1987; Whiten & Brown, 1998), it is not currently included on any instruments for detecting ASD. Accordingly, clinicians working with this population should be aware that this unique signing style could be indicative of ASD.

Nonmanual Markers

Signed languages use facial expressions and body movements (e.g., shoulder shifting) to signal types of questions (e.g., with raised or furrowed eyebrows; Baker, 1983), relative clauses (Liddell, 1978), conditionals (Liddell, 1986), topics (Coulter, 1979), and adverbial or lexical information (Anderson & Reilly, 1998). They may also be used for referential indexing and establishing linguistic agreement (Bahan, 1996). The ability to look at others' faces and bodies and deduce linguistic information from them is thus an important prerequisite for sign learning. Yet children with ASD have difficulty attending to the face (Dawson et al., 2005) and recognizing information transmitted by facial expressions (Grossman & Tager-Flusberg, 2008). Several studies have shown that individuals with ASD tend to fixate on the mouth rather than the eyes (Spezio et al., 2007) and have more difficulty recognizing emotions signaled by the eyes (Baron-Cohen et al., 1997). There is currently little work investigating whether D/HH children with ASD have challenges with the linguistic facial expressions and body movements of signed languages, but there is evidence that deaf children with ASD struggle to recognize emotions transmitted by facial expressions (Denmark et al., 2014) and produce fewer facial expressions (Denmark et al., 2019). Assessments of D/HH children with ASD should specifically test for children's ability to comprehend and produce affective and linguistic facial expressions and body movements.

Pointing and Gesture

Hearing children with ASD differ from neurotypical hearing children in their ability to use manual communicative gestures, which typically develop in tight connection with speech (Iverson & Goldin-Meadow, 2005). In particular, very young children with ASD show decreased pointing behavior, especially to share or comment on an object (Stone et al., 1997). In addition, the ability to use representational or conventional gestures is often impaired and is one of the factors considered in the diagnosis of ASD (American Psychiatric Association [APA], 2013). Impairment in the ability to point and gesture has obvious consequences for D/HH children acquiring a signed language. Index finger points are used in ASL for a number of purposes, especially for indicating present and nonpresent referents (pronouns). Shield, Meier, and Tager-Flusberg (2015) found that deaf children with ASD were significantly less likely to produce the ASL pronouns ME and YOU than a control group of neurotypical deaf children, suggesting that this could be a challenge for D/HH children with ASD. Clinicians assessing D/HH children for ASD should specifically test for children's ability to point, both in linguistic (i.e., pronominal) and nonlinguistic (i.e., to share, comment, and request objects) contexts.

Motor Skills

Although motor challenges are not included in the diagnostic criteria for ASD, approximately 50–80% of all children with ASD have motor deficits (Bhat et al., 2011), including impairments in gross and fine motor coordination (Green et al., 2009) and praxis/motor planning (Mostofsky et al., 2006). Since signed languages require both gross and fine motor control, as well as praxis/motor planning skills, such motor deficits could affect how D/HH children with ASD acquire and use sign. Two recent studies have shown that deaf signing children with ASD have significant problems with motor planning compared to neurotypical deaf children (Bhat et al., 2018; Shield et al., 2017). These studies found that the children with ASD were slower and less accurate in their production of fingerspelled words as well as in their imitation of nonsense gestures than neurotypical deaf children, showing that motor challenges affect both the production of linguistic signs as well as the more domain-general ability to imitate. Clinicians assessing D/HH children for ASD should be aware of the possibility that children could have comorbid motor disorders, including dyspraxia, and that such disorders could affect children's ability to produce signs. This also suggests that solely focusing on children's expressive language skills to the exclusion of their comprehension skills could yield an inaccurate assessment.

Thus, there are numerous areas of development that must be considered when evaluating language in D/HH children with ASD. In the next section, we discuss how clinicians should approach a language evaluation, starting with the selection of an appropriate instrument.

CHOOSING AN INSTRUMENT

When assessing a D/HH child with ASD, the choice of which tool(s) to use is a formidable task. First, very few language assessment batteries have been normed on D/HH children. Second, the clinician may want to assess the child's expressive and receptive language and their skills at the word (lexical), sentence (syntactic), and discourse (pragmatic) levels.

An assessment should target known areas of difficulty for children with ASD, as outlined earlier. Similarly, when assessing D/HH children previously diagnosed with ASD, assessment must consider known areas of difficulty in order to monitor progress and assist in intervention planning. Notably, assessment of *all* of these areas is necessary. If only vocabulary and syntax are tested, indicators of ASD that may be more obvious in connected language and pragmatic language could be missed.

What Are Clinicians Currently Using?

We, the authors of this chapter, all work in the American context; as such, the tests that we describe here refer specifically to English and ASL. Clinicians working in other countries are encouraged to consult the Sign Language Assessment Instruments website (http://www.

signlang-assessment.info/index.php/home-en.html) to find information about tools designed for assessment in other signed languages.

Most commercially available English-language tests have not been normed on D/HH children and should be avoided if possible. However, if they must be used, scores must be interpreted with caution and contextualized using all available data on the child. If accommodations or adaptations are used during testing (e.g., using a signed language interpreter), formal scores cannot be calculated or compared to normative data. Using a variety of standard language test batteries and dynamic assessments is essential for fully appreciating a child's overall language profile. If appropriate language assessments cannot be found, standardized assessment results should be de-emphasized in favor of other kinds of assessments (e.g., behavioral, narrative samples, criterion-referenced or curriculum-based measures).

Table 4.2.1 lists instruments that have been designed specifically for D/HH children. Since the field of signed language assessment is still very young, with most signed assessments being developed since 2008, not all of the assessments may meet clinical standards. Although these assessments are imperfect, it is preferable to use them whenever possible rather than attempting to modify, translate, or adapt a spoken/written assessment.

Notably, none of the ASL instruments listed here tests pragmatics, which is the domain of language that is typically the most affected in individuals with ASD. The Social Communication Skills Pragmatics Checklist (Goberis, 1999) is one tool for assessing pragmatic language skills that has been used with D/HH children. Goberis et al. (2012) found that D/HH children lagged significantly behind hearing children on a variety of pragmatic skills, though it should be noted that the D/HH children came from a variety of language backgrounds, and some may have experienced language deprivation (31.7% came from English-only homes). Although this instrument has been used in published research with D/HH children, it has not been adapted for use with them, nor does it contain items specifically addressing (Deaf) culturally relevant pragmatic skills.

We also highlight the use of receptive language tests, which are often administered with touch-screen devices and only require the child to point to items on the screen. An additional advantage of such instruments is that clinicians do not themselves have to ask questions in a signed language, and test administration is uniform over time.

When testing very young children or children who present with very limited formal language, standardized assessments may not be appropriate. In these cases, the child's communication skills should be observed during play or by using checklists such as the Visual Communication and Sign Language Checklist (VCSL; Simms et al., 2013). A skilled clinician who has experience working with D/HH

Table 4.2.1 Currently available American Sign Language (ASL) assessments

Assessment Tool	Age	Phonology	Lexicon	Syntax	Classifiers/ Depiction	Pragmatics	Type
Visual Communication and Sign Language Checklist (VCSL; Simms et al., 2013)	0;0–5;0		X	X	X		Normed Production Checklist (Criterion)
MacArthur Bates ASL-CDI (Anderson & Reilly, 2002)	0;0–3;0		X				Normed Production Checklist
American Sign Language Index of Productive Syntax (Lillo-Martin et al., 2017)	1;6–4;0		X	X	X		Criterion-Based Production Checklist
American Sign Language Receptive Skills Test (ASL RST; Enns et al., 2013)	3;0–13;0		(A vocabulary pretest is provided but it is not specifically a vocabulary assessment)	X	X		Normed Receptive
American Sign Language Phonological Awareness Test (McQuarrie et al., 2012)	4;0–7;0	X					Receptive (Not normed)
American Sign Language Assessment Instrument (ASLAI; Hoffmeister et al., 2013)	3;0–18;5	X	X	X	X		Normed Receptive
American Sign Language Sentence Reproduction Test (Hauser et al., 2006)	n/a						Normed Production (Global Language)

children will recognize how to use materials to interact with such children. In these instances, it is crucial to collect observational data to inform team members about the child's communication skills.

TEST ADMINISTRATION

In our experience, English-language test batteries designed for and normed on hearing children are often used to test the language skills of D/HH children, administered with adaptations and accommodations. This practice is contentious and is discouraged by researchers who study signed language assessments (Henner et al., 2018). A non-standard method of administration invalidates standard scores, so formal scores cannot be reported. We acknowledge the realities of daily clinical practice (budget constraints, personnel restrictions, geographic limitations, etc.) that lead to this practice. In Chapter 4.3, we make recommendations for ameliorating some of the problems that arise when English-language tests are used to assess language in signing D/HH children, as well as considerations regarding administration of assessments through an interpreter.

FUTURE DIRECTIONS

The field of signed language assessment is still very new, with most assessments only being designed from 2008 (see Table 4.2.1). More signed language assessments are needed, covering the full range of language functions from vocabulary to pragmatic skills. We especially emphasize the need for signed language assessments that focus on the unique pragmatic needs of signing D/HH children. Pragmatic language assessments for D/HH children should also include cultural adaptations that are not included on assessments for hearing children (e.g., sharing information, attention-getting strategies, use of appropriate sign space).

Too often in our school systems, when a particular developmental skill is not assessed (or is assessed poorly), little is done to intervene. Developing tools which provide valid and fair assessment of the pragmatic language skills of D/HH children is an essential first step toward understanding children's needs and developing targeted intervention. Anecdotally, some schools have started to incorporate pragmatic language skills (or soft skills) as part of an "expanded core curriculum" for D/HH children. However, some communities question whether soft-skill curricula could represent a form of ableism in that they encourage D/HH children to behave exactly like hearing children. We acknowledge the complexities raised by these objections while affirming that soft-skill curricula represent an effort to assess D/HH children's pragmatic language skills and provide intervention if delays are evident.

Future research should explore the impact of a soft-skill training approach on pragmatic language skill outcomes for D/HH children. We also need to know what professionals are doing around the world in order to come to a consensus about clinical best practice.

In addition to the assessments themselves, it is essential that more D/HH adults be trained as clinicians in the future. The relative shortage of D/HH professionals in the ASD field means that D/HH children are most often evaluated by professionals who do not share their language, cultural background (e.g., Deaf, or racial/ethnic), disability, or experience as a minority, which can lead to bias and misunderstanding. When assessing the language skills of D/HH children, D/HH and hearing professionals should work collaboratively, sharing expertise, ideas, and observations. It is also essential that D/HH professionals contribute to the field's understanding of how to provide an accurate assessment of D/HH children's language development in order to differentiate symptoms of ASD from language deprivation. This will likely require efforts to remove barriers preventing D/HH adults from pursuing advanced education in professions such as speech-language pathology, psychology, and developmental pediatrics.

Given the shortage of dually trained providers and D/HH professionals with the recognized credentials for assessment and treatment of ASD, it is also critical that we develop measures that can be used reliably by professionals to objectively screen for symptoms which distinguish features of ASD from expected developmental trajectories. Conversely, we must train people who work with D/HH populations to recognize the unique features of ASD and especially how these features manifest in a signed communication modality.

REFERENCES

American Psychiatric Association (APA). (2013). *Diagnostic and statistical manual of mental disorders, fifth edition*. American Psychiatric Publishing.

Anderson, D., & Reilly, J. (1998). PAH! The acquisition of adverbials in ASL. *Sign Language and Linguistics, 1*(2), 117–142. https://doi.org/10.1075/sll.1.2.03and

Anderson, D., & Reilly, J. (2002). *The MacArthur Communicative Development Inventory: Normative data for American Sign Language* (vol. 7). Oxford University Press.

Annamma, S. A., Boelé, A. L., Moore, B. A., & Klingner, J. (2013). Challenging the ideology of normal in schools. *International Journal of Inclusive Education, 17*(12), 1278–1294. https://doi.org/10.1080/13603116.2013.802379

Bahan, B. (1996). *Non-manual realization of agreement in ASL* (Unpublished doctoral dissertation). Boston University, Boston, MA.

Baker, C. (1977). Regulators and turn-taking in American Sign Language discourse. In L. Friedman (Ed.), *On the other hand: New perspectives on American Sign Language* (pp. 215–236). Academic Press.

Baker, C. L. (1983). A microanalysis of the nonmanual components of questions in American Sign Language. In P. Siple (Ed.), *Understanding language through sign language research* (pp. 27–57). Academic Press.
Baron-Cohen, S., Leslie, A. M., & Frith, U. (1985). Does the autistic child have a "theory of mind"? *Cognition, 21*(1), 37–46. https://doi.org/10.1016/0010-0277(85)90022-8
Baron-Cohen, S., Wheelwright, S., & Jolliffe, T. (1997). Is there a "language of the eyes"? Evidence from normal adults, and adults with autism or Asperger syndrome. *Visual Cognition, 4*(3), 311–331. https://doi.org/10.1080/713756761
Bhat, A. N., Landa, R. J., & Galloway, J. C. (2011). Current perspectives on motor functioning in infants, children, and adults with autism spectrum disorders. *Physical Therapy, 91*(7), 1116–1129. https://doi.org/10.2522/ptj.20100294
Bhat, A. N., Srinivasan, S. M., Woxholdt, C., & Shield, A. (2018). Differences in praxis performance and receptive language during fingerspelling between deaf children with and without autism spectrum disorder. *Autism, 22*(3), 271–282. https://doi.org/10.1177/1362361316672179
Coates, J., & Sutton-Spence, R. (2001). Turn-taking patterns in deaf conversation. *Journal of Sociolinguistics, 5*(4), 507–529. https://doi.org/10.1111/1467-9481.00162
Coulter, G. R. (1979). *American Sign Language typology* (Unpublished doctoral dissertation). University of California, San Diego, San Diego, CA.
Crowe, K., Fordham, L., McLeod, S., & Ching, T. Y. C. (2014). "Part of our world": Influences on caregiver decisions about communication choices for children with hearing loss. *Deafness & Education International, 16*(2), 61–85. https://doi.org/10.1179/1557069X13Y.0000000026
Dawson, G., Webb, S. J., & McPartland, J. (2005). Understanding the nature of face processing impairment in autism: Insights from behavioral and electrophysiological studies. *Developmental Neuropsychology, 27*(3), 403–424. https://doi.org/10.1207/s15326942dn2703_6
Denmark, T., Atkinson, J., Campbell, R., & Swettenham, J. (2014). How do typically developing deaf children and deaf children with autism spectrum disorder use the face when comprehending emotional facial expressions in British Sign Language? *Journal of Autism and Developmental Disorders, 44*(1), 2584–2592. https://doi.org/10.1007/s10803-014-2130-x
Denmark, T., Atkinson, J., Campbell, R., & Swettenham, J. (2019). Signing with the face: Emotional expression in narrative production in deaf children with autism spectrum disorder. *Journal of Autism and Developmental Disorders, 49*(1), 294–306. https://doi.org/10.1007/s10803-018-3756-x
Enns, C. J., Zimmer, K., Boudreault, P., Rabu, S., & Broszeit, C. (2013). *American Sign Language: Receptive skills test.* Northern Signs Research, Inc.
Gale, E., & Schick, B. (2009). Symbol-infused joint attention and language use in mothers with deaf and hearing toddlers. *American Annals of the Deaf, 153*(5), 484–503. https://doi.org/10.1353/aad.0.0066
Gallaudet Research Institute. (2011). *Regional and national summary report of data from the 2009–2010 annual survey of deaf and hard of hearing children and youth.* GRI, Gallaudet University.
Goberis, D. (1999). *Pragmatics Checklist (adapted from C. S. Simons, 1984).*
Goberis, D., Beams, D., Dalpes, M., Abrisch, A., Baca, R., & Yoshinaga-Itano, C. (2012). The missing link in language development of deaf and hard of

hearing children: Pragmatic language development. *Seminars in Speech and Language, 33*(4), 297–309. https://doi.org/10.1055/s-0032-1326916

Green, D., Charman, T., Pickles, A., Chandler, S., Loucas, T., Simonoff, E., & Baird, G. (2009). Impairment in movement skills of children with autistic spectrum disorders. *Developmental Medicine & Child Neurology, 51*(4), 311–316. https://doi.org/10.1111/j.1469-8749.2008.03242.x

Grossman, R. B., & Tager-Flusberg, H. (2008). Reading faces for information about words and emotions in adolescents with autism. *Research in Autism Spectrum Disorders, 2*(4), 681–695. https://doi.org/10.1016/j.rasd.2008.02.004

Hall, W. C., Levin, L. L., & Anderson, M. L. (2017). Language deprivation syndrome: A possible neurodevelopmental disorder with sociocultural origins. *Social Psychiatry and Psychiatric Epidemiology, 52*(6), 761–776. https://doi.org/10.1007/s00127-017-1351-7

Hamilton, A., Brindley, R., & Frith, U. (2009). Visual perspective taking impairment in children with autistic spectrum disorder. *Cognition, 113*(1), 37–44. https://doi.org/10.1016/j.cognition.2009.07.007

Hauser, P., Paludneviciene, R., Supalla, T. R., & Bavelier, D. (2006). *American Sign Language—Sentence reproduction test: Development & implications.* http://scholarworks.rit.edu/other/596

Henner, J., Novogrodsky, R., Reis, J., & Hoffmeister, R. (2018). Recent issues in the use of signed language assessments for diagnosis of language disorders in signing deaf and hard of hearing children. *Journal of Deaf Studies and Deaf Education, 23*(4), 307–316. https://doi.org/10.1093/deafed/eny014

Hoffmeister, R. (1996). What do Deaf kids know about ASL even though they 'see' MCE? In *Conference Proceedings, Deaf Studies IV: "Vision of the past-visions of the future"*, April 27–30, 1995 (pp. 273–308). Woburn, MA: Gallaudet University Press.

Hoffmeister, R., Henner, J., Benedict, R., Fish, S., & Rosenburg, P. (2013, February 22). *Current information on the American Sign Language assessment instrument (ASLAI).* Presented at the American Council of Educators for the Deaf and Hard of Hearing (ACEDHH), Santa Fe, NM.

Iverson, J. M., & Goldin-Meadow, S. (2005). Gesture paves the way for language development. *Psychological Science, 16*(5), 367–371. https://doi.org/10.1111/j.0956-7976.2005.01542.x

Liddell, S. K. (1978). Nonmanual signals and relative clauses in American Sign Language. In P. Siple (Ed.), *Understanding language through sign language research* (pp. 59–90). Academic Press.

Liddell, S. K. (1986). Head thrust in ASL conditional marking. *Sign Language Studies, 52*(1), 243–262. https://doi.org/10.1353/sls.1986.0003

Lieberman, A. M. (2015). Attention-getting skills of deaf children using American Sign Language in a preschool classroom. *Applied Psycholinguistics, 36*(4), 855–873. https://doi.org/10.1017/S0142716413000532

Lieberman, A. M., Hatrak, M., & Mayberry, R. I. (2014). Learning to look for language: Development of joint attention in young deaf children. *Language Learning and Development, 10*(1), 19–35. https://doi.org/10.1080/15475441.2012.760381

Lillo-Martin, D., Goodwin, C., & Prunier, L. (2017). ASL-IPSyn: A new measure of grammatical development. *Poster presentation, Boston University Conference on Language Development (BUCLD).* Boston, MA.

Lord, C., Rutter, M., DiLavore, P. C., Risi, S., Gotham, K., & Bishop, S. L. (2012). *Autism Diagnostic Observation Schedule, Second Edition (ADOS-2)*. Western Psychological Services.

Matson, J. L., Worley, J. A., Fodstad, J. C., Chung, K.-M., Suh, D., Jhin, H. K., . . . Furniss, F. (2011). A multinational study examining the cross cultural differences in reported symptoms of autism spectrum disorders: Israel, South Korea, the United Kingdom, and the United States of America. *Research in Autism Spectrum Disorders, 5*(4), 1598–1604. https://doi.org/10.1016/j.rasd.2011.03.007

McQuarrie, L., Abbott, M., & Spady, S. (2012). American Sign Language phonological awareness: Test development and design. In *Proceedings of the 10th annual Hawaii international conference on education* (pp. 1–17). Honolulu, HI.

Mitchell, R. E., & Karchmer, M. A. (2004a). Chasing the mythical ten percent: Parental hearing status of deaf and hard of hearing students in the United States. *Sign Language Studies, 4*(2), 138–163. https://doi.org/10.1353/sls.2004.0005

Mitchell, R. E., & Karchmer, M. A. (2004b). When parents are deaf versus hard of hearing: Patterns of sign use and school placement of deaf and hard-of-hearing children. *Journal of Deaf Studies and Deaf Education, 9*(2), 133–152. https://doi.org/10.1093/deafed/enh017

Mostofsky, S. H., Dubey, P., Jerath, V. K., Jansiewicz, E. M., Goldberg, M. C., & Denckla, M. B. (2006). Developmental dyspraxia is not limited to imitation in children with autism spectrum disorders. *Journal of the International Neuropsychological Society, 12*(3), 314–326. https://doi.org/10.1017/S1355617706060437

Norbury, C. F., & Sparks, A. (2013). Difference or disorder? Cultural issues in understanding neurodevelopmental disorders. *Developmental Psychology, 49*(1), 45–58. https://doi.org/10.1037/a0027446

Ohta, M. (1987). Cognitive disorders of infantile autism: A study employing the WISC, spatial relationship conceptualization, and gesture imitations. *Journal of Autism and Developmental Disorders, 17*(1), 45–62. https://doi.org/10.1007/BF01487259

Reed, T., & Peterson, C. C. (1990). A comparative study of autistic subjects' performance at two levels of visual and cognitive perspective taking. *Journal of Autism and Developmental Disorders, 20*(4), 555–567. https://doi.org/10.1007/BF02216060

Schick, B., de Villiers, P., de Villiers, J., & Hoffmeister, R. (2007). Language and theory of mind: A study of deaf children. *Child Development, 78*(2), 376–396. https://doi.org/10.1111/j.1467-8624.2007.01004.x

Schick, B., Williams, K., & Bolster, L. (1999). Skill levels of educational interpreters working in public schools. *Journal of Deaf Studies and Deaf Education, 4*(2), 144–155. https://doi.org/10.1093/deafed/4.2.144

Shield, A., Knapke, K., Henry, M., Srinivasan, S. M., & Bhat, A. N. (2017). Impaired praxis in gesture imitation by deaf children with autism spectrum disorder. *Autism & Developmental Language Impairments, 2*, 1–14. https://doi.org/10.1177/2396941517745674

Shield, A., & Meier, R. P. (2012). Palm reversal errors in native-signing children with autism. *Journal of Communication Disorders, 45*(6), 439–454. https://doi.org/10.1016/j.jcomdis.2012.08.004

Shield, A., Meier, R. P., & Tager-Flusberg, H. (2015). The use of sign language pronouns by native-signing children with autism. *Journal of Autism and Developmental Disorders, 45*(7), 2128–2145. https://doi.org/10.1007/s10803-015-2377-x

Shield, A., Pyers, J., Martin, A., & Tager-Flusberg, H. (2016). Relations between language and cognition in native-signing children with autism spectrum disorder. *Autism Research, 9*(12), 1304–1315. https://doi.org/10.1002/aur.1621

Simms, L., Baker, S., & Clark, M. D. (2013). The standardized visual communication and sign language checklist for signing children. *Sign Language Studies, 14*(1), 101–124. https://doi.org/10.1353/sls.2013.0029

Spencer, P. E. (2000). Looking without listening: Is audition a prerequisite for normal development of visual attention during infancy? *Journal of Deaf Studies and Deaf Education, 5*(4), 291–302. https://doi.org/10.1093/deafed/5.4.291

Spencer, P. E., & Meadow-Orlans, K. P. (1996). Play, language, and maternal responsiveness: A longitudinal study of deaf and hearing infants. *Child Development, 67*(6), 3176–3191. https://doi.org/10.2307/1131773

Spezio, M. L., Adolphs, R., Hurley, R. S. E., & Piven, J. (2007). Analysis of face gaze in autism using "Bubbles." *Neuropsychologia, 45*(1), 144–151. https://doi.org/10.1016/j.neuropsychologia.2006.04.027

Stone, W. L., Ousley, O. Y., Yoder, P. J., Hogan, K. L., & Hepburn, S. L. (1997). Nonverbal communication in two- and three-year-old children with autism. *Journal of Autism and Developmental Disorders, 27*(6), 677–696. https://doi.org/10.1023/A:1025854816091

Szarkowski, A., Mood, D., Shield, A., Wiley, S., & Yoshinaga-Itano, C. (2014). A summary of current understanding regarding children with autism spectrum disorder who are deaf or hard of hearing. *Seminars in Speech and Language, 35*(4), 241–259. https://doi.org/10.1055/s-0034-1389097

Szymanski, C. A., Brice, P. J., Lam, K. H., & Hotto, S. A. (2012). Deaf children with autism spectrum disorders. *Journal of Autism and Developmental Disorders, 42*(10), 2027–2037. https://doi.org/10.1007/s10803-012-1452-9

Whiten, A., & Brown, J. (1998). Imitation and the reading of other minds: Perspectives from the study of autism, normal children and non-human primates. In S. Bråten (Ed.), *Intersubjective communication and emotion in early ontogeny* (pp. 260–280). Cambridge University Press.

Wilbur, R. B., & Petersen, L. (1998). Modality interactions of speech and signing in simultaneous communication. *Journal of Speech, Language, and Hearing Research, 41*(1), 200–212. https://doi.org.10.1044/jslhr.4101.200

4.3

Discussion of Issues Related to Assessment of Signed or Spoken Language Development in Children with Autism Spectrum Disorder

Amy Kissel Frisbie, Aaron Shield, Deborah Mood, Nicole Salamy, and Jonathan Henner

ASPECTS OF SIGNED LANGUAGE ASSESSMENT THAT COULD BE APPLIED TO SPOKEN LANGUAGE ASSESSMENT

Many aspects of signed language assessment raised in Chapter 4.2 are relevant to spoken language assessment. One example is the use of interpreters to assess language in deaf and/or hard of hearing (D/HH) children. There are several precautions to bear in mind about assessments obtained via an interpreter. Some of these precautions apply solely to D/HH children, while others are applicable to assessments with hearing children in multilingual contexts (see Crowley, 2004; Langdon & Saenz, 2016). This is especially relevant when evaluating communication skills in a person with autism spectrum disorder (ASD).

With regard to assessments of D/HH children conducted through a signed language interpreter, it is important to determine whether the child has the ability to shift their visual attention between the clinician and the interpreter. An assessment with a child, clinician, and interpreter involves a triadic interaction, involving three people, rather than a dyadic interaction, which involves only two individuals. Adding a third person to what is typically a two-person dynamic requires additional shifting of gaze and attention, which is known to be impaired in ASD (e.g., Landry & Bryson, 2004). This introduces a level of complexity to the interaction that could make it more difficult for some children to respond to test questions. Although hearing children do not need to gaze-shift to perceive spoken language from a home language interpreter, it is important to consider that children may find the triadic

Amy Kissel Frisbie, Aaron Shield, Deborah Mood, Nicole Salamy, and Jonathan Henner, *Discussion of Issues Related to Assessment of Signed or Spoken Language Development in Children with Autism Spectrum Disorder* In: *The Handbook of Language Assessment Across Modalities.* Edited by: Tobias Haug, Wolfgang Mann, and Ute Knoch, Oxford University Press. © Oxford University Press 2022. DOI: 10.1093/oso/9780190885052.003.0013 interaction more complex or confusing than a typical two-person interaction.

Other aspects of interpreted assessments apply equally to signed and spoken language interpreters. For example, data acquired from an interpreted assessment may be invalid if it is unclear how the interpreter may have changed individual test items during the translation process (we use 'translation' here following Haug & Mann (2007). 'Translation' is also the appropriate term for English print to ASL, however, spoken stimuli are considered 'interpreted' rather than translated. Some practitioners prefer to use 'modify' rather than 'translate'). This presents a risk to ensuring test item integrity during translation Clinicians should also remember that interpreters are trained to mediate between two languages; they are not trained to assess language production. Therefore, clinicians should refrain from asking interpreters to identify and diagnose specific features of ASD as they manifest in language use. However, it is useful to inform the interpreter of specific features of ASD before the evaluation begins (e.g., for sign and speech: use of jargon, echolalia, pronoun avoidance, stereotyped signs or words; for sign only: palm reversals, inappropriate use of signing space, use of nonmanual markers, and visual-spatial referencing) so that the interpreter can inform the clinician if these are produced in a way that could suggest ASD. However, this information should be treated as external commentary and not as a clinical identification of features.

Another relevant recommendation from the field of signed language assessment is the importance of expanding the evaluation process beyond standardized testing alone. Diagnostics for people with ASD can be quite complicated as there are often co-occurring factors that impact spoken or signed language. Information should be gathered from professionals familiar with the child's communication in order to supplement the evaluation. Case studies have been recommended as a valuable tool for the diagnosis of language disorders in complex situations (e.g., Henner et al., 2018; Quinto-Pozos et al., 2013, 2017), and we extend the same suggestion here. If a valid, fair language assessment cannot be obtained due to a lack of representation in standardization samples, it should be de-emphasized in favor of other kinds of data collection, such as language samples or behavioral observations. In this regard, it is important to note that many professionals who work with D/HH populations (e.g., teachers of the deaf) may not have training in ASD, so it is not sufficient merely to ask if they have concerns about ASD in general. This can be true for special educators and early interventionists as well when evaluating spoken language abilities of children suspected of having ASD.

Finally, a very important consideration for both signed and spoken language development is highlighted in both chapters: motor planning/

praxis skills. Just as in verbal speech, precise motor movements are required to produce signs. The literature has highlighted difficulty with motor planning in both hearing and deaf children with ASD. This is important for speech-language pathologists (SLPs) to be aware of when determining the best communication modality (i.e., signed or spoken language) for children with ASD, whether hearing or not.

Aspects of Spoken Language Assessment That Could Be Applied to Signed Language Assessment

Chapter 4.1 highlights several aspects of language assessment of children with ASD which are equally applicable for D/HH children. First, Chapter 4.1 emphasizes the difficulty of assessing pragmatic language, the area of communicative development most commonly impaired in ASD, and the same is true for D/HH children, as described in Chapter 4.2.

Similarly, multiple areas of language development (e.g., expressive/receptive, lexicon, syntax, etc.) should be considered in the assessment of hearing and D/HH children with ASD. In doing so, standardized assessments should be complemented by more naturalistic observations and by dynamic assessments.

The author of Chapter 4.1 raises the issue of differentiating between ASD diagnosis and other developmental disorders, such as childhood apraxia of speech (CAS). In Chapter 4.2, we have similarly underscored the importance of differentiating between the effects of language deprivation, which can mimic ASD symptoms, and true signs of ASD. We have also pointed out that motor planning issues can affect signed language production, although CAS does not by definition apply to signing children. Nonetheless, clinicians assessing language in children with ASD who are hearing or D/HH should be aware of the potential complications involved in motor planning which could affect expressive language in particular and be sure to include measures that do not require the child to produce language, such as receptive language assessments.

Finally, the language evaluation of both D/HH and hearing children must be completed within a developmental framework. ASD symptoms may appear differently in early childhood than in adolescence. Several early symptoms of ASD typically improve over time. For example, hearing children with ASD typically develop response to joint attention skills by school age (Malesa et al., 2013; Mundy & Jarrold, 2010), and early symptoms such as echolalia (McEvoy et al., 1988; Roberts, 1989) and palm reversals (Shield & Meier, 2012) may disappear or diminish over time. Therefore, when assessing for the purpose of a differential diagnosis, one must consider whether these symptoms were ever present and, if so, at what stage of developmental functioning.

Indications that a child's language presents signs of ASD should be followed up by a skilled clinician. In addition to considering classic language features which are commonly associated with ASD, it is important to attend to whether children are able to spontaneously generalize use of words/signs across a variety of settings (e.g., can the word "more" or the sign MORE be used to request *more* food as well as *more* of an activity). It is often helpful to consider the function of the child's behavior and language. For example, does the child appear motivated to communicate for a variety of purposes? Are they interested in a reciprocal exchange rather than just gathering information? Do they support a limited language repertoire with prosocial behaviors such as eye contact, gestures, posturing for communication?

Suggestions for Spoken Language Assessment

The discussion of different cultural norms in the Deaf community raises parallel issues for clinicians assessing hearing children with ASD. Just as the American Deaf community has its own cultural norms for politeness, which can differ significantly from the dominant middle-class white, American culture, so, too, may hearing children from sociocultural minority groups be socialized with behavioral expectations that differ from the dominant culture. Clinicians should thus be aware of potential cultural differences and have a thorough understanding of what is required to administer a culturally competent assessment.

Similarly, intersectional differences may affect hearing and D/HH children alike. For example, in the American context, black Deaf people may identify as black first and Deaf second. Accordingly, it cannot be assumed that any outward behavior shown by D/HH children is due to their membership in the larger Deaf community; their behavior may be acceptable in their home culture, too. We suggest that clinicians assessing hearing children with ASD be aware of the possibility of such intersectional differences. Of course, each country or community has different sociocultural milieus; some countries are more homogeneous and some more heterogeneous. We cannot make blanket recommendations here due to the diversity of contexts in which these assessments may take place. Rather, we suggest that clinicians take stock of the various factors which may be at work in the background of an assessment and which may appear invisible unless consciously considered.

Suggestions for Signed Language Assessment

The authors of Chapter 4.2 correctly point out the importance of evaluating joint attention abilities in children with ASD who use signed language. Limited joint attention skills (i.e., the ability to shift one's eye gaze between objects and people) are well documented in the ASD literature. Their confirmation that this could also be a limitation for children with ASD who are D/HH is relevant to our understanding of the acquisition of spoken language by hearing children with ASD. While hearing children do have access to auditory input when those around them use spoken language, they, too, could be at risk for reduced vocabulary development if they are not able to look at the indicated object, action, or person when named. Importantly, the authors also go on to hypothesize that "the sign-learning task may be more difficult if the ability to engage in joint attention . . . is compromised" (see Shield et al., this volume Chapter 4.2). Among SLPs in the United States, it is a common practice to teach young, hearing, emerging communicators with ASD a few signs as their first words. Intervention models such as the Early Start Denver Model suggest this practice when spoken words are slow to come (Rogers & Dawson, 2010), but emphasize that joint attention skills must also be taught. Ongoing research must consider if the use of signs is warranted for hearing children when they have persistent deficits in joint attention skills.

Another key point in signed language development raised by the authors in Chapter 4.2 is the importance of early intervention and education occurring in appropriate learning environments. In the United States, children with ASD who use spoken language are often educated in a classroom with other children with ASD. While matching children by diagnosis or cognitive abilities may be appropriate for some children, their communication modalities and language level should also be taken into consideration. It is vital that children with ASD have access to a rich language environment; this may include considerations about their home language as well (especially if bilingual or exposed to more than one language in their family).

Finally, an ongoing question related to both hearing and D/HH children with ASD is which communication modality(ies) lead(s) to the best outcomes. Many clinicians and families in both fields are exploring the use of augmentative and alternative communication (AAC) systems, which may combine gestures, eye pointing, vocalizations, and pointing to symbols, for people with limited speech. While considered a long-standing best-practice option for individuals who are minimally verbal with other diagnoses, more recent research has supported the use of AAC for people with ASD (see American Speech Language Hearing Association [ASHA], n.d.). Schlosser and Wendt (2008) highlight the research summary findings that 25–61% of hearing children with ASD have limited to no functional speech, thus making them good candidates for the use of AAC. They conclude that the use of AAC does not impede the development of spoken language (a fear often expressed by parents of hearing children with ASD) and may actually increase speech production for some children, especially those who had vocalizations before starting to use AAC. Future research and clinical efforts should include bringing together professionals from all areas of ASD treatment, including D/HH professionals and SLPs, to consider the benefits of incorporating AAC into intervention plans for both hearing and D/HH children with ASD.

REFERENCES

American Speech-Language-Hearing Association (ASHA). (n.d.). *Autism*. https://www.asha.org/Practice-Portal/Clinical-Topics/Autism/

Crowley, C. J. (2004). The ethics of assessment with culturally and linguistically diverse populations. *ASHA Leader*, *9*(5), 6–7. https://doi.org/10.1044/leader.FTR5.09052004.6

Haug, T., & Mann, W. (2007). Adapting tests of sign language assessment for other sign languages: A review of linguistic, cultural, and psychometric problems. *Journal of Deaf Studies and Deaf Education*, *13*(1), 138–147. https://doi.org/10.1093/deafed/enm027

Henner, J., Novogrodsky, R., Reis, J., & Hoffmeister, R. (2018). Recent issues in the use of signed language assessments for diagnosis of language disorders in signing deaf and hard of hearing children. *Journal of Deaf Studies and Deaf Education*, *23*(4), 307–316. https://doi.org/10.1093/deafed/eny014

Landry, R., & Bryson, S. E. (2004). Impaired disengagement of attention in young children with autism. *Journal of Child Psychology and Psychiatry*, *45*(6), 1115–1122. https://doi.org/10.1111/j.1469-7610.2004.00304.x

Langdon, H. W., & Saenz, T. I. (2016). *Working with interpreters and translators: A guide for speech-language pathologists and audiologists*. Plural Publishing.

Malesa, E., Foss-Feig, J., Yoder, P., Warren, Z., Walden, T., & Stone, W. L. (2013). Predicting language and social outcomes at age 5 for later-born siblings of children with autism spectrum disorders. *Autism*, *17*(5), 558–570. https://doi.org/10.1177/1362361312444628

McEvoy, R. E., Loveland, K. A., & Landry, S. H. (1988). The functions of immediate echolalia in autistic children: A developmental perspective. *Journal of Autism and Developmental Disorders*, *18*(4), 657–668. https://doi.org/10.1007/BF02211883

Mundy, P., & Jarrold, W. (2010). Infant joint attention, neural networks and social cognition. *Neural Networks*, *23*(8-9), 985–997. https://doi.org/10.1016/j.neunet.2010.08.009

Quinto-Pozos, D., Singleton, J. L., & Hauser, P. C. (2017). A case of specific language impairment in a deaf signer of American Sign Language. *Journal of Deaf Studies and Deaf Education*, *22*(2), 204–218. https://doi.org/10.1093/deafed/enw074

Quinto-Pozos, D., Singleton, J. L., Hauser, P. C., Levine, S. C., Garberoglio, C. L., & Hou, L. (2013). Atypical signed language development: A case study of challenges with visual–spatial processing. *Cognitive Neuropsychology*, *30*(5), 332–359. https://doi.org/10.1080/02643294.2013.863756

Roberts, J. M. (1989). Echolalia and comprehension in autistic children. *Journal of Autism and Developmental Disorders*, *19*(2), 271–281. https://doi.org/10.1007/BF02211846

Rogers, S. J., & Dawson, G. (2010). *Early Start Denver Model for young children with autism: Promoting language, learning, and engagement*. Guilford Press.

Schlosser, R. W., & Wendt, O. (2008). Effects of augmentative and alternative communication intervention on speech production in children with autism: A systematic review. *American Journal of Speech-Language Pathology*, *17*(3), 212–230. https://doi.org/10.1044/1058-0360(2008/021)

Shield, A., & Meier, R. P. (2012). Palm reversal errors in native-signing children with autism. *Journal of Communication Disorders*, *45*(6), 439–454. https://doi.org/10.1016/j.jcomdis.2012.08.004

Topic 5

Assessing Language Development in L1 Children with Developmental Language Disorder

5.1

Developmental Language Disorder and the Assessment of Spoken Language

Carol-Anne Murphy, Pauline Frizelle, and Cristina McKean

Assessment serves several overlapping objectives in the context of supporting children with developmental language disorder (DLD). These may include identifying children at risk of DLD; determining the presence of a speech, language, and communication need; differential diagnosis of DLD from other conditions; generating a detailed profile of strengths and needs across domains to inform appropriate intervention goals and methods; and measuring progress in attaining intervention goals (Denman et al., 2017; Paul et al., 2018). However, assessment of children with DLD is not without its challenges. In this chapter, we begin by outlining recent changes in diagnostic criteria and core features of DLD and their implications for assessment. We then critique approaches to assessment of children with DLD in light of the requirements of the bio-psychosocial model of disability and meeting the needs of diverse populations. We do not specifically address multilingual populations, as this is discussed in detail in Chapters 6.1–6-3.

The majority of the chapter addresses assessment methods and their purposes and areas where further development is required. We conclude by outlining current and promising directions in the assessment of children with DLD.

DIAGNOSTIC CRITERIA FOR DEVELOPMENTAL LANGUAGE DISORDER AND THEIR RELATIONSHIP TO ASSESSMENT

Due to long-standing inconsistencies in diagnostic criteria and their application, assessment of DLD is increasingly informed by the recommendations of the Criteria and Terminology Applied to Language Impairments: Synthesizing the Evidence (CATALISE) consortium (Bishop et al., 2016, 2017). This described new criteria for identification

Carol-Anne Murphy, Pauline Frizelle, and Cristina McKean, *Developmental Language Disorder and the Assessment of Spoken Language* In: *The Handbook of Language Assessment Across Modalities.* Edited by: Tobias Haug, Wolfgang Mann, and Ute Knoch, Oxford University Press. © Oxford University Press 2022. DOI: 10.1093/oso/9780190885052.003.0014 of DLD, terminology for describing the child's profile, and labels that might be applied to different profiles. These represent a significant departure from long-standing criteria for specific language impairment (SLI; the term being replaced by DLD). Key differences are illustrated in Table 5.1.1.

A number of developments in theory and empirical research since SLI was coined have driven these changes (these are fully explored in Reilly, Tomblin et al., 2014). Neuro-constructivist perspectives challenge the notion of "residual normality" in developmental conditions wherein nonverbal cognition and language are entirely separable. Neuroconstructivism suggests that children are born with a set of biological constraints but that these constraints are domain-general rather than domain-specific. Domain specificity emerges across development as a result of learning and processing. The infant is not a blank slate but rather certain structures in the neocortex are more relevant to processing one kind of input over another, and so these domain-relevant systems are the most likely to be harnessed for processing particular types of input. These systems are likely to also be usable for other types of processing, albeit often with suboptimal outcomes allowing for plasticity and compensation to be possible. Atypical developmental profiles are the result of subtle differences in early domain-relevant abilities, which then—in interaction with the child's experience and through processes of plasticity and compensation—disrupt the process of emergent neurobiological, functional specialization (see Thomas, 2003; Thomas & Karmiloff-Smith, 2003). It is highly unlikely therefore that entirely "specific" deficits can exist. As Thomas and Karmiloff-Smith (2002) state, "when marked behavioral deficits arise in a single domain, it is likely

Table 5.1.1 Key differences in definition and diagnosis between specific language impairment (SLI) and developmental language disorder (DLD)

SLI	DLD
• A discrepancy between language and nonverbal ability required for diagnosis – Language skills below age-related expectations; particular cut-off scores (e.g., falling >1.25 standard deviations [SD] or 2 SD below the mean) for access to certain services – Nonverbal IQ in the average range • Exclusionary criteria for diagnosis (language difficulties in the absence of . . .) • Restrictive—excludes co-occurring conditions	• No longer require nonverbal IQ in the average range for diagnosis • Language score below age-related expectations but no specific "cutoffs" required • Impact on communicative and educational functioning recognized and necessary for diagnosis • Inclusionary rather than exclusionary criteria for diagnosis (language difficulties in the presence of . . .) • Presence of co-occurring conditions allowed • Recognition of persistence/endurance

that the cognitive processes underlying apparently intact performance in other domains are also atypical in subtle ways—which may go undetected without sensitive testing of abilities outside of the behavioral impairment" (p. 6).

DLD criteria have moved away, therefore, from widely applied discrepancy and exclusionary criteria, such that nonverbal IQ in the average range is no longer a criterion (Bishop et al., 2017).

The criteria also incorporate the presence of co-occurring conditions and acknowledge that the needs of the child may not be exclusive to language. DLD is subsumed in a wider category of language disorder characterized by *persistence* of language difficulties into middle childhood and beyond, which have an impact on academic and social/communicative *functioning*. These criteria of persistence and limitations in functioning are challenging for assessment practice: the former due to the fluid nature of language development, particularly in the preschool years, and the latter due to the imprecision of the construct of social/communicative functioning. Change over time and variability in profiles reflect the fluid nature of language impairment and question the validity of descriptions and diagnoses of language impairment derived from assessment at one point in time. In the preschool years, children's language trajectories vary substantially such that it is difficult to predict which children will have persisting difficulties and which will resolve. Although this remains an inexact science, research efforts to develop reliable identification methods for children at risk in these early years continue. Current knowledge and practice are described next.

As children move through primary and secondary school, the severity of their language difficulties will likely be more stable; however, their qualitative profiles in terms of the affected language domains vary substantially over time (Conti-Ramsden & Botting, 1999). This aligns with emergentist (Evans, 2001) and developmental neuro-constructivist perspectives on impairment (Thomas & Karmiloff-Smith, 2003), which predict interactivity between domains of language (McKean et al., 2013a) and a dynamic and changing system over time (McKean et al., 2013b). This interactivity is one driver for the CATALISE consortium's recognition that there is no agreed taxonomy of subtypes of DLD. However, the characterization of the child's strengths and weaknesses across the core domains of language (phonology, morphosyntax, pragmatics/social communication, and vocabulary) and language modalities (receptive and expressive) remains critical to effective intervention planning. Thus, the consortium recommends comprehensive assessment (Bishop et al., 2017). Furthermore, the use of a range of assessment methods including standardized and nonstandardized testing with caregiver reports, observation, and consideration of the language-learning context is encouraged. However, discussions of assessment practice have not foregrounded the perspective of children with language disorders, nor is the role of the environment considered.

BIO-PSYCHOSOCIAL MODELS OF DISABILITY AND THEIR RELATIONSHIP TO ASSESSMENT

Although functioning is invoked by the CATALISE criteria, and diagnosing DLD requires identifying the impact of the presumed language difficulties on functioning, the construct of "functioning" is underspecified. This distinction between an underlying impairment and an individual's functioning draws from bio-psychosocial models of disability, in particular, the World Health Organization (WHO) model of functioning and disability in children and young people: the International Classification of Functioning-Children and Youth (ICF-CY) (WHO, 2007). In this framework, a person's experience of disability is recognized as emerging as a function of interactions between their underlying impairment (i.e., the health condition and its effects), their environment, and personal factors such as gender and psychological assets. An individual's activity and participation describe the individual in terms of how they can execute tasks (activity) and how these affect real-life situations (participation).

Assessment via the ICF involves assessing the speech and language disorder at the level of impairment (in morphosyntax, phonology, pragmatics, semantics) and across the activities affected (expressive speech and language, oral and reading comprehension, written language, etc.) and considering the contexts of participation and functioning (reflected academically in, e.g., ability to follow classroom instructions and in navigating social communication with peers) (Westby & Washington, 2017).

Standardized assessments typically focus on linguistic representations and knowledge but at a remove from conversational language or use in an academic environment. For example, approaches to elicitation of grammatical structures often involve sentence completion tasks (e.g., examiner points to a picture and says "this boy is running" and to the next saying "this girl is. . . . " requiring the child to complete the sentence); assessment of comprehension typically involves forced-choice picture pointing tasks. Activity and participation restrictions tend to be assessed through less formal approaches (e.g., observation checklists used while the child is playing/interacting with others), and the development of measures of personal and environmental factors has attracted still less attention.

ASSESSMENT METHODS AND PURPOSES

Creating a comprehensive and holistic profile of impairment and functioning, as well as personal and environmental factors required for appropriate intervention planning, necessarily involves the use of multiple assessment methods. Approaches, varying with the age of the child and purpose, can include validated parent/caregiver reports of language and/or communication skills, self-report of functioning, quality of life and well-being, direct behavioral assessments using standardized or informal clinician-generated testing procedures, and observational methods again using recognized formal tools or less formal methods.

Screening and Identification

Language trajectories in the preschool years are highly variable (Bornstein et al., 2016, Reilly, McKean, et al., 2014). Almost 70% of children identified at the age of 2 as late talkers go on to have typical language profiles by the time they turn 4, comprising only half of children with low language at 4, the remaining half having typical language scores at age 2. If services for the child were targeted using late talker status alone as an indicator of risk, there would be considerable over- and underservicing of need. Identifying assessment approaches and tools that might more accurately predict those children in need of follow-up and support is crucial. There is not as yet a "gold standard" diagnostic screening tool for children who might present with or be at risk of language impairment (Wallace et al., 2015).

Application of a public health approach to DLD (Law et al., 2017) moves assessment beyond a clinical, "case"-based lens and increases the focus on prevention. McKean et al. (2016) reported an approach integrating child, family, and home-learning environment factors measured at 12 months to predict language skills at 4 years. The resulting model provided moderate predictive validity and greater accuracy than late talker status at 2 years. Although work remains to make such approaches ready for clinical practice, the development of "risk prediction models" is a promising avenue for future research.

Recent longitudinal studies indicate relative stability in language profiles for most children from 4 years (McKean et al., 2015; McKean, Wraith, et al., 2017). Although large changes in relative language abilities are unlikely, clinically meaningful changes can still occur and be invoked by interventions. Difficulties are more likely to persist if pervasive (i.e., where low language scores are combined with poor nonverbal ability or multiple areas of language are impaired), and present at school entry (Bishop & Edmundson, 1987). Children with receptive language difficulties have a poorer prognosis in terms of persistence and outcome, with some suggesting that this profile indicates severity of language difficulties rather than a separate subgroup (Tomblin & Zhang, 2006).

However, a relatively stable language profile does not imply that "one-off" assessments suffice in identifying need and monitoring progress. The school years may also see the identification of children with a range of social, emotional, mental health, and/or behavioral difficulties masking previously undetected language disorders (Hollo et al., 2014; Hopkins et al., 2018). Late emerging subgroups with language disorder have been identified: McKean and colleagues (2017) found children with greater socioemotional-behavioral difficulties more likely to be in this group, and Snowling et al. (2016) found that a family history of language or literacy difficulties made this trajectory more likely. High rates of language disorder are identified in populations of children accessing child and adolescent mental health services or those involved in the youth justice system (Im-bolter et al., 2013; Winstanley et al., 2019), suggesting that vulnerable groups such as these should routinely be assessed for presence of undetected DLD.

Standardized Tests

Standardized assessments, which are widely used by speech and language therapists to differentially diagnose DLD (Denman et al., 2017), can be administered reliably across children and on repeated occasions, allowing for the generation of standard scores or percentile ranks derived from a normative sample and for the child's performance to be compared against same-age peers. Commonly used tests include the New Reynell Developmental Language Scales (Edwards et al., 2011) and the Expressive Receptive and Recall of Narrative Instrument (ERRNI; Bishop, 2004). Denman et al.'s recent review (2017) identified 76 standardized tests with normative data for use with monolingual English-speaking children aged 4–12 years. However, available tests vary substantially in psychometric properties, including level of diagnostic accuracy (Denman et al., 2017; Spaulding et al., 2006). For instance, incomplete reporting of confidence intervals and diagnostic validity may mean that practitioners place too much confidence in individual test scores or make erroneous assumptions regarding improvement in scores over time. Further difficulties emerge when clinicians use such tests to identify specific aspects of language processing and knowledge requiring remediation. In many cases, the purpose of a test or test battery is to identify the presence of an impairment, giving only broad indicators of which linguistic domains are most affected. They are not necessarily sufficiently sensitive or detailed to inform intervention planning. This raises the question of validity more broadly.

A valid test of language does not confound the knowledge being measured with other factors. However, this is not always achieved. Testing expressive morphology in typically developing children and those with language impairment using two standardized tests, Merrell and Plante (1997) found inconsistent pass/fail rates between the tests and low point-to-point agreement on items targeting the same morphosyntactic structure. Frizelle and colleagues (2017, 2019a) have highlighted considerable difficulties with multiple-choice picture tasks in comprehension assessment. Children could repeat sentences that they did not understand in a study comparing their performance on a multiple-choice comprehension task of relative clauses, with repetition of the same sentences using a sentence recall task (Frizelle et al., 2017). Frizelle and colleagues (2017) attributed the discrepancy to the additional processing load of multiple-choice picture-selection comprehension tasks. They subsequently examined (Frizelle et al., 2019a) the effect of multiple-choice sentence-picture matching and an animated sentence verification task on typically developing children's complex sentence understanding. Here, children performed better on the animated task than on the multiple-choice task. Each testing method revealed a different order of difficulty in children's complex sentence comprehension. Both studies raise concerns about the linguistic assumptions and cognitive demands placed on the child using picture-choice methodology. By presenting one image representing the target sentence and three foils or distractors reflecting different interpretations, only children with a deep understanding of the sentence will respond correctly. However, there are issues with the semantic plausibility of each distractor and the premise that distractors for each target sentence are equally plausible. Additionally, in some tests, distractors are pragmatically implausible (e.g., a picture of a key under a cup) and designed such that the correct answer can be achieved without understanding the specific sentence structure. Cognitively, the presence of three distractors requires the child to rule out three alternative interpretations of the sentence, thus increasing the processing and memory load considerably and requiring the child to engage in a process far removed from what occurs in natural discourse. This is particularly concerning since multiple-choice picture-selection comprehension tasks are among the most common assessment paradigms for evaluating children's sentence comprehension within a standardized framework. Of even greater concern is that if typically developing children display these differences, they will be more pronounced for children with additional difficulties, as was the case with a group of children with Down syndrome (Frizelle et al., 2019b). Next steps involve looking specifically at the effect of different methodologies on children with DLD.

Most standardized tests distinguish between children who have an expressive language disorder only versus those with receptive-expressive difficulties. Tests with multiple subtests are categorized according to either domain and allow for the calculation of both expressive and receptive composite scores. This distinction has also been formalized in the *Diagnostic and Statistical Manual of Mental Disorders* (DSM-5, text revision; American Psychiatric Association, 2013). However, there are considerable diagnostic and treatment limitations in using this division. A psychometrically defined gap between expressive and receptive scores will depend on the specific areas of language tested and the accurate measurement of items. Deevy and Leonard (2004), for example, reported on a group of children with DLD (aged 4; 01–6;10) who scored poorly on expressive language tests but in the low average range on a receptive vocabulary measure, suggesting an expressive disorder. However, testing on wh- question comprehension showed significant difficulties relative to younger typically developing children and thus difficulties in both domains. Also concerning is the fact that areas of expressive language with which children with DLD evince particular difficulty, such as subject-verb agreement, are problematic to assess receptively (Leonard, 2009) without invoking confounds such as metalinguistic awareness (Rice & Wexler, 2001). Consistent with this argument, Tomblin and Zhang (2006) used factor analysis to identify separable dimensions in children's performance on standardized language tests. They found that considering language as a single dimension was a better model fit than one treating expressive and receptive language scores as individual factors. Additionally, as children got older, grammatical and vocabulary skills could be differentiated, but a receptive/expressive language distinction did not emerge. When assessing language, a global construct of "language knowledge" may be a more helpful approach that is in keeping with empirical data and theories of language impairment. Errors are usually made, whatever the domain, due to limitations in children's language knowledge. Given the interdependency of expressive and receptive language skills (evident in sentence recall tasks and priming studies), limitations in language knowledge are likely to impact on both language domains to varying degrees depending on task constraints.

Roy, Chiat, and Dodd (2014) argue that some children, ostensibly those from low socioeconomic status (SES) backgrounds, are less familiar with the testing context and accompanying demands than those from high SES backgrounds. Certain standardized assessments can favor language "experience" and world knowledge, with subtests favoring meta-linguistic skills and prior exposure to a structured learning environment. Thus, for example, the testing method may underestimate the abilities of children who have not yet had consistent exposure to a structured, school-based environment.

This underscores the need to use an appropriate normative sample to derive valid standard scores and centile ranks. Clearly, a sample needs to be sufficiently large for valid comparisons and reflect the nature of the population for which clinical use is intended, considering key criteria such as gender, SES, and cultural diversity. Despite multilingualism being the norm globally, a major challenge for clinicians and researchers alike is the development of tests that are valid for children growing up in multilingual contexts (also see Chapters 6.1–6.3).

Elicited or Spontaneous Language Sample Analysis

Language sampling is a crucial component of the assessment toolkit, providing information not captured in the sentence elicitation formats of many standardized assessments (Paul et al., 2018). Because it bridges contrived clinical assessment procedures and real-world communicative functioning, it gives a more valid representation of functioning. Adding standardization supports reliable measurement and comparison. Considering the ICF, this "language in action" can be conceptualized as a measure of activity rather than impairment. Furthermore, the elicitation approach (e.g., using story retell procedures) can potentially stress the system to identify impairments that spontaneous conversation may mask (Westerveld & Vidler, 2016). While time constraints limit clinicians' use of language sampling (Kemp & Klee, 1997), valuable clinical information has been identified from even relatively short language samples (Heilmann et al., 2010).

Criterion-Referenced Tests

Unlike norm-referenced tests designed to identify deficits more broadly, criterion-referenced assessment tools are constructed to identify children with a level of proficiency in a particular knowledge area. Such tests are more descriptive, usually with multiple opportunities to estimate children's progress, thereby allowing for the characterization of children's advancement over time. They may be particularly suited to assessing morphosyntactic development in preschool children, since typically developing preschoolers have usually mastered most elements of morphosyntax at this age (Oetting & Hadley, 2017).

Constructs such as communicative functioning, perceived well-being, and quality of life, which do not relate to child age, where the concept of "typicality" is somewhat moot and where subjectivity is unavoidable or indeed preferred, are also often measured using such scales. The Functional Outcomes in Children Under Six (FOCUS; (Thomas-Stonnell et al., 2013) is notable as one of the few validated measures of children's communicative functioning (Washington et al., 2013) with the capacity to measure change over time and in response to interventions. It contains 50 items covering communication and related participation skills derived from a content analysis of parental descriptions of their children's communication. The FOCUS can be completed by either speech-language therapists or parents and captures change in areas such as socialization, independence, communication intent, and intelligibility(Thomas-Stonnell et al 2013). Development of such tools across childhood is vital to the application of the new DLD criteria to research and practice.

Dynamic Assessment

The variety of reasons why children perform poorly on a test may have important implications for intervention planning. Dynamic assessment (DA) approaches offer an alternative to standardized assessments, seeking to assess potential for learning or "modifiability" and progress (see also Chapters 3.1–3.3). They may be used either to extend standardized testing or instead of it. Typically, DA involves a mediated learning experience, or test-teach-retest, and may include elements of graduated prompting or scaffolding. It is argued that such approaches can demonstrate knowledge of grammar that is not captured in standardized tests, evaluate the potential for progress, identify prompts and learning strategies that may be most effective for intervention, and, in some cases, provide insight into metalinguistic and metacognitive skills (Lidz, 1991). Further work is needed to develop reliable and valid DA approaches for child language assessment.

BEST PRACTICE FOR ASSESSMENT OF CHILDREN WITH DEVELOPMENTAL LANGUAGE DISORDER

Considering the nature of DLD, the strength and weaknesses of differing assessment approaches, and the goal of interventions, a comprehensive and holistic approach to assessment is recommended. Diagnosis must not be based on a single standardized test result but must integrate knowledge from less formal assessment approaches and consider real-world functioning and change over time. Interventions must be devised with detailed knowledge of specific domains of impairment and strategies that promote change for the individual child identified through detailed criterion-referenced testing and DA of hypothesized areas of need. Furthermore, goals should be devised with reference to the child's communicative functioning to ensure interventions have maximum "real-world" effect, the child's environment is considered, and barriers and enablers to their participation are assessed and addressed. Finally, it is crucial that assessment of children with language disorder captures the voice and views of children themselves. This is not only consistent with ensuring their human rights, but also important given some recent studies indicating that the perspectives of children may depart from the views of parents and other adults familiar with the children (e.g., Gallagher et al., 2019).

FUTURE DIRECTIONS

The use of technology: Clinical assessment in DLD has yet to embrace the possibilities of technology but there are promising developments in this area. The limitations of using static pictures to assess dynamic scenes might be overcome through the use of computer-based animation as demonstrated by Frizelle et al. (2019a, 2019b); technology may support automating language transcription and analysis or inform DA through, for example, evaluating the "dosage" of language models required to achieve mastery of a construct.

Accounting for language exposure in multilingual contexts: A promising innovation is the design of an algorithm taking into account language exposure and bilingualism to determine whether a child's Communicative Development Inventory (CDI) score (Fenson, 2007)—a checklist of words or statements the child understands and/or produces—across two languages (English plus 1 of 13 additional languages) is typical for children aged 2 years given the exposure received (Floccia et al., 2018). There is much to do to generalize this approach to different sociocultural contexts, ages, and language domains; however, it is an encouraging first step in the development of valid assessment approaches for multilingual children.

Use of risk models in screening: Future research needs to test whether the combination of assessment approaches may provide more robust screening methods (e.g., combining broad-based language assessments with tests of specific clinical markers such as non-word repetition and sentence repetition and exploring the presence of risk factors in the child's profile and case history such as gesture and play skills; O'Neill et al., 2019).

Stressing the system: Tests actively incorporating items that are particularly sensitive to a specific disorder are becoming more common. Within assessments yielding composite scores, subtests should be weighted so that when each score is combined and multiplied by its weighting, there is an increased chance of achieving high sensitivity and specificity and accurately identifying those with DLD.

Assessing "functioning" and listening to the voice of the child: Assessments that reliably capture a child's communicative functioning are rare, with implications for diagnosis and intervention planning. This should therefore be a priority for future research alongside the need to find methods to include the child's voice in goal-setting and intervention delivery decisions.

REFERENCES

American Psychiatric Association (2013). *Diagnostic and statistical manual of mental disorders (5th ed.).* http://dsm.psychiatryonline.org/doi/abs/10.1176/appi.books.9780890425596.dsm01

Bishop, D. V. M. (2004). *Expression, reception and recall of narrative instrument.* Pearson.

Bishop, D. V. M., & Edmundson, A. (1987). Language impaired 4-year-olds: Distinguishing transient from persistent impairment. *Journal of Speech and Hearing Disorders, 52*(2), 156–173. https://doi.org/10.1044/jshd.5202.156

Bishop, D. V. M., Snowling, M. J., Thompson, P. A., Greenhalgh, T., & CATALISE-2 consortium (2017). Phase 2 of CATALISE: A multinational and multidisciplinary Delphi consensus study of problems with language development: Terminology. *Journal of Child Psychology and Psychiatry, 58*(10), 1068–1080. https://doi.org/10.1111/jcpp.12721

Bishop, D. V. M., Snowling, M. J., Thompson, P. A., Greenhalgh, T., & CATALIAE consortium (2016). CATALISE: A multinational and multidisciplinary Delphi

consensus study. Identifying language impairments in children. *PLOS One, 11*(7), 1–26. https://doi.org/10.1371/journal.pone.0158753
Bornstein, M. H., Hahn, C.-S., & Putnick, D. L. (2016). Long-term stability of core language skill in children with contrasting language skills. *Developmental Psychology, 52*(5), 704–716. https://doi.org/10.1037/dev0000111
Conti-Ramsden, G., & Botting, N. (1999). Classification of children with specific language impairment: Longitudinal considerations. *Journal of Speech Language and Hearing Research, 42*(5), 1195–1204. https://doi.org/10.1044/jslhr.4205.1195
Deevy, P., & Leonard, L. (2004). The comprehension of wh-questions in children with specific language impairment. *Journal of Speech, Language, and Hearing Research, 47*(4), 802–815. https://doi.org/10.1044/1092-4388(2004/060)
Denman, D., Speyer, R., Munro, N., Pearce, W. M., Chen, Y.-W., & Cordier, R. (2017). Psychometric properties of language assessments for children aged 4–12 years: A systematic review. *Frontiers in Psychology, 8*. https://doi.org/10.3389/fpsyg.2017.01515
Edwards, S., Letts, C., & Sinka, I. (2011). *New Reynell Developmental Language Scales* (4th ed.). GL Assessment.
Evans, J. L (2001). An emergent account of language impairments in children with SLI: Implications for assessment and intervention. *Journal of Communication Disorders, 34*(1–2), 39–54. https://doi.org/10.1016/S0021-9924(00)00040-X
Fenson, L. (2007). *MacArthur-Bates communicative development inventories*. Paul H. Brookes.
Floccia, C., Sambrook T. D., Delle Luche, C., Kwok, R., Goslin, J., White, L., Cattani, A., Sullivan, E., & Abbot-Smith, K. (2018). IV: Results for studies 2 and 3: The UKBTAT model and its application to non-target additional language learners. *Monographs of the Society for Research in Child Development, 83*(1), 61–67. https://doi.org/10.1111/mono.12351
Frizelle, P., O'Neill, C., & Bishop, D. V. M. (2017). Assessing understanding of relative clauses: A comparison of multiple-choice comprehension versus sentence repetition. *Journal of Child Language, 44*(6), 1435–1457. https://doi.org/10.1017/S0305000916000635
Frizelle, P., Thompson, P., Duta, M., & Bishop, D. V. M. (2019a). Assessing children's understanding of complex syntax: A comparison of two methods. *Language Learning, 69*(2), 255–291. https://doi.org/10.1111/lang.12332
Frizelle P., Thompson, P., Duta, M., & Bishop D. V. M. (2019b). The understanding of complex syntax in children with Down syndrome. *Wellcome Open Research, 3*, 1–34. https://doi.org/10.12688/wellcomeopenres.14861.2
Gallagher, A. L., Murphy, C. A., Conway, P. F., & Perry, A. (2019). Engaging multiple stakeholders to improve speech and language therapy services in schools: An appreciative inquiry-based study, *BMC Health Services Research, 19*(1), 1–17. https://doi.org/10.1186/s12913-019-4051-z
Heilmann, J., Nockerts, A., & Miller, J. F. (2010). Language sampling: Does the length of the transcript matter? *Language, Speech & Hearing Services in Schools, 41*(4), 393–404. https://doi.org/10.1044/0161-1461(2009/09-0023)
Hollo, A., Wehby, J. H., & Oliver, R. M. (2014). Unidentified language deficits in children with emotional and behavioral disorders: A meta-analysis. *Exceptional Children, 80*(2), 169–186. https://doi.org/10.1177/001440291408000203

Hopkins, T., Clegg, J., & Stackhouse, J. (2018). Examining the association between language, expository discourse and offending behaviour: An investigation of direction, strength and independence. *International Journal of Language & Communication Disorders*, *53*(1), 113–129. https://doi.org/10.1111/1460-6984.12330

Im-Bolter, Cohen, N. J., & Farnia, F. (2013). I thought we were good: social cognition, figurative language, and adolescent psychopathology. *Journal of Child Psychology and Psychiatry*, *54*(7), 724–732. https://doi.org/10.1111/jcpp.12067

Kemp, K., & Klee, T. (1997). Clinical language sampling practices: Results of a survey of speech-language pathologists in the United States. *Child Language, Teaching and Therapy*, *13*(2), 161–176. https://doi.org/10.1177/026565909701300204

Law, J., Levickis, P., McKean, C., Goldfeld, S., Snow, P., & Reilly, S. (2017). *Child language in a public health context*. Centre of Research Excellence in Child Language, Murdoch Children's Research Institute.

Leonard, L. B. (2009). Is expressive language disorder an accurate diagnostic category? *American Journal of Speech and Language Pathology*, *18*(2), 115–123. https://doi.org/10.1044/1058-0360(2008/08-0064)

Lidz, C. (1991). *Practitioner's guide to dynamic assessment*. Guilford Press.

McKean, C., Law, J., Mensah, F., Cini, E., Eadie, P., Frazer, K., & Reilly, S. (2016). Predicting meaningful differences in school-entry language skills from child and family factors measured at 12 months of age. *International Journal of Early Childhood*, *48*(3), 329–351. https://doi.org/10.1007/s13158-016-0174-0

McKean, C., Letts, C., & Howard, D. (2013a). Functional reorganization in the developing lexicon: Separable and changing influences of lexical and phonological variables on children's fast-mapping. *Journal of Child Language*, *40*(2), 307–335. https://doi.org/10.1017/S0305000911000444

McKean, C., Letts, C., & Howard, D. (2013b). Developmental change is key to understanding primary language impairment: The case of phonotactic probability and nonword repetition. *Journal of Speech, Language, and Hearing Research*, *56*(5), 1579–1594. https://doi.org/10.1044/1092-4388(2013/12-0066)

McKean, C., Mensah, F., Eadie, P., Bavin, E., Bretherton. L., Cini, E., & Reilly S. (2015). Levers for language growth: Characteristics and predictors of language trajectories between 4 and 7 years. *PLOS ONE*, *10*(8), 1–21. https://doi.org/10.1371/journal.pone.0134251

McKean, C., Wraith, D., Eadie, P., Cook, F., Mensah, F., & Reilly, S. (2017). Subgroups in language trajectories from 4 to 11 years: The nature and predictors of stable, improving and decreasing language trajectory groups. *Journal of Child Psychology and Psychiatry*, *58*(10), 1081–1091. https://doi.org/10.1111/jcpp.12790

Merrell, A. W., & Plante, E. (1997). Norm-referenced test interpretation in the diagnostic process. *Language, Speech and Hearing Services in Schools*, *28*(1), 50–58. https://doi.org/10.1044/0161-1461.2801.50

Oetting, J. B., & Hadley, P. A. (2017). Morphosyntax in child language disorders. In R. G. Schwartz (Ed.), *Handbook of child language disorders* (2nd ed., pp. 365–391). Taylor and Francis.

O'Neill, H., Murphy, C. A., & Chiat, S. (2019). What our hands tell us: A two-year follow-up investigating outcomes in subgroups of children with language delay. *Journal of Speech, Language, and Hearing Research*, *62*(2), 356–366. https://doi.org/10.1044/2018_JSLHR-L-17-0261

Paul, R., Norbury, C., & Gosse, C. (2018). *Language disorders from infancy through adolescence: Listening, speaking, reading, writing, and communicating*. Elsevier Mosby.

Reilly, S., Tomblin, B., Law, J., McKean, C., Mensah, F., Morgan, A., Goldfeld, S., Nicholson, J., & Wake, M. (2014). Specific language impairment: A convenient label for whom? *International Journal of Language & Communication Disorders*, *49*(4), 416–451. https://doi.org/10.1111/1460-6984.12102

Reilly, S., McKean, C., & Levickis P. (2014). *Late talking: Can it predict later language difficulties?* Centre for Research Excellence in Child Language.

Rice, M., & Wexler, K. (2001). *Rice/Wexler test of early grammatical impairment*. The Psychological Corporation.

Roy, P., Chiat, S., & Dodd, B. (2014). *Language and socioeconomic disadvantage: From research to practice*. City University London. http://openaccess.city.ac.uk/4989/

Snowling, M. J., Duff, F. J., Nash, H. M., & Hulme, C. (2016). Language profiles and literacy outcomes of children with resolving, emerging, or persisting language impairments. *Journal of Child Psychology and Psychiatry*, *57*(12), 1360–1369. https://doi.org/10.1111/jcpp.12497

Spaulding, T. J., Plante, E., & Farinella, K. A. (2006). Eligibility criteria for language impairment: Is the low end of normal always appropriate? *Language, Speech and Hearing Services in Schools*, *37*(1), 61–72. https://doi.org/10.1044/0161-1461(2006/007)

Thomas, M. S. C. (2003). Multiple causality in developmental disorders: Methodological implications from computational modelling. *Developmental Science*, *6*(5), 537–556. https://doi.org/10.1111/1467-7687.00311

Thomas, M. S. C., & Karmiloff-Smith, A. (2002). Are developmental disorders like cases of adult brain damage? Implications from connectionist modelling. *Behavioural and Brain Sciences*, *25*, 727–788.

Thomas, M. S. C., & Karmiloff-Smith, A. (2003). Modeling language acquisition in atypical phenotypes. *Psychological Review*, *110*(4), 647–682. https://doi.org/10.1037/0033-295X.110.4.647

Thomas-Stonell, N., Washington, K., Oddson, B., Robertson, B., & Rosenbaum, P. (2013). Measuring communicative participation using the FOCUS©: Focus on the outcomes of communication under six. *Child Care Health and Development*, *39*(4), 474–480. https://doi.org/10.1111/cch.12049

Tomblin, J. B., & Zhang, X. (2006). The dimensionality of language ability in school-age children. *Journal of Speech, Language and Hearing Research*, *49*(6), 1193–1208. https://doi.org/10.1044/1092-4388(2006/086)

Wallace, I. F., Berkman, N. D., Watson, L. R., Coyne-Beasley, T., Wood, C. T., Cullen, K., & Lohr, K. N. (2015). Screening for speech and language delay in children 5 years old and younger: A systematic review. *Pediatrics*, *136*(2), e448–462. https://doi.org/10.1542/peds.2014-3889

Washington, K., Thomas-Stonell, N., Oddson, B., McLeod, S., Warr-Leeper, G., Robertson, B., & Rosenbaum, P. (2013). Construct validity of the FOCUS© (Focus on the Outcomes of Communication Under Six): A communicative participation outcome measure for preschool children. *Child: Care, Health and Development*, *39*(4), 481–489. https://doi.org/10.1111/cch.12043

Westby, C., & Washington, K. N. (2017). Using the International Classification of Functioning, Disability and Health in assessment and intervention of school-aged children with language impairments. *Language, Speech, and Hearing Services in Schools, 48*(3), 137–152. https://doi.org/10.1044/2017_LSHSS-16-0037

Westerveld, M. F., & Vidler, K. (2016). Spoken language samples of Australian children in conversation, narration and exposition. *International Journal of Speech-Language Pathology,* 18(3), 288–298. https://doi.org/10.3109/17549507.2016.1159332

Winstanley, M., Webb, R. T., & Conti-Ramsden, G. (2019). Psycholinguistic and socioemotional characteristics of young offenders: Do language abilities and gender matter? *Legal and Criminological Psychology, 24*(2), 195–214. https://doi.org/10.1111/lcrp.12150

World Health Organisation (WHO). (2007). ICF-CY: *International classification of functioning, disability and health. Children & youth version*. WHO Press.

5.2

Developmental Language Disorder and the Assessment of Signed Language

David Quinto-Pozos

It is common for professionals and researchers who work with deaf and/or hard-of-hearing children (D/HH) who use a signed language to have many questions about assessment. Such experts often want to know about typical developmental trends for D/HH children (including language and other aspects of development), and whether the children with whom they are working deviate from such patterns. The quest for norms of development for D/HH children is strong despite knowledge by professionals and researchers that there exists notable variation in D/HH children, influenced largely by the age at which they receive robust exposure to a signed language. In a growing number of cases, professionals are also devising ways to provide signed language intervention and track progress over time. Unfortunately, the number of assessment instruments that can be used with such children are few by comparison, but professionals and researchers are aware of this limitation and have devised assessment approaches that consider multiple aspects of childhood development. In this chapter, I outline some of the challenges of assessing signing D/HH children who are suspected of exhibiting a developmental language disorder (DLD). Similarly, various assessment instruments are highlighted along with some of the approaches that have been adopted by researchers who work with D/HH children. Different aspects of language are considered separately for organizational purposes, even though professionals and researchers are aware of how linguistic processes interact in development. Suggestions are provided for professionals and researchers who work with D/HH signing children, and various recommendations for future research on assessment are proposed.

David Quinto-Pozos, *Developmental Language Disorder and the Assessment of Signed Language* In: *The Handbook of Language Assessment Across Modalities.* Edited by: Tobias Haug, Wolfgang Mann, and Ute Knoch, Oxford University Press. DOI: 10.1093/oso/9780190885052.003.0015

DEVELOPMENTAL SIGNED LANGUAGE DISORDER

The first decade of this millennium ushered in various published studies of D/HH signing children believed to present with a developmental signed language disorder (Marshall et al., 2006, 2015; Morgan et al., 2007; Quinto-Pozos et al., 2017, among others).[1] According to criteria that have traditionally been used to diagnose hearing children in research studies (e.g., Leonard, 1998), D/HH children have been excluded from consideration for a DLD diagnosis, especially one of *specific language impairment* (SLI), because of their audiological deafness. Recently, Quinto-Pozos, Singleton, and Hauser (2017) proposed modifications to the SLI diagnostic criteria that would apply to D/HH signing children. Even so, researchers who work on signed language have been considering DLD/SLI as a valid categorization of the signed language comprehension and/or production of some D/HH children for more than a decade. The vast majority of studies in this area focus on D/HH children in the United Kingdom who sign British Sign Language (BSL) or D/HH children in the United States who are users of American Sign Language (ASL). Throughout the remainder of the chapter, "DLD" will be used more generally to encompass children who have been labeled with a developmental signed language disorder or SLI concerning their signed language.

Researchers in this area of inquiry have relied heavily on the judgments of language professionals (teachers, speech and language therapists, signed language specialists) at bilingual schools for deaf children when considering children for involvement in their studies (e.g., Quinto-Pozos et al., 2011). For example, in Mason and colleagues' group study of D/HH signers of BSL (Mason et al., 2010), the researchers used a screening questionnaire that was sent to schools for the deaf in order to identify possible children for the study. The questionnaire contained items about language comprehension (e.g., child exhibits difficulty understanding signed sentences, questions, and stories, asks for repetition often, etc.) and language production (e.g., child shows hesitation and/or frustration when signing, sometimes cannot remember correct sign to use, etc.). Quinto-Pozos and colleagues (2013, 2017) also relied on the judgments of language professionals for their case study projects, coupled with the opinions of the deaf parents of those children suspected of having a language disorder. Interestingly, Novogrodsky et al. (2017) discuss data that were collected using the American Sign Language Assessment Instrument (ASLAI; Hoffmeister et al., 2015), and they note that the judgments of educators accurately predict the grammatical judgments of D/HH children who were exposed to ASL early by their deaf parents, but the same adult judgments were not predictive of the performance of the non-native signers who were exposed to ASL later.

This last point touches on an important theme that concerns the language assessment of D/HH children suspected to be candidates for a DLD diagnosis: there is much variability in the signed language development of D/HH children who are not exposed to their signed language at an early age. More than 90% of D/HH children are born to hearing, non-signing parents, which means they do not generally receive early exposure to a signed language (Mitchell & Karchmer, 2004). Many—though not all—of those children are later exposed to a signed language, and the months or years delay in language exposure results in much variability in the acquisition, processing, and competency in that signed language (Mayberry, 1993; Mayberry & Fischer, 1989; Novogrodsky et al., 2017, among others).

One of the challenges of working with D/HH children suspected of having a developmental signed language disorder is the availability of standardized assessment instruments, which is influenced by the small numbers of native signers who can participate in the norming of such tests and inform what researchers know to be "typical" in terms of language development (Mann & Haug, 2014). Various tests—ranging from language comprehension to language production—have been created for research purposes, but the vast majority of those instruments have not been normed on large populations of language users.[2] Because of this, the assessments might be best considered as partial metrics for examining suspected cases of DLD rather than complete diagnostic instruments. With this in mind, researchers have adopted methodologies that combine multiple sources of information about a child in order to decide on his or her categorization as either typically developing (TD) or as a child who presents with a DLD. This chapter will discuss some of the state of the art, as it were, of working with D/HH signing children suspected of having a developmental signed language disorder, and the focus will be on the various assessments that have been used with such children. For more complete discussions of signed language assessments used with D/HH children, see Haug (2005), Singleton and Supalla (2011), Mann and Haug (2014), Enns et al. (2016), and Henner et al. (2017).

ASSESSING SIGNED LANGUAGE SKILLS

In this section focusing on D/HH signing children, language assessments that are used with school-aged children will be highlighted since that is the population of language users that is most often the focus of studies of DLD and language disorders more broadly. The collection of conversational language samples has been useful to researchers in this area, and that is covered first. Then, language comprehension assessments will be discussed followed by language production assessments. As complements to language assessment, the chapter will also discuss cognitive and neuropsychological assessment and the assessment of motor skills. The skills and knowledge of administrators of the assessments and those who analyze the data is covered next, followed by a section on proposed future directions in this area.

Assessing Conversational Language Skills

Language assessments often target specific lexical items or grammatical constructions, but they often ignore a child's ability to converse with adults or with his or her peers. One approach for examining a child's general communication abilities that has been employed with school-aged D/HH children is to allow a child to converse with adults and age-matched peers in a casual interview-type setting. The American Sign Language Proficiency Assessment (ASL-PA) calls for matching the child with adult and peer interlocutors over two sessions that are video recorded for later analysis (Maller et al., 1999). The protocol also includes having the child recount the *Tortoise and the Hare* narrative in signed language (see Supalla et al., unpublished). Quinto-Pozos and colleagues have employed the use of the ASL-PA with their case study participants who have been reported to exhibit some type of DLD (Quinto-Pozos et al., 2013, 2017). This instrument, which can be used with D/HH signing children aged 6–12, allows researchers to consider how a child might perform with language use when in everyday conversation with others. Whereas the ASL-PA is an omnibus measure of language ability rather than a diagnostic tool, the analysis of the video-recorded data is designed to scrutinize a child's language production for the presence of 23 target structures across eight morphosyntactic features of ASL. ASL-PA scores reflect overall general proficiency and can be categorized into low, moderate, and high ASL Levels. The use of such an instrument provides important information for the researcher, which can be used to complement the results of other more targeted assessments when considered a child's overall abilities.

Assessing Comprehension and/or Language Processing

Various instruments have been created that target the comprehension of a signed language by a D/HH child. Most of the tests are used only for research purposes (i.e., cannot be purchased or otherwise used by educators and language specialists at schools with D/HH children), with a few exceptions (e.g., Herman et al., 1999, 2004; Quinto-Pozos & Hou, 2010; Quinto-Pozos et al., 2010). Instruments that focus on single signs, sentences, and visual-spatial scenes will be described. These tests generally use language prompts followed by picture responses (typically three or four options).

The comprehension of sentences and grammatical structures of varying levels of complexity has been the focus of various instruments that have been developed over the past two decades. Herman,

Holmes, and Woll (1999) created the British Sign Language Receptive Skills Test (BSL-RST), which has been adapted for multiple signed languages (one example is the ASL-RST: Enns & Herman, 2011). Researchers in the United Kingdom have used the BSL-RST for several of their studies on D/HH children with DLD (e.g., Mason et al., 2010; Marshall et al., 2015). In these studies, the DLD children perform at least *1.3 standard deviations* below age-matched norms. Tests that have been developed for ASL grammatical knowledge, which are subtests of the ASLAI (Hoffmeister et al., 2015), have been used to examine grammatical correctness (Novogrodsky et al., 2017) and analogy reasoning (Henner et al., 2016). One report of child case-study data from the ASLAI can be found in a conference poster presentation, which addresses the longitudinal performance of two deaf children with DLD (Novogrodsky, Hoffmeister, et al., 2014). Finally, Quinto-Pozos and colleagues have created ASL comprehension tests that focus on perspective-taking skills (Quinto-Pozos & Hou, 2010; Quinto-Pozos et al., 2010). These tests have been used in case study work that examines D/HH native signers suspected of having a DLD (e.g., Quinto-Pozos et al., 2013).

Assessing Language Production

Some tests necessarily include the testing of both language processing/comprehension and language production, and they are included first in this section. Signs and nonsense signs have been the targeted by multiple researchers since the testing of such items generally taps into phonological awareness and phonological processing. In perhaps the first of its kind, Marshall, Denmark, and Morgan (2006) created a test with 48 BSL signs; the nonsense signs were phonologically possible signs in BSL, but not actual lexical items. For this instrument, the researchers manipulated phonological complexity by systematically varying handshape (marked and unmarked) and movement (hand-internal or path versus hand-internal and path). The authors tested 15 TD D/HH children aged 4–10 (both native and non-native signers) as a pilot study to examine whether such an instrument could be sensitive to phonological complexity. The results included a strong correlation of age and performance and an increase in errors as a function of phonological complexity. Mann et al. (2010) followed this work in the United Kingdom with another test focusing on phonological processing. This instrument consisted of 40 nonsense signs which varied in handshape and contained either two movements or, for single movements, a single path or hand-internal movement. This instrument was tested on children suspected of having a DLD, although such children did not perform as expected; most of the DLD children performed well. Marshall et al. (2011) suggest that this was possibly due to low task difficulty (resulting in low means and large standard deviations even for TD children) and/or due to greater phonological unpredictability of sign phonotactics compared to spoken language phonotactics, which, they argue, places a greater load on short-term memory for meaningless signs.

Semantic fluency has also been the target of assessment concerning D/HH children suspected of having a DLD. Marshall et al. (2013) devised a semantic fluency task for D/HH signers, following similar tests that have been used with hearing users of spoken language, that requires retrieval of words within semantic categories (e.g., animals, foods, etc.). A small group of children with DLD in BSL were tested, and they did not differ from the control group of TD signers of BSL on any measure related to the number of responses produced (whether correct or incorrect), types of responses, or to anything related to semantic clusters. As such, it remains to be seen whether a semantic fluency test of the type employed by Marshall and colleagues is useful for identifying children with DLD.

Sentence repetition has been used as a measure to assess D/HH children suspected of exhibiting features of DLD. In the United Kingdom, Marshall et al. (2015) showed that D/HH children ages 7;4–12;9 and grouped into the DLD category were significantly less accurate on an overall accuracy score, and they repeated various devices (lexical items, sign order, facial expressions, and verb morphological structures) significantly less accurately than TD children. The DLD children also had more problems with overall sentence meaning. Quinto-Pozos and colleagues used the ASL Sentence Reproduction Test (ASL-SRT; Hauser et al., 2008) in their case study work with deaf children suspected of having a developmental signed language disorder. In one case (Quinto-Pozos et al., 2013), the adolescent performed well, and it was later shown that she did not possess a deficit that affected her ASL skills in a general sense, but rather that her impairment was confined to visual-spatial processing and perspective taking. In another case (Quinto-Pozos et al., 2017), the authors showed that the ASL-SRT could reliably identify linguistic structures that the deaf adolescent struggled with, which they suggested was due to a deficit with sequential processing. In this latter case, the instrument that targets conversational language use (the ASL-PA, discussed in the section "Assessing Conversational Language Skills") was not precise enough to capture the adolescent's processing deficit since he had likely developed ways to circumvent that weakness during conversational language use (in particular, the comprehension of fingerspelling). Nonetheless, the combination of both instruments (along with others) provided a more complete picture of the adolescent's language skills. Quinto-Pozos and Cooley (2020) also used ASL-SRT data to examine phonological productions by a child with an expressive signed language disorder.

Finally, researchers have also used narrative production as part of their focus on D/HH children's signed language skills in order to understand the abilities of children suspected of having a DLD. Herman et al. (2014) analyzed D/HH children's narratives for global structure, information content, and local level grammatical devices, especially verb morphology. The DLD children ages 5;0–14;8 produced shorter, less structured, and grammatically simpler narratives than the TD children, and verb morphology was particularly problematic for the language impaired children. In the United States, Quinto-Pozos and colleagues used the narrative portion of the ASL-PA as a measure of the language abilities with their case study participants. In the case of the adolescent with a visual-spatial deficit (Quinto-Pozos et al., 2013), the ASL-PA correctly identified a linguistic structure that possessed difficulties. And, as expected, that adolescent performed well on other ASL structures that were coded.

ASSESSING NEUROPSYCHOLOGICAL AND COGNITIVE DEVELOPMENT

As with most studies of signing D/HH children suspected of having a developmental language disorder, the researcher generally wants to be able to rule out cases where the children might demonstrate atypicality in areas other than language. For some of the case study work performed in the United States (Quinto-Pozos et al., 2013, 2017), the researchers also administered a battery of cognitive and neuropsychological assessments, most of which are standardized measures, in order to understand various aspects of development. Hauser and colleagues (2015; Quinto-Pozos et al., 2014) describe the battery of measures as tests of general cognitive ability; processing of facial cues; vision and visual-spatial processing; hands, fingers, and psychomotor skills; executive functioning; visual working memory; and social-emotional functioning. See Hauser et al. (2015) and Quinto-Pozos et al. (2014) for names and references of the tests. Of course, these tests are in addition to assessments of receptive and expressive language skills. Studies performed in the United Kingdom with D/HH children suspected of exhibiting a DLD have also used standardized assessments to examine children's nonverbal abilities, including those testing memory and pattern recognition/construction (Mason et al., 2010).

ASSESSING MOTOR SKILLS

The testing of (manual) motor skills is important for signing D/HH children suspected of having a DLD because of the main articulators (i.e., the hands) used for language production. Apart from this, researchers have identified links between language skills and motor skills in DLD children (DiDonato Brumbach & Goffman, 2014).

In the proposed modifications to the SLI diagnostic criteria to be used with D/HH children, Quinto-Pozos, Singleton, and Hauser (2017) suggest that motor skills must be examined. For example, the authors suggest that no structural anomalies that impede language production should be present for face, arm, hand, and finger structure. In addition, they suggest that no impairments that impede language production should be present for gross and fine motor function. These recommendations are made for D/HH children who use signed language and in place of the criteria that focus on oral motor function from the original criteria for diagnosis of SLI (Leonard, 1998). Because of this, for D/HH children suspected of having a developmental signed language disorder, a researcher or clinician should not use utilize motor skills assessments such as the Clinical Assessment of Oropharyngeal Motor Development (St. Louis & Ruscello, 1987), as cited in DiDonato Brumbach and Goffman (2014) for hearing children with SLI, a type of DLD.

Motor skills have been tested on the D/HH children in studies from both sides of the Atlantic. Quinto-Pozos and colleagues employed gross and fine motor control assessments in their case studies, including tests of grip strength and fingertapping (Quinto-Pozos et al., 2013, 2017), and Mason and colleagues used a bead-threading task in their group study (Mason et al., 2010).

SKILLS REQUIRED OF RESEARCHERS AND OTHER TESTERS

There are a number of skills that professionals who assess D/HH children should likely possess, some of which align with the skills needed for testing hearing children. Among those skills are language ability and linguistic knowledge for assessment scoring (also see Chapters 1.2 and 11.1–11.3).

With regard to language skills, ensuring that the child understands the task is vital (Quadros & Cruz, 2011, among others). Ideally, a person who administers any test to D/HH signing children would be a fluent signer. In the absence of signed language fluency, a qualified interpreter would expected to be used, although this introduces its own challenges with regard to language testing (e.g., ensuring that the interpreter does not provide the D/HH child with the expected response based on their interpretation of the spoken language). When possible, fluent D/HH signers should administer tests with D/HH children, since they are often more aware of language and communication practices within the D/HH signing population, and they can provide their views on the nuances of a D/HH child's communication strategies—some of which may be overlooked by a nonfluent signer who is administering a test.

Some of the signed language assessment instruments require a sophisticated knowledge of linguistics in order to accurately score a child's responses (e.g., see Singleton & Supalla, 2011, for a discussion). In such cases, locating qualified people to score the tests is necessary. Related to this point is that some assessments require a significant amount of time for scoring, which needs to be taken into account.

FUTURE DIRECTIONS

In the past couple of decades there has been a welcome addition of multiple signed language assessments, and these additions, along with previously developed measures, have proved useful in examining suspected cases of signed language impairment among D/HH children. However, there is much work that remains in the area of signed language assessments, especially considering developmental signed language disorders. The areas of future work proposed here are the following: distinguishing language disorder from late or less-than-optimal exposure to a signed language (this includes understanding the variation that exists among non-native signers), considering literacy development by distinguishing language disorder from an impairment of reading (dyslexia), and, from a theoretical point of view, understanding modality influences on language development, which could provide a model for language structures that serve as targets for language testing across modalities.

One of the main concerns of many educators and researchers with respect to D/HH children relates to the age at which a D/HH child is regularly exposed to robust signed language models. The issue is that D/HH children born to hearing, non-signing parents are at risk of language delay, which can impact development more generally, because they are generally not exposed to rich models of visually accessible language. The picture is complicated by cochlear implant technology, which presents an option for parents that may or may not result in successful spoken language acquisition for a D/HH child. The main point is that some children are not regularly exposed to robust signed language models until late in development from a language acquisition point of view. This could be as late as the late teens (or early adulthood) for some D/HH people. These D/HH learners who are not exposed to a signed language early exhibit noticeable differences from those who are native or early signers (Mayberry, 1993; Novogrodsky et al., 2017; Supalla et al., 2014). However, what is not known is whether the acquisition patterns of late-exposed children mirror those of children with a language impairment. It may be that late exposure looks similar to early exposure, but with a later developmental period, whereas D/HH children with a language impairment might pattern differently. Interestingly, educators of the D/HH are not necessarily able to accurately predict who might do well on tests of syntax in this group of late signers, although they can generally do so for native signers (Novogrodsky et al., 2017; Quinto-Pozos et al., 2013, 2017). Work on distinguishing delayed exposure from language disorder is needed.

D/HH people who use signed language are bilingual by default since they are also readers (and possibly speakers) of the ambient spoken language of their country. Because of this, considering a D/HH child's second language (L2) development and how it relates to their signed language development is vital. It may be that a D/HH child's first language (L1) influences their L2 development, even though they are in different modalities and have different grammars and lexical items. One device that has been described as a bridge to literacy development for D/HH children is fingerspelling (Haptonstall-Nykaza & Shick, 2007; Humphries & MacDougall, 1999). If a child's ability to perceive, process, or produce fingerspelling is impaired, their literacy development might suffer (see Quinto-Pozos et al., 2017). However, signed language assessments considering literacy development are important for understanding the development of the whole bilingual child, especially in cases where a D/HH child may only read and write (and not speak) in their developing L2. This area of research should consider interactions between the two languages for the D/HH child and whether an impairment in one language would be reflected with comparable challenges or deficits in the other language.

Finally, continued work on signed languages allows researchers to understand how languages and acquisition are similar regardless of the modality of acquisition, while also realizing that there exist differences across modalities. Some robust methods for testing hearing children who acquire spoken language might not be as reliable for D/HH children acquiring a signed language (e.g., a semantic fluency task: Marshall et al., 2013; a nonsense sign repetition task: Mann et al., 2010). Likewise, there may be signed language structures that could present challenges for D/HH learners of a signed language but not hearing learners of a spoken language (e.g., visual perspective taking: Quinto-Pozos et al., 2013). Future work should continue to consider differences across modalities that could result in different ways of testing D/HH children.

NOTES

1. The term "deaf" will be used to refer to children and adolescents who use a signed language and who do not have the hearing ability to perceive speech without amplification or the use of a cochlear implant. This group includes those persons who are hard of hearing but still use a signed language for daily communication.
2. One notable exception is the ASLAI (Hoffmeister et al., 2015). Various subtests of the ASLAI have been normed on more than 500 deaf children,

including native and non-native signers. While there exist analyses of the lexical and semantic knowledge of deaf children on the ASLAI (Novogrodsky, Caldwell-Harris, et al., 2014; Novogrodsky, Fish, et al., 2014), there are no published studies from the ASLAI that report data from children with DLD, but see Novogrodsky, Hoffmeister, et al., 2014 for data reported in a conference poster.

REFERENCES

DiDonato Brumbach, A. C., & Goffman, L. (2014). Interaction of language processing and motor skill in children with specific language impairment. *Journal of Speech, Language, and Hearing Research*, *57*(1), 158–171. https://doi.org/10.1044/1092-4388(2013/12-0215)

Enns, C., Haug, T., Herman, R., Hoffmeister, R., Mann, W., & McQuarrie, L. (2016). Exploring signed language assessment tools in Europe and North America. In M. Marschark, V. Lampropoulou, & E. K. Skordilis (Eds.), *Diversity in deaf education* (pp. 171–218). Oxford University Press.

Enns, C. J., & Herman, R. C. (2011). Adapting the Assessing British Sign Language Development Receptive Skills test into American Sign Language. *Journal of Deaf Studies and Deaf Education*, *16*(3), 362–374. https://doi.org/10.1093/deafed/enr004

Haptonstall-Nykaza, T. S., & Schick, B. (2007). The transition from fingerspelling to English print: Facilitating English de- coding. *Journal of Deaf Studies and Deaf Education*, *12*(2), 172–183. https://doi.org/1093/deafed/enm003

Haug, T. (2005). Review of sign language assessment instruments. *Sign Language & Linguistics*, *8*(1/2), 61–98. https://doi.org/10.1075/sll.8.1.04hau

Hauser, P. C., Paludneviciene, R., Supalla, T., & Bavelier, D. (2008). American Sign Language-Sentence Reproduction Test: Development and implications. In R. M. de Quadros (Ed.), *Sign language: Spinning and unraveling the past, present and future* (pp. 160–172). Editora Arara Azul.

Hauser, P. C., Quinto-Pozos, D., & Singleton, J. L. (2015). Studying sign language disorders: Considering neuropsychological data. In E. Orfanidou, B. Woll, & G. Morgan (Eds.), *Research methods in sign language studies: A practical guide* (pp. 336–351). Wiley-Blackwell.

Henner, J., Caldwell-Harris, C. L., Novogrodsky, R., & Hoffmeister, R. J. (2016). American Sign Language syntax and analogical reasoning skills are influenced by early acquisition and age of entry to signing schools for the deaf. *Frontiers in Psychology*, *7*, 1–14. https://doi.org/10.3389/FPSYG.2016.01982

Henner, J., Hoffmeister, R., & Reis, J. (2017). Developing sign language assessments for the deaf and hard-of-hearing. In S. Cawthon & C. Lou Garberoglio (Eds.), *Research methodology in deaf education* (pp. 141–160). Oxford University Press.

Herman, R., Grove, N., Holmes, S., Morgan, G., Sutherland, H., & Woll, B. (2004). *Assessing BSL Development: Production test (narrative skills)*. City University Publication.

Herman, R., Holmes, S., & Woll, B (1999). *Assessing British Sign Language development: Receptive Skills Test*. Forest Bookshop.

Herman, R., Rowley, K., Mason, K., & Morgan, G. (2014). Deficits in narrative abilities in child BSL signers with specific language impairment. *International Journal of Language and Communication Disorders*, *49*(3), 343–353. https://doi.org/10.1111/1460-6984.12078

Hoffmeister, R., Fish, S., Benedict, R., Henner, J., Novogrodsky, R., & Rosenburg, P. (2015). *American Sign Language Assessment Instrument (ASLAI): Revision 4*. Boston University Center for the Study of Communication and the Deaf.

Humphries, T., & MacDougall, F. (1999). "Chaining" and other links: Making connections between American Sign Language and English in two types of school settings. *Visual Anthropology Review*, *15*(2), 84–94. https://doi.org/10.1525/var.2000.15$1$2

Leonard, L. (1998). *Children with specific language impairment*. MIT Press.

Maller, S. J., Singleton, J. L., Supalla, S. J., & Wix, T. (1999). The development and psychometric properties of the American Sign Language Proficiency Assessment (ASL-PA). *Journal of Deaf Studies and Deaf Education*, *4*(4), 249–269. https://doi.org/10.1093/deafed/4.$1$2

Mann, W., & Haug, T. (2014). Mapping out guidelines for the development and use of sign language assessments: Some critical issues, comments and suggestions. In D. Quinto-Pozos (Ed.), *Multilingual aspects of signed language communication and disorder* (pp. 123–142). Multilingual Matters.

Mann, W., Marshall, C. R., Mason, K., Morgan, G. (2010). The acquisition of sign language: The impact of phonetic complexity on phonology. *Language Learning and Development*, *6*(1), 60–86. https://doi.org/10.1080/15475440903245951

Marshall, C. R., Denmark, T., & Morgan, G. (2006). Investigating the underlying causes of SLI: A non-sign repetition test in British Sign Language. *Advances in Speech-Language Pathology*, *8*(4), 347–355. https://doi.org/10.1080/14417040600970630

Marshall, C. R., Mann, W., & Morgan, G. (2011). Short term memory in signed languages: Not just a disadvantage for serial recall. *Frontiers in Psychology*, *2*, 1–2. https://doi.org/10.3389/fpsyg.2011.00102

Marshall, C. R., Mason, K., Rowley, K., Herman, R., Atkinson, J., Woll, B., & Morgan, G. (2015). Sentence repetition in deaf children with specific language impairment in British Sign Language. *Language Learning and Development*, *11*(3), 237–251. https://doi.org/10.1080/15475441.2014.917557

Mason, K., Rowley, K., Marshall, C. R., Atkinson, J. R., Herman, R., Woll, B., & Morgan, G. (2010). Identifying specific language impairment in deaf children acquiring British Sign Language: Implications for theory and practice. *British Journal of Developmental Psychology*, *28*(1), 33–49. https://doi.org/10.1348/026151009X484190

Marshall, C. R., Rowley, K., Mason, K., Herman, R., & Morgan, G. (2013). Lexical organization in deaf children who use British Sign Language: Evidence from a semantic fluency task. *Journal of Child Language*, *40*(1), 193–220. https://doi.org/10.1017/S0305000912000116

Mayberry, R. I. (1993). First language acquisition after childhood differs from second language acquisition: The case of American Sign Language. *Journal of Speech, Language, and Hearing Research*, *36*(6), 1258–1270. https://doi.org/10.1044/jshr.3606.1258

Mayberry, R. I., & Fischer, S. D. (1989). Looking through phonological shape to lexical meaning: The bottleneck of nonnative sign language processing. *Memory and Cognition, 17*(6), 740–754. https://doi.org/10.3758/BF03202635

Mitchell, R., & Karchmer, M. (2004). Chasing the mythical ten percent: Parental hearing status of deaf and hard of hearing students in the United States. *Sign Language Studies, 4*(2), 138–163. https://doi.org/10.1353/sls.2004.0005

Morgan, G., Herman, R., & Woll, B. (2007). Language impairments in sign language: Breakthroughs and puzzles. *International Journal of Language and Communication Disorders, 42*(1), 97–105. https://doi.org/10.1080/13682820600783178

Novogrodsky, R., Caldwell-Harris, C., Fish, S., & Hoffmeister, R. (2014). The development of antonym knowledge in American Sign Language (ASL) and its relationship to reading comprehension in English. *Language Learning, 64*(4), 749–770. https://doi.org/10.1111/lang.12078

Novogrodsky, R., Fish, S., & Hoffmeister, R. (2014). The development of synonyms in American Sign Language (ASL): Toward a further understanding of the components of ASL vocabulary knowledge. *Sign Language Studies, 14*(2), 225–249. https://doi.org/10.1353/sls.2014.0003

Novogrodsky, R., Henner, J., Caldwell-Harris, C., & Hoffmeister, R. (2017). The development of sensitivity to grammatical violations in American Sign Language: Native signers versus nonnative. *Language Learning, 67*(4), 791–818. https://doi.org/10.1111/lang.12245

Novogrodsky, R., Hoffmeister, R., Fish, S., Benedict, R., Henner, J., Rosenburg, P. Conlin-Luippold, F., & Caldwell Harris, C. (2014). Two case studies of SLI in American Sign Language (ASL). A poster presented at a workshop of Specific Language Impairment, Experimental Psycholinguistics Conference (ERP), Madrid, Spain.

Quadros, R. M., & Cruz, C. R. (2011). *Língua de Sinais. Instrumentos de Avaliação.* Artmed Editora S. A.

Quinto-Pozos, D., & Cooley, F. (2020). A developmental disorder of signed language production in a native deaf signer of ASL. *Languages, 5*(40), 1–18.

Quinto-Pozos, D., Forber-Pratt, A., & Singleton, J. (2011). Do developmental communication disorders exist in the signed modality? Perspectives from professionals. *Language, Speech, and Hearing Services in Schools, 42*(4), 423–443. https://doi.org/10.1044/0161-1461(2011/10-0071)

Quinto-Pozos, D., & Hou, L. (2010). *American Sign Language Perspective Taking Spatial Orientation Test (ASL-PTSO).* Unpublished assessment, University of Texas at Austin.

Quinto-Pozos, D., Hou, L., & Garberoglio, C. L. (2010). *American Sign Language Perspective Taking Comprehension Test (ASL-PTCT).* Unpublished assessment, University of Texas at Austin.

Quinto-Pozos, D., Singleton, J., & Hauser, P. (2017). A case of Specific Language Impairment in a native deaf signer of American Sign Language. *Journal of Deaf Studies and Deaf Education, 22*(2), 204–218. https://doi.org/10.1093/deafed/enw074

Quinto-Pozos, D., Singleton, J., Hauser, P., & Levine, S. (2014). A case-study approach to investigating developmental signed language disorders. In D. Quinto-Pozos (Ed.), *Multilingual aspects of signed language communication and disorder* (pp. 70–89). Multilingual Matters.

Quinto-Pozos, D., Singleton, J., Hauser, P., Levine, S., Garberoglio, C. L., & Hou, L. (2013). Atypical signed language development: A case study of challenges with visual-spatial processing. *Cognitive Neuropsychology, 30*(5), 332–359. https://doi.org/10.1080/02643294.2013.863756

Singleton, J. L., & Supalla, S. (2011). Assessing children's proficiency of natural signed languages. In M. Marschark & P. Spencer (Eds.), *Oxford handbook of deaf studies, language, and education* (2nd ed., pp. 306–321). Oxford University Press.

Supalla, T., Hauser, P. C., & Bavelier, D. (2014). Reproducing American Sign language sentences: Cognitive scaffolding in working memory. *Frontiers in Psychology, 5*, 1–16. https://doi.org/10.3389/fpsyg.2014.00859

Supalla, T., Newport, E., Singleton, J., Supalla, S., Coulter, G., & Metlay, D. (unpublished). *The test battery for American Sign Language morphology and syntax.*

St. Louis, K. O., & Ruscello, D. M. (1987). *Oral speech mechanism screening examination revised*. Pro-Ed.

5.3

Discussion of Issues Related to Assessing Signed or Spoken Language in Children with Developmental Language Disorder

Carol-Anne Murphy, Pauline Frizelle, Cristina McKean, and David Quinto-Pozos

ASPECTS OF SIGNED LANGUAGE ASSESSMENT THAT COULD BE APPLIED TO SPOKEN LANGUAGE ASSESSMENT

Points made by Quinto-Pozos regarding assessment of the deaf and hard-of-hearing (D/HH) child with developmental language disorder (DLD) have implications for the assessment of the child with DLD who is not D/HH. Of note are the suggestions regarding literacy, the potential for semantic fluency assessment to contribute to identification of DLD, the use of standardized protocols to support assessment at the conversational level, and the necessary skills of those completing assessments.

Literacy

The particular challenge of literacy development for the D/HH child with DLD, who is both "bilingual by default" and linguistically impaired, was especially striking. In the field of DLD in the hearing population, literacy assessment research has tended to focus on decoding skills, phonological awareness, and reading comprehension, and several standardized assessments are available to probe these abilities (e.g., the Preschool and Primary Inventory of Phonological Awareness [PIPA], Dodd et al., 2000; York Assessment of Reading Comprehension [YARC], Hulme et al., 2009). These assessment practices are underpinned by the simple view of reading, which sees reading comprehension as a product of oral language comprehension abilities and decoding, and clearly inform both intervention planning and differential diagnosis (Nation,

Carol-Anne Murphy, Pauline Frizelle, Cristina McKean, and David Quinto-Pozos, *Discussion of Issues Related to Assessing Signed or Spoken Language in Children with Developmental Language Disorder* In: *The Handbook of Language Assessment Across Modalities.* Edited by: Tobias Haug, Wolfgang Mann, and Ute Knoch, Oxford University Press. © Oxford University Press 2022. DOI: 10.1093/oso/9780190885052.003.0016

2019). Tools to assess written language and spelling for hearing children with DLD are noticeably absent and reflect a paucity of both theoretical and intervention research in this area (cf. Joye et al., 2019).

Semantic Fluency

Consistent with the suggestion for D/HH children with DLD by Quinto-Pozos, the potential for semantic fluency assessment to support identification in DLD is unknown. While captured in some phonological awareness batteries (e.g., the Phonological Assessment Battery by Frederickson et al., 1997) used in assessments of dyslexia and considered an outcome measure in assessment and intervention for word-finding difficulties (e.g., Best, 2005; Ebbels et al., 2011), semantic fluency is not routinely measured among children with DLD. Rapid automatic naming is included as a supplementary subtest in some test batteries. Semantic fluency is not included among the clinical markers for DLD, where typically verb tense marking, non-word repetition skills, and sentence repetition are considered and for which tests have been identified (e.g., Early Repetition Battery; Seeff-Gabriel et al., 2008; Grammar and Phonology Screening Test, Van Der Lely et al., 2007). This is despite the fact that children with DLD are commonly found to have difficulties with vocabulary acquisition (McGregor et al., 2013) and sparse or poorly developed semantic networks.

Standardized Protocols for Functional Communication Assessment

The use of standardized protocols for the assessment of different language domains within functional conversation in D/HH children as described by Quinto-Pozos (Chapter 5.2) would also fulfil an important role in the assessment of children with DLD, but few such tools exist. The focus on communicative functioning in the new DLD criteria bring a welcome impetus for development in this area. Specific protocols that have been developed aim to assess conversation skills, identify pragmatic deficits, and differentiate between children with social pragmatic communication disorder and those with autistic spectrum disorder. The Manchester Inventory for Playground Observation (MIPO; Gibson et al., 2011) measures children's competence in peer social interaction in the school playground. Similarly, the Targeted Observation of Pragmatics in Children's Conversation (TOPICC; Adams et al., 2011) requests the child to complete semi-structured tasks that allows the clinician to derive an overall rating of the quality of interaction in conversation. While narrative assessments provide a breakdown of macro- versus microstructural components, there are no protocols that support clinicians to capture these elements in conversation. Standardized protocols for these areas would fulfil an important purpose.

The Skills of the Assessor

The preceding approaches point out the vital consideration of the skills necessary to assess children with DLD (see Chapters 11.1–11.3). In the area of child language disorder, research has tended to focus on assessor decision-making rather than on skills. For example, in work examining clinicians' test selection, clinicians were found not to examine test psychometric properties when choosing standardized assessments (Betz et al., 2013) and to lack clarity regarding the purpose of the tool (Merrell & Plante, 1997), with specific challenges regarding the assessment of children with identified DLD (Lyons et al., 2008).

Future Developments

As is the case with hearing individuals with DLD, a number of promising technological developments could be applied to the assessment of children who are D/HH with language disorder and that could help reduce variation between assessors and improve reliability (also see Chapters 12.1–12.3). The use of computer-based animations to assess sentence comprehension could be applied universally with both hearing and signing populations. Through machine learning, progress is being made in the development of hand signing readers that translate sign to speech and which would allow for automated language transcription and analysis. Video technology makes it possible for signers to see each other (particularly significant for a visual language) and to be assessed with more than one interlocuter present, albeit in cyberspace; the assessment of signed discourse and interactions can therefore take place remotely and account for varying cultural norms and contexts.

The Voice of the Child

With a growing recognition of the lifelong nature of DLD and its implications for social and societal inclusion, the focus on delivering interventions that bring "functional gains" which are clinically meaningful to the individual and which could potentially prevent the most adverse long-term consequences has increased. For the D/HH child with DLD there is the risk of exclusion potentially from both the hearing and signing communities and, with that, a compounding risk of social isolation. We are at the start of a journey in developing methods to integrate the voice of the hearing child with DLD into the assessment process and would encourage a parallel development to be considered for D/HH children with DLD.

ASPECTS OF SPOKEN LANGUAGE ASSESSMENT THAT COULD BE APPLIED TO SIGNED LANGUAGE ASSESSMENT

The writings by colleagues who report on hearing children with DLD (see Chapter 5.1) provide insight into ways in which assessment of

D/HH children could benefit from developments in the larger field. Among the points highlighted here are recent suggestions concerning diagnosis criteria and terminology for children with language problems; consideration of the presence of co-occurring conditions during the process of assessment, diagnosis, and intervention; and methods of assessment that take into account dynamic processes of learning. Each of these is expanded on below.

Language Assessment Criteria and Terminology

One exciting area of development in spoken language is the number of large-scale discussions focused on long-standing issues in the field concerning language assessment criteria and the terminology used for children with language problems (see Chapter 5.1). Of particular importance for work with D/HH children is that the suggested criteria depart from long-standing approaches of using exclusionary criteria for diagnosis of a language disorder. For example, the recent Criteria and Terminology Applied to Language Impairments: Synthesizing the Evidence (CATALISE) recommendations for inclusion of children (Bishop et al., 2016) regardless of level of nonverbal ability, which was previously a common exclusionary criterion, are a welcome change for those working with D/HH children.

Murphy and colleagues (Chapter 5.1) also highlight the fact that the revised criteria for diagnosis take into account the presence of co-occurring conditions that may not be exclusive to language. These conditions, they suggest, could also be fluid in nature, which means that a single assessment might not be equipped to capture the complexity of a particular child's dynamic profile. Rather, comprehensive assessment is needed to understand how a child's abilities vary over time across receptive and productive modalities. This novel approach for considering children's language problems is well-suited for the population of D/HH children, which could be described as notably heterogenous in nature. The vast majority of D/HH children are not exposed to a signed language at birth, and such delayed exposure could influence their language development tremendously. Furthermore, rates of diagnosis with a co-occurring condition (e.g., attention deficit disorder or attention deficit hyperactivity disorder) are significant among this population (Guardino, 2008; Mitchell & Karchmer, 2006). As such, recommendations from CATALISE will allow clinicians and researchers to work with a broader segment of the population in the process of diagnosis and intervention.

Consideration of Co-Occurring Conditions

Unfortunately, D/HH children have traditionally been excluded from being considered for a diagnosis of a DLD (e.g., such as specific language impairment; Leonard, 1998) because of their lack of typical hearing. As part of our work with single case studies of D/HH children from signing households, my colleagues and I have suggested ways to address such exclusionary criteria (Quinto-Pozos et al., 2017). Our argument has been that a deaf child with early exposure to a signed language could exhibit a developmental signed language disorder just as a hearing child with early exposure to a spoken language. This sentiment is echoed by the authors of the revised CATALISE criteria, who note that "Most children with hearing impairment demonstrate normal language skills in the visual modality if exposed to a sign language early in life. Nonetheless, it is possible to have an impairment in acquiring sign language, just as in spoken language" (Bishop et al., 2016, p. 16). They also indicate that "some children have language abilities—in spoken and/or signed language—that are well below those of their hearing-impaired peer group, and may be regarded as having a disproportionate language impairment that is not secondary to hearing loss" (p. 16). These acknowledgments are important for those who work with D/HH children suspected of having language problems.

Dynamic Assessment

Murphy and colleagues also referred in Chapter 5.1 to dynamic assessment (DA) as a way to examine a child's linguistic abilities and their abilities to exhibit their potential for learning. Such techniques for assessment have been used in an empirical study with D/HH children (Mann et al., 2014, also see Chapter 3.2), but it is unclear to what extent they have been adopted by clinicians who work with D/HH children. Due in part to the lack of normed assessment tools for assessing D/HH childhood signers, DA could be leveraged as a valuable tool for working with children who have been identified as having language problems.

Future directions could include leveraging technology for language assessment, as suggested by the authors of the chapter on spoken language assessment. While signed language assessment has long benefited from computer technology for test administration (e.g., to deliver video-based prompts for child responses), advancements in online administration could make sign-based assessments accessible to a larger population of clinicians and researchers. Various online portals have been created in recent years for accessing signed language assessments, such as the following (just to name a few):

1. American Sign Language: https://vl2.gallaudet.edu/labs/early-education-literacy-lab/vl2-assessment-portal/
2. British Sign Language: https://www.ucl.ac.uk/dcal/assessment/dcal-assessment-portal
3. Sign Language of the Netherlands: http://www.signlang-assessment.info/index.php/home-en.html

Final Remarks

Considering both spoken and signed language assessment within a single chapter allows unique aspects of each field to be highlighted while also pointing out similarities between the approaches. There is much to be learned from understanding the perspectives of colleagues in a related area, and we hope that our content can benefit researchers and clinicians who work with children with various linguistic needs.

REFERENCES

Adams, C., Gaile, J., Lockton, E., & Freed, J. (2011). Targeted observation of pragmatics in children's conversations (TOPICC): Adapting a research tool into a clinical assessment profile. *Speech and Language Therapy in Practice*, Spring, 7–10.

Best, W. (2005). Investigation of a new intervention for children with word-finding problems. *International Journal of Language and Communication Disorders*, *40*(3), 279–318. https://doi.org/10.1080/13682820410001734154

Betz, S., Eickhoff, J., & Sullivan, S. (2013). Factors influencing the selection of standardized tests for the diagnosis of Specific Language Impairment. *Language, Speech, and Hearing Services in Schools*, *44*(2), 133–146. https://doi.org/10.1044/0161-1461(2012/12-0093)

Bishop, D., Snowling, M., Thompson, P., & Greenhalgh, T. (2016). CATALISE: A multinational and multidisciplinary Delphi consensus study. Identifying Language Impairments in children. *Plos One*, *11*(7), e0158753. https://doi.org/10.1371/journal.pone.0158753

Dodd, B., Crosbie, S., McIntosh, B., Teitzel, T., & Ozanne, A. (2000). *Preschool and primary inventory of phonological awareness (PIPA)*. Pearson Clinical.

Ebbels, S. H., Nicoll, H., Clark, B., Eachus, B., Gallagher, A. L., Horniman, K., Jennings, M., McEvoy, K., Nimmo, L., & Turner, G. (2012). Effectiveness of semantic therapy for word-finding difficulties in pupils with persistent language impairments: a randomized control trial. *International Journal of Language & Communication Disorders*, *47*, 35–51. https://doi.org/10.1111/j.1460-6984.2011.00073.x

Frederickson, N., Frith, U., & Reason, R. (1997). *Phonological Assessment Battery (manual and test materials)*. NFER-Nelson.

Gibson, J., Hussain, J., Holsgrove, S., Adams, C., & Green, J. (2011). Quantifying peer interactions for research and clinical use: The Manchester Inventory for Playground Observation. *Research in Developmental Disabilities*, *32*(6), 2458–2466. https://doi.org/10.1016/j.ridd.2011.07.014

Guardino, C. A. (2008). Identification and placement for students with multiple disabilities: Choosing the path less followed. *American Annals of the Deaf*, *153*, 55–64. https://doi.org/10.1353/aad.0.0004

Hulme, C., Stothard, S. E., Clarke, P., Bowyer-Crane, C., Harrington, A., Truelove, E., & Snowling, M. J. (2009). *York Assessment of Reading for Comprehension (YARC): Early Reading*. GL Assessment.

Joye, N., Broc, L., Olive, T., & Dockrell, J. (2019). Spelling performance in children with developmental language disorder: A meta-analysis across

European languages. *Scientific Studies of Reading, 23*(2), 129–160. https://doi.org/10.1080/10888438.2018.1491584
Leonard, L. (1998). *Children with specific language impairment*. MIT Press.
Lyons, R., Byrne, M., Corry, T., Lalor, L., Ruane, H., Shanahan, R., & McGinty, C. (2008). An examination of how speech and language therapists assess and diagnose children with specific language impairment in Ireland. *International Journal of Speech-Language Pathology, 10*(6), 425–437. https://doi.org/10.1080/17549500802422569
Mann, W., Peña, E., & Morgan, G. (2014). Exploring the use of dynamic assessment with deaf children, who use American Sign Language: Two case studies. *Journal of Communication Disorders, 52*, 16–30. https://doi.org/10.1016/j.jcomdis.2014.05.002
McGregor, K., Oleson, J., Bahnsen, A., & Duff, D. (2013). Children with developmental language impairment have vocabulary deficits characterized by limited breadth and depth. *International Journal of Language and Communication Disorders, 48*(3), 307–319. https://doi.org/10.1111/1460-6984.12008
Merrell, A., & Plante, E. (1997). Norm-referenced test interpretation in the diagnostic process. *Language, Speech, and Hearing Services in Schools, 28*(1), 50–58. https://doi.org/10.1044/0161-1461.2801.50
Mitchell, R., & Karchmer, M. (2006). Demographics in deaf education: More students in more places. *American Annals of the Deaf, 152*, 95–103. https://doi.org/10.1353/aad.2006.0029
Nation, K. (2019). Children's reading difficulties, language, and reflections on the simple view of reading. *Australian Journal of Learning Difficulties, 24*(1), 47–73. https://doi.org/10.1080/19404158.2019.1609272
Quinto-Pozos, D., Singleton, J., & Hauser, P. (2017). A case of Specific Language Impairment in a native deaf signer of American Sign Language. *Journal of Deaf Studies and Deaf Education, 22*, 204–218. https://doi.org/10.1093/deafed/enw074
Seeff-Gabriel, B. K., Chiat, S., & Roy, P. (2008). *The early repetition battery*. Pearson.
Van der Lely, H., Gardner, H., McClelland, A. G. R., & Froud, K. E. (2007). *Grammar and Phonology Screening Test (GAPS)*. DLDCN.com.

Topic 6

Issues Related to Assessing the Oral Language Skills of Hearing Bi/Multilingual Children

6.1

Assessing the Oral Language Skills of Bi-/Multilinguals

Lisa M. Bedore, Elizabeth D. Peña, Kathleen Durant, and Stephanie McMillen

BEST PRACTICES IN DEVELOPING ASSESSMENTS FOR BILINGUAL/MULTILINGUAL CHILDREN

When children are acquiring language in bilingual/multilingual contexts their knowledge of semantics and morphosyntax in each language tends to be more variable than that of their monolingual peers. As a result, bilingual and multilingual children are more likely than their monolingual peers to be under- or overdiagnosed as having language and/or learning difficulties. Underdiagnosis occurs when educators wait to assess language learning concerns in order to provide children with extended time to learn the language of schooling. Overdiagnosis, or diagnoses that are relatively more severe than expected based on population norms, happens when testers treat all differences in communicative behaviors as if they reflected language disorder. Best practices for educators and researchers include understanding the impacts of bilingual (or divided) language experience on language development and developing procedures that can be used to accurately differentiate children with and without developmental language disorders (DLD). Here we focus on how understanding the variability in language knowledge that results from divided input can be applied to known best practices in order to differentiate children with and without DLD (for assessment of children with DLD in spoken or signed languages, see Chapters 5.1–5.3).

For educators to develop and apply an understanding of the variability inherent in bilingual/multilingual language learning, documenting language experiences that support learning and identifying the differences in language knowledge that are robust markers of DLD are essential. Questionnaires can be used to guide our judgments about how much a child might be expected to know in each of their languages. In turn, this information guides decisions about the assessment plan in each

Lisa M. Bedore, Elizabeth D. Peña, Kathleen Durant, and Stephanie McMillen, *Assessing the Oral Language Skills of Bi-/Multilinguals* In: *The Handbook of Language Assessment Across Modalities*. Edited by: Tobias Haug, Wolfgang Mann, and Ute Knoch, Oxford University Press. © Oxford University Press 2022. DOI: 10.1093/oso/9780190885052.003.0017 language that is needed to make clinical decisions about children's ability to learn and their educational or intervention plan if needed.

LANGUAGE EXPERIENCE QUESTIONNAIRES

The amount of experience children have with each of their languages is systematically related to their level of proficiency in each. For example, current input and output account for about 60% of the variance in semantics and morphosyntax knowledge in kindergarten (Bedore et al., 2012). The role of continued experience becomes increasingly apparent in the early school years. Within a US Spanish-English (SE) speaking population, English performance increases in a linear fashion but Spanish increases only when children continue hearing and using Spanish (Bedore et al., 2016). The findings of researchers working with children from other language backgrounds (e.g., Arabic, Turkish, French, Cantonese) validate the predictive value of language experience across bilingual populations (Chondrogianni & Marinis, 2011; Paradis & Jia, 2017). As such, documenting language experience is a good first step in planning language of testing for clinical purposes. For example, Peña and colleagues have shown that children need to use each language about 30% of the time if they are to have sufficient depth of knowledge to respond (Peña et al., 2018). However, accurate decisions about children's language skills can be made with children who use a language as little as 20% of the time (Gillam et al., 2013).

Questions about how to most effectively obtain information about language experience focus on the utility of parent and teacher judgments versus queries that elicit descriptions. For example, parents' ratings of children's vocabulary knowledge correspond with test performance in the semantics domain on the Bilingual English Spanish Assessment (BESA; Peña et al., 2018), while teacher's ratings correspond best to performance in the area of language form (Bedore et al., 2011; Gutiérrez–Clellen & Kreiter, 2003). Work with monolingual English-speaking children has shown that parents can accurately describe their children's current behaviors but that it is more difficult to obtain reliable accounts of past behavior (Massa et al., 2008). Several questionnaires have built successfully on these principles. The BESA includes a questionnaire about language use (Bilingual Input Output Survey [BIOS]) and another about language ability (Inventory to Assess Language Knowledge [ITALK]). These target very specific questions around input and output that tie into children's daily schedules or focus on specific examples of language domains that parents or teachers are expected to rate. Another example is the Alberta Language Development Questionnaire (Paradis et al., 2010). This questionnaire uses a language broker to ask parents specific questions about development and home language use patterns that are the basis of behavioral ratings. In all of these cases, responses are scored and the summary scores are the source of information about dominance and concern. Evidence of the reliability of such approaches is strongly based on their internal validity and their classification accuracy. Furthermore, the interpretation of the questionnaire is based on an external delimitation of concern rather than responses to individual questions that might be interpreted differently by parents of different cultural and linguistic groups and thus more difficult to interpret at the individual level.

Another important point is that these questionnaires use scripted oral interviews. These are advantageous when parents do not read in the languages of community or when they may benefit from opportunities to clarify interview questions. Furthermore, under such circumstances, a written questionnaire may not be returned at high rates. This procedure may seem time-intensive, but the questionnaires center on the most discriminating questions. The needed information may be obtained in 15 minutes or less, so many parents are willing to complete them when interviewed by phone or in person (Peña et al., 2018).

DEVELOPING ASSESSMENTS

In addition to language of testing, we need to select language structures for testing that reliably differentiate children with and without language impairment. Children with DLD have extreme difficulties in morphosyntax (Leonard, 2014). For monolingual children, clinicians rely on developmental milestones and standardized tests focused on clinical markers to make diagnostic decisions. Because bilinguals are much more variable in their English (second language; L2) performance due to differences in age of English acquisition and experience with the two languages, the current best practice is to test children in both languages. Another aspect of best practice is to identify those forms or clinical markers that best differentiate children with DLD. Here we provide examples from the development of the BESA as an example of assessment conducted in Spanish and English around clinical markers.

BESA Semantics as an Example of Best Practice

Children with DLD demonstrate deficits in vocabulary learning, establishing lexical connections, and expressing vocabulary breadth and depth (Brackenbury & Pye, 2005 also see Chapters 5.1–5.3). For bilingual children, variable language exposure results in divided lexical-semantic knowledge across multiple lexicons; this poses a challenge for assessing whether bilingual children have a disorder or a difference. In developing assessments, finding semantic forms that accurately classify children with and without impairment is an important contributor to good classification.

Breadth and Depth of Semantic Knowledge

Bilinguals—regardless of language ability—tend to have lower vocabulary scores in each language compared with their monolingual peers (e.g., Bialystok et al., 2010; Pearson et al., 1993, 1997) secondary to their distributed lexical knowledge (Oller et al., 2007). For example, a bilingual child may know the word "sticker" in English and "pelota" (ball) in Spanish but lack the translation equivalents for these words due to context-specific vocabulary exposure (i.e., school and home). Although children with DLD tend to have delayed word-learning and reduced vocabulary size in comparison to their typically developing (TD) peers (Gray, 2004; Rice, Buhr, & Nemeth, 1990), scores on single-word vocabulary tests do not tend to differentiate monolingual or bilingual children (Anaya et al., 2018; Gray et al., 1999; McGregor, 2009; Peña et al., 2006). More challenging tasks are needed to differentiate. For example, children with DLD often lack the semantic depth necessary for language comprehension and use (Gray, 2004; Hick et al., 2002). As such, assessing depth of semantic knowledge, or the connectivity between semantic information that drives efficient lexical access and retrieval, supports accurate diagnosis of DLD.

The BESA taps into lexical-semantic knowledge using concepts and word associations based on research demonstrating patterns of differences in lexical organization and retrieval across bilingual children with and without DLD. For example, bilingual children with DLD exhibit difficulty producing responses, especially for categorically related items (e.g., fruit: strawberry, forest: trees) in comparison to their TD peers during a word association task (Sheng et al., 2012). This work illustrates how children with DLD have sparse semantic networks resulting in poorer lexical organization and processing. The six tasks comprising the BESA semantics subtest on the BESA include analogies, associations, descriptions, functions, linguistic concepts, and similarities and differences.

Peña et al. (2015) examined the classification accuracy of the BESA semantics test. This measure effectively differentiated functionally monolingual groups of Spanish- or English-speaking children with 81% classification accuracy, while the balanced bilinguals had 76% and 90% classification accuracy, respectively, for the English and Spanish subtests. The difference between these discriminant scores may be due to children's sociolinguistic experiences across cultural contexts (Peña et al., 2015). A study by Peña, Bedore, and Zlatic-Guinta (2002) showed that during a category generation task, bilingual children often produced items unique to each language. For example, when children were asked to name birthday foods, "cake" was commonly generated in both Spanish and English; however, it was also common for children to produce words such as "arroz" (rice) and "frijoles" (beans) in

Spanish and "hamburger" and "hot dog" in English (Peña et al., 2002). This example reflects children's language-specific knowledge across cultural contexts.

Cultural Sensitivity in Assessment Practices

Bilingual children's performance on semantic measures is directly related to their second language (L2) exposure (Bedore et al., 2016; Bohman et al., 2010; Hoff et al., 2012). As language is bound to cultural contexts, the semantic knowledge learned in those environments directly influences how familiar children will be with a variety of tasks. For example, Peña and Quinn (1997) found that tasks that were more familiar to preschool children who were Puerto Rican or dialect speakers of African American English (e.g., description tasks: describing functions, answering simple and complex wh- questions) were better when used to classify children who were TD to those with poorer language skills than were unfamiliar tasks (e.g., labeling tasks: expressive vocabulary). Thus, best practice for assessing children with linguistically diverse backgrounds must also include culturally sensitive measures because task familiarity is influenced by children's cultural experiences.

For instance, the BESA semantics subtest includes concepts and word associations that are familiar to bilingual children across sociolinguistic contexts. As children have a wide range of individual experiences across various linguistic contexts, they are able to respond to test stimuli in different ways and still receive credit for their knowledge. For example, if the child was asked to describe the difference between two squares of the same size, the child would receive credit for stating "colors" or specifying the color of each square (e.g., "green and blue"). These responses represent the child's ability to accurately identify and express differences between to similar items, while the test question maintains consideration for the child's cultural and linguistic knowledge.

Morphosyntactic Assessment for Spanish-English Bilingual Children

Morphosyntactic deficits are indicative of DLD cross-linguistically. For SE bilinguals the BESA reliably assesses morphosyntactic ability by targeting language-specific grammatical constructions that discriminate between bilingual children with TD and DLD. The impact of language experience and cross-linguistic patterns of morphosyntactic development will be explored in more depth next.

LANGUAGE EXPERIENCE AND MORPHOSYNTACTIC ASSESSMENT

Assessing morphosyntactic performance in only one language is likely to give a biased profile of a bilingual's morphosyntactic ability. Depth of L1 knowledge may be influenced by divided L1 and L2 input, limiting access to complex structures in both languages. Forms that are present in Spanish but not English may be acquired at a slower rate, with partial knowledge, resulting in limited use. For example, desires and possibilities are produced with the subjunctive mood in Spanish (e.g., *La mamá quiere que laven los dientes después de la comida* [The mother wants the children to brush (subjunctive) their teeth after dinner]). Monolingual Spanish-speaking children master the subjunctive by 4–7 years of age, a time period associated with starting school and subsequent L2 immersion in the United States. As a result, sequential SE bilingual children in the United States may have delayed acquisition of the subjunctive or, in the case of some heritage speakers, may not acquire it at all (Baron et al., 2018). SE bilinguals' L2 morphosyntactic production may reflect L1 interference. For example, a continued or repeated action in the past is expressed through obligatory imperfect tense marking in Spanish but not in English. Consequently, SE bilinguals are more likely to use past progressive constructions to describe past actions in comparison to monolingual English speaker's use of the simple past tense (e.g., "he was dancing at the park" versus "he danced at the park") (Bedore & Peña, 2008).

Typical Bilingual Development Informs Morphosyntactic Assessment

The separate English and Spanish morphosyntactic subtests on the BESA are informed by the research on monolingual, simultaneous, and sequential bilingual morphosyntactic developmental patterns (Peña et al., 2018). Grammatical constructions are acquired in language-specific sequences by bilingual children as a consequence of the differences in frequency, complexity, and saliency of L1 and L2 grammatical morphemes (Bedore & Peña, 2008). For example, the unstressed final consonants that mark past tense in English (e.g., -ed in /lʊkt/) are low in phonological salience, while high-salience stressed syllabic forms mark the preterite tense in Spanish (e.g., stressed -e in the final position in /ayudé/ "I helped). These dissimilarities are reflected in the production of past tense in Spanish-speaking children at age 3 compared to age 4 in English speakers. (Bedore & Peña, 2008; Sebastián & Slobin, 1994). Likewise, the presence of articles during early lexical production in Spanish-speaking children is indicative of high-frequency co-occurring articles and nouns in Spanish (López Ornat, 1997). English-speaking children produce articles regularly in Brown's (1973) Stage 3, which children reach between about 27 and 30 months of age. The BESA targets developmentally appropriate constructions of equal difficulty in both Spanish (e.g., articles) and English (e.g., tense markers), yielding psychometrically valid results.

Clinical Markers of Morphosyntactic Impairment

Bilingual/multilingual children's morphosyntactic production during L2 English acquisition can appear similar to those of English monolingual children with DLD. For example, for SE bilinguals, the cognitive demands of acquiring English may result in reduced complexity in Spanish use and delays in developing later acquired syntactic structures, such as the subjunctive mood (Bedore et al., 2012). Incomplete L2 English knowledge may be demonstrated through the omission of English tense markers in TD SE bilingual children, a pattern similar to difficulties with tense marked forms, low-frequency plurals, and possessives exhibited by English-speaking children with DLD. Spanish-speaking children with DLD have less difficulty with tense and aspect marking and more difficulty with inflected articles and direct object clitic forms that need to match their referent noun in number and gender (Bedore & Leonard, 2001, 2005). This is because for children with DLD in Spanish it is phonologically illegal to omit the syllabic tense and aspect markings (e.g., present and preterite) resulting in an overreliance on a limited range of markers (e.g., third-person form).

A morphosyntactic assessment translated from English to Spanish would improperly target tense marking as a clinical marker of DLD in Spanish, where articles or clitics would be more informative. Consequently, the BESA targets English verb morphology markers including third-person singular present tense verbs, regular and irregular past-tense verbs, copula verbs, negations with auxiliaries, and passive-voice constructions, as well as noun morphology shown to reliably differentiate plural nouns and possessives (Peña et al., 2018). The Spanish section of the morphosyntactic subtest targets articles, preterite tense verb forms, clitics, and subjunctive verb forms. The BESA yields high levels of classification accuracy by combining information about language experience and performance accuracy on clinical markers in English and Spanish to identify bilingual children with DLD.

FUTURE DIRECTIONS: EXTENDING BEYOND SPANISH-ENGLISH BILINGUALS

In applying the approach discussed here to other bilingual/multilingual groups it is important to understand how learners of different language backgrounds acquire English and how they respond to items that tap the most reliable markers of DLD in English. For children who regularly use English (balanced bilinguals and English-dominant bilinguals), performance on clinical markers reliably differentiates groups (Bedore et al., 2018). Spanish-dominant bilinguals score in the same range as their peers with DLD on these markers. Instead, performance on grammatical constructions, such as negatives or passives, that were demanding in terms of memory more reliably differentiated the performance of Spanish-dominant bilingual children with and without DLD. Given that language experience accounts for a significant amount of the variance in children's performance (e.g., Bedore et al., 2012), it would be useful to explore this approach to understanding English acquisition with other populations.

Lexical acquisition for bilingual/multilinguals is twofold: it depends on the child's exposure to each language as well as his or her language-learning ability. While young children with DLD are slower to acquire words and require more exposures than their TD peers (Rice et al., 1994), this deficit remains stable over time (McGregor et al., 2013). Given these characteristic deficits of DLD across languages (e.g., English, Spanish, Mandarin; Sheng et al., 2006, 2012), tasks that tap into lexical acquisition would be useful for identifying impairment across languages. For example, dynamic assessment (also see Chapters 3.1–3.3), which is a method that uses a mediated learning experience to evaluate children's language-learning ability, effectively differentiates children with DLD from their typical peers for SE bilingual children (Peña & Iglesias, 1992). This assessment method has been extended to other language pairs, including Swiss-German (Maragkali & Hessels, 2017), as well as other culturally and linguistically diverse groups (Hasson et al., 2013), including signing deaf children (Mann et al., 2015). Future research should continue evaluating unbiased assessment measures that tap into language-learning ability.

Regardless of the languages spoken, understanding the precise nature of the relationship between exposure, including thresholds needed for continued development across languages, and language development, will inform research and clinical decision-making. For example, SE bilingual children demonstrated variations in individuals; however, children overall demonstrated limited growth in the production of English language sample measures during the summer period when children were receiving less input in that language (Rojas & Iglesias, 2013). Additionally, experience can be quantified in a number of ways. Knowing if a composite of current exposure/use and age of first English exposure (which we call "experience") is the best predictor of production or if exposure/use and experience + home language is the best predictor of performance will determine the most efficacious path toward English language testing. For identifying bilingual/multilingual children with DLD, determining typical developmental trajectories of language across domains in the face of diverse language exposure and extending this to determine where trajectories diverge for children with language impairment is an important step for informing test development and intervention.

Grammatical production data from other language groups show that the same kinds of difficulties with vocabulary use and grammatical forms are evident in learners from multiple language backgrounds. However, in qualitatively evaluating language production patterns in children from other groups it is evident that error types across languages may interact. For example, Blom and Paradis (2013) find that that children who speak tense-marking languages (e.g., Gujarati, Somali, Italian) as an L1 tend to demonstrate accelerated acquisition of English past tense relative to delayed acquisition by children who speak languages that do not mark tense (Mandarin, Cantonese, Vietnamese). In an experimental comparison, Lu (2016) found Spanish-speaking preschoolers were relatively more accurate in their production of regular past tense, while Mandarin-speaking children were more accurate on irregular verbs. Each of these examples illustrates how interactions between the languages children speak potentially influence their developmental trajectories around reliable markers of language impairment. Future work should focus on understanding how these forms emerge and their potential utility as clinical markers.

REFERENCES

Alt, M., Plante, E., & Creusere, M. (2004). Semantic features in fast-mapping: Performance of preschoolers with specific language impairment versus preschoolers with normal language. *Journal of Speech, Language, and Hearing Research*, *47*(2), 407–420. doi:10.1044/1092-4388(2004/033)

Anaya, J. B., Peña, E. D., & Bedore, L. M. (2018). Conceptual scoring and classification accuracy of vocabulary testing in bilingual children. *Language, Speech, and Hearing Services in Schools*, *49*(1), 85–97. https://doi.org/10.1044/2017_LSHSS-16-0081

Baron, A., Bedore, L. M., Peña, E. D., Logren, S., Lopez, A., & Villagran, E. (2018). Developmental patterns of Spanish grammar in Spanish-English bilingual children. *American Journal of Speech Language Pathology*, 1–13. http://hdl.handle.net/2152/22395

Bedore, L. M., & Leonard, L. B. (2001). Grammatical morphology deficits in Spanish-speaking children with specific language impairment. *Journal of Speech, Language, and Hearing Research*, *44*(4), 905–924. https://doi.org/10.1044/1092-4388(2001/072)

Bedore, L. M., & Leonard, L. B. (2005). Verb inflections and noun phrase morphology in the spontaneous speech of Spanish-speaking children with specific language impairment. *Applied Psycholinguistics*, *26*(02). https://doi.org/10.1017/S0142716405050149

Bedore, L. M., & Peña, E. D. (2008). Assessment of bilingual children for identification of language impairment: Current findings and implications for practice. *International Journal of Bilingual Education and Bilingualism*, *11*(1), 1–29. https://doi.org/10.2167/beb392.0

Bedore, L. M., Peña, E. D., Anaya, J. B., Nieto, R., Lugo-Neris, M. J., & Baron, A. (2018). Understanding disorder within variation: Production of English grammatical forms by English language learners. *Language, Speech, and Hearing Services in Schools*, *49*(2), 277–291. doi:10.1044/2017_LSHSS-17-0027

Bedore, L. M., Peña, E. D., Griffin, Z. M., & Hixon, J. G. (2016). Effects of age of English exposure, current input/output, and grade on bilingual language performance. *Journal of Child Language, 43*(3), 687–706. https://doi.org/10.1017/S0305000915000811

Bedore, L. M., Peña, E. D., Joyner, D., & Macken, C. (2011). Parent and teacher rating of bilingual language proficiency and language development concerns. *International Journal of Bilingual Education and Bilingualism, 14*(5), 489–511. https://doi.org/10.1080/13670050.2010.529102

Bedore, L. M., Peña, E. D., Summers, C., Boerger, K., Greene, K., Resendiz, M., & Gillam, R. B. (2012). The measure matters: Language dominance profiles across measures in Spanish English bilingual prekindergarten students. *Bilingualism: Language and Cognition, 15*(3), 616–629. https://doi.org/10.1017/S1366728912000090

Bialystok, E., Luk, G., Peets, K. F., & Yang, S. (2010). Receptive vocabulary differences in monolingual and bilingual children. *Bilingualism (Cambridge, England), 13*(4), 525–531. https://doi.org/10.1017/S1366728909990423

Blom, E., & Paradis, J. (2013). Past tense production by English second language learners with and without language impairment. *Journal of Speech, Language, and Hearing Research, 56*(1), 281–294. https://doi.org/10.1044/1092-4388(2012/11-0112)

Bohman, T. M., Bedore, L. M., Peña, E. D., Mendez-Perez, A., & Gillam, R. B. (2010). What you hear and what you say: Language performance in Spanish English bilinguals. *International Journal of Bilingual Education and Bilingualism, 13*(3), 325–344. https://doi.org/10.1080/13670050903342019

Brackenbury, T., & Pye, C. (2005). Semantic deficits in children with language impairments: Issues for clinical assessment. *Language, Speech, and Hearing Services in Schools, 36*(1), 5–16. https://doi.org/10.1044/0161-1461(2005/002)

Brown, R. (1973). *A first language: The early stages*. Harvard University Press.

Chondrogianni, V., & Marinis, T. (2011). Differential effects of internal and external factors on the development of vocabulary, tense morphology and morpho-syntax in successive bilingual children. *Linguistic Approaches to Bilingualism, 1*(3), 318–345. https://doi.org/10.1075/lab.1.3.05cho

Gillam, R. B., Peña, E. D., Bedore, L. M., Bohman, T. M., & Pérez, A. M. (2013). Identification of specific language impairment in bilingual children, Part 1: Assessment in English. *Journal of Speech, Language, and Hearing Research, 56*, 1813–1823. https://doi.org/10.1044/1092-4388(2013/12-0056)

Gray, S. (2004). Word learning by preschoolers with specific language impairment: Predictors and poor learners. *Journal of Speech, Language, and Hearing Research, 47*(5), 1117–1132. https://doi.org/10.1044/1092-4388(2004/083)

Gray, S., Plante, E., Vance, R., & Henrichsen, M. (1999). The diagnostic accuracy of four vocabulary tests administered to preschool-age children. *Language, Speech, and Hearing Services in Schools, 30*(2), 196–206. https://doi.org/10.1044/0161-1461.3002.196

Gutiérrez–Clellen, V. F., & Kreiter, J. (2003). Understanding child bilingual acquisition using parent and teacher reports. *Applied Psycholinguistics, 24*(02), 267–288. https://doi.org/10.1017/S0142716403000158

Hasson, N., Camilleri, B., Jones, C., Smith, J., & Dodd, B. (2013). Discriminating disorder from difference using dynamic assessment with bilingual children. *Child Language Teaching and Therapy, 29*(1), 57–75. https://doi.org/10.1177/0265659012459526

Hick, R. F., Joseph, K. L., Conti-Ramsden, G., Serratrice, L., & Faragher, B. (2002). Vocabulary profiles of children with specific language impairment. *Child Language Teaching and Therapy, 18*(2), 165–180. https://doi.org/10.1191/0265659002ct233oa

Hoff, E., Core, C., Place, S., Rumiche, R., Señor, M., & Parra, M. (2012). Dual language exposure and early bilingual development. *Journal of Child Language, 39*(1), 1–27. https://doi.org/10.1017/S0305000910000759

Leonard, L. B. (2014). *Children with specific language impairment* (2nd ed.). MIT Press.

López Ornat, S. (1997). What lies between a pre-grammatical and a grammatical representation? Evidence on nominal and verb form-function mapping in Spanish from 1;7 to 2;1. In A. Peréz-Leroux & W. Glass (Eds.), *Contemporary perspectives on the acquisition of Spanish. Volume 1: Developing grammars* (pp. 3–20). Cascadilla Press.

Lu, Y. (2016). *The acquisition of past tense in bilingual children*. Unpublished doctoral dissertation. University of Texas at Austin.

Mann, W., Peña, E. D., & Morgan, G. (2015). Child modifiability as a predictor of language abilities in deaf children who use American Sign Language. *American Journal of Speech-Language Pathology, 24*(3), 374–385. https://doi.org/10.1044/2015_AJSLP-14-0072

Maragkali, I., & Hessels, M. G. (2017). A pilot study of dynamic assessment of vocabulary in German for bilingual preschoolers in Switzerland. *Journal of Studies in Education, 7*(1), 32–49. https://doi.org/10.5296/jse.v7i1.10392

Massa, J., Gomes, H., Tartter, V., Wolfson, V., & Halperin, J. M. (2008). Concordance rates between parent and teacher clinical evaluation of Language Fundamentals Observational Rating Scale. *International Journal of Language & Communication Disorders, 43*(1), 99–110. https://doi.org/10.1080/13682820701261827

McGregor, K. K. (2009). Semantics in child language disorders. In R. G. Schwartz (Ed.), *Handbook of child language disorders* (pp. 365–387). Psychology Press.

McGregor, K. K., Oleson, J., Bahnsen, A., & Duff, D. (2013). Children with developmental language impairment have vocabulary deficits characterized by limited breadth and depth. *International Journal of Language & Communication Disorders/Royal College of Speech & Language Therapists, 48*(3), 307–319. https://doi.org/10.1111/1460-6984.12008

Oller, D. K., Pearson, B. Z., & Cobo-Lewis, A. B. (2007). Profile effects in early bilingual language and literacy. *Applied Psycholinguistics, 28*(2), 191–230. https://doi.org/10.1017/S0142716407070117

Paradis, J., Emmerzael, K., & Duncan, T. S. (2010). Assessment of English language learners: Using parent report on first language development. *Journal of Communication Disorders, 43*(6), 474–497. https://doi.org/10.1016/j.jcomdis.2010.01.002

Paradis, J., & Jia, R. (2017). Bilingual children's long-term outcomes in English as a second language: Language environment factors shape individual differences in catching up with monolinguals. *Developmental Science, 20*(1), e12433. https://doi.org/10.1111/desc.12433

Pearson, B. Z., Fernandez, S. C., Lewedeg, V., & Oller, D. K. (1997). The relation of input factors to lexical learning by bilingual infants. *Applied Psycholinguistics, 18*(01), 41–58. https://doi.org/10.1017/S0142716400009863

Pearson, B. Z., Fernández, S. C., & Oller, D. K. (1993). Lexical development in bilingual infants and toddlers: Comparison to monolingual norms. *Language Learning*, *43*(1), 93–120. https://doi.org/10.1111/j.1467-1770.1993.tb00174.x

Peña, E. D., Bedore, L. M., & Kester, E. S. (2015). Discriminant accuracy of a semantics measure with Latino English-speaking, Spanish-speaking, and English-Spanish bilingual children. *Journal of Communication Disorders, 53*, 30–41. https://doi.org/10.1016/j.jcomdis.2014.11.001

Peña, E. D., Bedore, L. M., & Zlatic-Giunta, R. (2002). Category-generation performance of bilingual children: The influence of condition, category, and language. *Journal of Speech, Language, and Hearing Research*, *45*(5), 938–947. https://doi.org/ 10.1044/1092-4388(2002/076)

Peña, E. D., Gutierrez-Clellen, V. F., Iglesias, A., Goldstein, B. A., & Bedore, L. M. (2018). *Bilingual English Spanish Assessment (BESA)*. MD: Brookes.

Peña, E. D., & Iglesias, A. (1992). The application of dynamic methods to language assessment: A nonbiased procedure. *The Journal of Special Education*, *26*(3), 269–280. https://doi.org/10.1177/002246699202600304

Peña, E. D., Spaulding, T. J., & Plante, E. (2006). The composition of normative groups and diagnostic decision making: Shooting ourselves in the foot. *American Journal of Speech-Language Pathology / American Speech-Language-Hearing Association*, *15*(3), 247–254. https://doi.org/10.1044/1058-0360(2006/023)

Peña, E. D., & Quinn, R. (1997). Task familiarity: Effects on the test performance of Puerto Rican and African American children. *Language, Speech, and Hearing Services in Schools*, *28*(4), 323–332. https://doi.org/10.1044/0161-1461.2804.323

Rice, M. L., Buhr, J. C., & Nemeth, M. (1990). Fast mapping word learning abilities of language-delayed preschoolers. *Journal of Speech and Hearing Disorders*, *55*, 33–42. doi:10.1044/jshd.5501.33

Rice, M. L., Oetting, J. B., Marquis, J., Bode, J., & Pae, S. (1994). Frequency of input effects on word comprehension of children with specific language impairment. *Journal of Speech, Language, and Hearing Research*, *37*(1), 106–122. https://doi.org/10.1044/jshr.3701.106

Rojas, R., & Iglesias, A. (2013). The language growth of Spanish-speaking English language learners. *Child Development*, *84*(2), 630–646. https://doi.org/10.1111/j.1467-8624.2012.01871.x

Sebastián, E., & Slobin, D. I. (1994). Development of linguistic forms: Spanish. In R. Berman & D. Slobin (Eds.), *Relating events in narrative: A cross-linguistic developmental study* (pp. 239–284). Lawrence Erlbaum.

Sheng, L., McGregor, K. K., & Marian, V. (2006). Semantic organization in young Mandarin-English bilingual children: L1, L2 and best performance. *Journal of Speech, Language and Hearing Research*, *49*(3), 572–589. https://doi.org/10.1044/1092-4388(2006/041)

Sheng, L., Peña, E. D., Bedore, L. M., & Fiestas, C. E. (2012). Semantic deficits in Spanish–English bilingual children with language impairment. *Journal of Speech, Language, and Hearing Research*, *55*(1), 1–15. https://doi.org/10.1044/1092-4388(2011/10-0254)

6.2

Assessing Signed Language Skills in Bi-/Multilingual, Deaf and Hard of Hearing Children

Kathryn Crowe

The assessment of bilingual children—that is, children who use two or more languages—must come from an understanding of two fundamental concepts. This is true regardless of a child's hearing status. First, a bilingual child is not the sum of two monolingual children (Grosjean, 1989). A bilingual child does not have separate, homogeneous languages but instead a unique linguistic profile in which the languages interact in ways that can positively and negatively interfere with different aspects of speech and language performance (Kohnert, 2010). Assessment of each language as if for two monolingual children will misrepresent a bilingual child's language competence and knowledge, with poor language proficiency compared to monolingual peers not being a reliable indicator of language competence or disorder (Cruz-Ferreira, 2018). Second, *balanced bilinguals*, children who have equal skills in all of the languages they use, are rare (Grosjean, 1989) and renders any comparison of performance between a child's languages not meaningful. Identifying relative strengths and weaknesses between languages, examining the mechanisms underlying acquisition and use of all languages, and understanding the child's linguistic environment are components of good assessment practice. Assessment is further complicated by the inherent diversity of the population of bilingual deaf and/or hard-of-hearing (D/HH) children, the lack of assessment tools, and mismatches between the languages that professionals and children use. Due to these difficulties, professionals working with D/HH children must look to assessment methods that hold promise for hearing bilingual D/HH children. Combining assessment approaches and triangulating assessment information leads to a richer and more accurate picture of a bilingual D/HH child's speech, spoken language, and signed language, upon which informed intervention decisions can be made.

Kathryn Crowe, *Assessing Signed Language Skills in Bi-/Multilingual, Deaf and Hard of Hearing Children* In: *The Handbook of Language Assessment Across Modalities*. Edited by: Tobias Haug, Wolfgang Mann, and Ute Knoch, Oxford University Press. © Oxford University Press 2022. DOI: 10.1093/oso/9780190885052.003.0018

ASSESSING LISTENING AND SPEAKING

D/HH children are now more likely than at any time in the past to acquire listening and speaking skills in two or more spoken languages. This is due to advances in healthcare (e.g., routinely screening newborns for hearing loss), technology (e.g., digital hearing aids and cochlear implants), and intervention (e.g., earlier fitting of hearing aids and cochlear implants, improved education services for very young D/HH children and their families). The cochlear implant, a device which transmits sound directly to the auditory nerve, provides many D/HH children who have significant hearing loss with access to the sounds of spoken language. For many D/HH children, access to spoken language through a cochlear implant increases their ability to acquire one or more spoken languages.

The acquisition of speech and listening skills requires skilled perception and production of the consonants, vowels, consonant clusters, and tones and an understanding of the phonological rules of a language (McLeod & Crowe, 2018). Knowledge of how speech is acquired by typically developing children across languages is a powerful tool for assessing the listening and speaking skills of bilingual D/HH children. An understanding of typical development provides a frame of reference against which professionals can monitor skills and changes in skills over time and, if possible, view children's progress in terms of expected milestones for children of a similar chronological age, developmental stage, and combination of languages used (also see Chapter 5.2). However, professionals often feel unprepared and less confident in providing services to children who are bilingual and/or use a language that they do not use themselves (Guiberson & Atkins, 2012; Williams & McLeod, 2012). This may be associated with a lack of assessment materials and normative data that clearly define the expected developmental steps in a specific language and/or for bilingual children and a lack of knowledge about appropriate assessment approached. As a guide, the following considerations are suggested.

Linguistic Diversity and Speech Sounds

Bilingual D/HH children may use more than one spoken language. Spoken languages are composed from a set of consonants and vowels, with each language having a unique phonetic inventory. The size of phonetic inventories varies across languages: Rotokas uses just 11 phonemes (Firchow & Firchow, 1969) and the West !Xoon dialect of Taa uses more than 100 phonemes (Naumann, 2016). Symbols for the description and transcription of sounds in all languages are laid out in the International Phonetic Alphabet (International Phonetic Association, 2015) and supplemental symbol sets (Ball, Esling, et al.,

2018; Ball, Howard, et al., 2018). Assessment of a D/HH child's access to, discrimination of, and production of speech sounds relies on a professional being informed about the phonetic, phonemic, and phonological features of the language the child uses and possible interactions between these languages. While the assessor may not be familiar with the sound systems of the languages a child uses, information is available from sources such as the Multilingual Children's Speech website (McLeod, 2018; http://www.csu.edu.au/research/multilingual-speech), the International Guide to Speech Acquisition (McLeod, 2007), and the Multicultural Topics in Communications Sciences and Disorders website (https://www.pdx.edu/multicultural-topics-communication-sciences-disorders/languages). For those not comfortable with transcription of speech sounds, tutorials describing phonetic/phonemic transcription (Howard & Heselwood, 2002), narrow transcription (Ball, Muller, Klopfenstein, et al., 2009), transcription of non-English sounds (Ball, Muller, Rutter, et al., 2009), and transcription of D/HH speech (Teoh & Chin, 2009) are available.

Accessing and Using Speech Sounds

Speech Perception

The ability to perceive, discriminate, and identify speech sounds in isolation, words, phrases, and connected speech is key to the development of listening, speech, and spoken language skills and often difficult for D/HH children. Audiologists have few options for formally assessing the speech perception skills of bilingual D/HH children due to the scarcity of reliable assessments in different languages and a lack of normative data for bilingual language users (Hapsburg & Peña, 2002). While formal assessments are lacking, informal assessment sensitive to the unique needs of bilingual D/HH children is possible. For example, detection and identification of speech sounds is frequently assessed using the Ling Sound Test (Ling, 1989). Administering the test requires an adult to say sounds, one at a time, and for the child to indicate they heard a sound (detection) or point to a picture corresponding to each sound (identification). In English, the phonemes /m/, /u/, /a/, /i/, /ʃ/, and /s/ are used, as together they represent the full spectrum of frequencies used for speech. When working with D/HH children, the appropriateness of these sounds needs to be carefully considered in relation to whether these sounds occur in the child's language/s and are produced similarly to the sounds in the original American English test. If the answer is *yes*, then it may appropriate to use the Ling Sounds. In Finnish, there is no /ʃ/ phoneme and no long open front vowel (i.e., /a/) meaning that the Ling Sounds are not part of the phonetic inventory that the D/HH child is acquiring as part of Finnish. Sounds within the language with similar spectral properties should be used instead. In Finnish, the sounds /m/, /u/, /i/, and /s/ are used, /ʃ/ is used as it is an allophone of /s/ although it is not phonemic in Finnish, and the low back vowel /ɑ/ is used as it has shared spectral characteristics to /a/. Med-El provides resources for the Ling Sounds in a variety of languages (http://www.medel.com/media-gallery-print-materials-rehab/).

Languages differ greatly in the ways that they use sound to create meaning, and this needs to be considered when assessing the speech perception skills of bilingual D/HH children. Two such examples are discussed here: *lexical tone* and *contrastive sounds versus allophones*. Lexical tone is the systematic use of pitch patterns (changes in fundamental frequency) to make distinctions in meaning and is a feature of more than half of the world's languages (Yip, 2002). Hearing children exposed to tonal languages develop tone perception and discrimination in the first months of life, with accurate production occurring much earlier than for vowels and consonants (Hua & Dodd, 2000; Singh & Fu, 2016). The acquisition of tone has been frequently investigated for D/HH children, particularly in regard to cochlear implant users, who show difficulties with tone compared to hearing peers (e.g., Xu et al., 2011). While some formal assessments of tone are available, such as the Cantonese Tone Identification Test (Lee et al., 2017), for the majority of tonal languages informal assessment in collaboration with parents, linguists, and/or native speakers is the only option.

All languages vary meaning by changing sounds in words. *Contrastive sounds* are those which affect a change in meaning when they are exchanged; for example, in English, /t/ and /d/ are contrastive, changing "tab" /tæb/ into "dab"/dæb/. *Allophones* are sounds that are phonetically different but considered to be the same phoneme within the language, so exchanging them does not impact on the meaning of a word. In American English, the /t/ has six allophones that are realized as [t], [tʰ], [t̚], [ɾ], [ʔ], and [ø] without changing the meaning of a word (Eddington, 2007). The boundaries that divide contrastive sounds and allophones vary across languages, as do the features that are important to making sounds contrastive. As an example, voicing is an important feature in English, as just seen in the /t/ and /d/ distinction, but degree of aspiration, not voicing, is contrastive in Icelandic. The sounds [t] and [tʰ] are allophones in English but contrastive in Icelandic. In English [tæb] and [tʰæb] both mean "tab," but the same difference in the Icelandic words "to judge" /taima/ [taiːma] and "to empty" /tʰaima/ [tʰaiːma] changes their meaning. Understanding the tonal, phonetic, phonemic, and phonological rules of the language/s that bilingual D/HH children use is therefore extremely important for informing the selection of meaningful content for assessing speech perception.

Speech Production

Assessing the speech production of bilingual children is challenging for professionals, especially when assessing languages that the professional does not use. Helpful resources provide comprehensive information on the assessment (McLeod et al., 2017) and transcription (Lockart & McLeod, 2013) of languages that assessors do not use themselves. Further studies of typical development in many languages (http://www.csu.edu.au/research/multilingual-speech) and cross-linguistic comparisons (McLeod & Crowe, 2018) may be helpful resources.

A goal of aural habilitation for D/HH children, including bilingual children, is intelligible speech. Speech intelligibility is the degree to which a person's speech production is able to be understood by a listener. Gaining a complete picture of the speech intelligibility of bilingual D/HH children in all of the languages they use is important. To this end, the use of reliable and validated rating scales that can be completed by people familiar with the child in a range of contexts is a good strategy. A tool such as the Intelligibility in Context Scale (ICS; McLeod et al., 2012), which is freely available, has been translated into more than 60 languages and also evaluated in a number of languages (e.g., Vietnamese; Phạm et al., 2017) and with hearing bilingual children (McLeod et al., 2015).

Assessment of the speech production of bilingual children where there is no assessment available in the target language is challenging; however, developing an assessment from scratch is often a more effective and reliable strategy than adapting a resource developed for a different language (Pascoe & Norman, 2011). Developing an informal assessment requires knowledge of the phonemic, tonal, phonotactic, and prosodic features of the language and working with a native speaker to develop a list of age- and culturally appropriate words that address the phonemes, tones, and structures important in that language (McLeod et al., 2017). Children's production of these words should be recorded, transcribed, and compared to the adult production for correctness, intelligibility, and acceptability (McLeod et al., 2017). Stimulability should be checked for sounds the child did not produce and any systemic errors and/or phonological processes (patterns of errors) noted. If information about the ages or order of typical speech sound acquisition or phonological process in the language are available, these should be consulted. Reviews of consonant acquisition across languages (McLeod & Crowe, 2018) may be a helpful resource. For D/HH children, the relationship between speech perception and speech production skills should be carefully considered.

Interpreting the results of speech production assessments for bilingual children is challenging and is different from monolingual children. A systematic review of the acquisition of speech sounds by typically developing bilingual children found little evidence that bilingual children developed speech more slowly than monolingual peers, but there were qualitative differences between these groups (Hambly et al., 2013). Bilingual children also showed transfer between their languages, which had both positive and negative effects. In light of this, and the impact that having a hearing loss may have on the speech production of bilingual D/HH children, comparison of children's speech production performance to normative data for monolingual children is not advisable.

LANGUAGE ASSESSMENT FOR BILINGUAL USERS OF SIGNED AND SPOKEN LANGUAGES

Diversity Considerations in Language Assessment

Bringing a monolingual view of bilingualism to the assessment of bilingual D/HH children, rather than a wholistic view of bilingualism, leads to underestimation of the quality and quantity of children's language competence and performance. Assessment of the language skills of typically developing bilingual hearing children is complex; however, additional layers of complexity exist in the assessment of children who are D/HH and children who use signed languages. Such children may be bilingual across modalities (bimodal bilingual), in either modality (spoken or signed), or use one language across two modalities (bimodal monolinguals). When selecting assessment approaches, important factors in assessment planning should be the language/s and modalities used by the child, the assessment resources available, and the purpose of the assessment. Assessment considerations for a range of bilingual situations are described here, but bilingualism in D/HH children is often not this simple. Consider a child from Ethiopia with a post-lingual hearing loss. He spent the first years of life speaking Amharic and learned English at school. After becoming deaf, he learned Ethiopian Sign Language and then moved to the United States, where he now uses American Sign Language (ASL) and often uses ASL and Ethiopian signs while speaking in English. Thus, reality can be far more complex than the scenarios presented here.

- *Unimodal bilingualism*: Best practice in assessing bilingual D/HH children who use spoken language or signed languages closely mirrors that for bilingual hearing children. One difference is that there are few assessment tools and little research guiding clinical or educational assessment of signed languages. Assessment tools and approaches that may be informative for planning appropriate assessments for bilingual D/HH children will be described later.
- *Bimodal bilingualism*: Bilingual D/HH children who are bimodal bilinguals use two different languages, one in an aural,

spoken, or written modality and one in a manual modality. Hearing children of deaf adults (CODAs) are often viewed as having weaker English skills than monolingual peers and weaker signed language skills than D/HH monolingual peers (Baker & van den Bogaerde, 2014). This likely reflects the same observation that is often made of typically developing bilingual hearing children, where dividing linguistic resources across two languages may be confused with language delay or disorder. Similarly to spoken language bilinguals, the quality and quantity of input and use of each language during development should be considered in assessment as well as the impact that this may have on assessment results (see the later section on "Sociocultural Approaches"). Finally, *code switching* should also be considered. This is a common and typical feature of spoken language bilingual children's communication that looks different for the bimodal bilingual, who may also use elements of both their languages simultaneously.

- *Bimodal monolingualism*: Some D/HH children communicate using a transliterated form of a spoken language, such as Cued Speech, simultaneous communication signing systems (e.g., Signed Exact English), signing in English word order, or key word signing. These children are using one language in two modalities. Assessment of bimodal monolingual children requires consideration of skills in each modality and understanding how modalities interact to support their expressive and receptive communication.

Assessment Approaches

Five assessment approaches are discussed here, along with the possibilities and caveats of each approach as it relates to bilingual D/HH children. The meaningful assessment of these children usually requires the use of more than one approach to consider skills in all languages a child uses. Here, discussion focuses on different approaches to how assessments can be conducted, rather than particular assessments that will be relevant only to a particular language or combination of language (such as English-Spanish bilinguals).

Norm-Referenced Standardized Measures

Norm-referenced standardized measures are the most commonly used method of language assessment and considered by many to be fundamental in the diagnosis of atypical language development (De Lamo White & Jin, 2011). Standardized assessments provide a measurement of a child's language performance that can be directly compared to the performance of a large group of children in a specific population (also see Chapter 2.1). This assumes test administration occurs in the prescribed way to make results valid, reliable, and comparable to the normative sample. Standardized assessments are usually inadequate and inappropriate for use with bilingual children (both D/HH and hearing) because they consider performance in one language, not general language competence, and comparison to the norm group does not account for the different language development trajectories or experiences of these groups (Bedore & Peña, 2008; Thordardottir et al., 2006). Guzman-Orth et al. (2017) describe considerations for assessment of Spanish-English bilinguals, and Enns et al. (2016) provides an overview of signed language assessments.

Criterion-Referenced Measures

Criterion-referenced measures examine a child's performance on a specific skill, and performance is compared to a prespecified criteria of appropriate behaviors, rather than to the performance of a peer group (De Lamo White & Jin, 2011). Criterion-referenced assessments are usually less formal and more flexible than standardized assessments and include methods such as checklists and language sampling. Criterion-referenced measures may also be *conceptually scored*. As bilingual children have their linguistic knowledge distributed over two or more languages, conceptual scoring allows for responses with the correct meaning to be scored as correct regardless of the language of the response (Bedore et al., 2005). Examples of criterion-references approaches include the following:

- The MacArthur-Bates Communicative Development Inventory (Fenson et al., 2007) is an early vocabulary checklist that has been adapted into more than 100 languages/dialects, including signed languages (https://mb-cdi.stanford.edu/adaptations.$1$2
- The American Sign Language Proficiency Interview is one example of a signed language criterion-referenced assessment (Maller et al., 1999).
- The Student Oral Language Observation Matrix (SOLOM; Montebello Unified School District Instructional Division, 1978) is a freely available rubric that defines skill in comprehension, fluency, vocabulary, production, and grammar. A signed language version has also been developed (Crowe et al., 2019).
- Language samples analysis requires professional skills (or skilled assistance) in the target language/s. Analyses can include lexical density, mean length of utterance in words, and checklists such as the Index of Productive Syntax, which has been used with bilingual children (e.g., Washington et al., 2019) and would be appropriate for use with D/HH children.

Language-Processing Measures

Language-processing measures evaluate children's ability to process language, with tasks assessing the integrity of the systems and processes that underlie language acquisition and minimize the impact of language knowledge on results (De Lamo White & Jin, 2011; Kohnert & Medina, 2009). Two examples of language-processing measures are described here.

- *Nonword/Nonsign repetition tasks* are process-based measures sensitive to differentiating children with typical and atypical language skills. These measures involve the child repeating nonsense words/signs of different levels of complexity, which taps into phonological processing and executive function mechanisms used in language acquisition. Tasks should be selected that minimize language bias for bilingual children (e.g., the Quasi-Universal NWR test; Chiat, 2015).
- *Verbal fluency tasks* are a quick and informal means of qualitatively assessing lexico-semantic skills related to lexical organization and retrieval. In fluency tasks, the child is asked to name as many exemplars of a semantic or phonological category as possible within a limited response time, usually 1 minute. Fluency tasks have been used to describe the language skills of D/HH children (e.g., Marshall et al., 2018).

Dynamic Assessment

Dynamic assessment (DA) considers children's language learning potential rather than their language knowledge (De Lamo White & Jin, 2011; Kohnert & Medina, 2009). DA commonly occurs in test-teach-retest paradigms that provide information about the child's current use of a linguistic feature and the effect that different intervention strategies have on supporting the child in using that linguistic feature at a higher developmental level. It is appropriate for use with bilingual children and has been used with D/HH children (e.g., Mann et al., 2015; also see Chapters 3.1–1.3).

Sociocultural Approaches

Sociocultural approaches provide a holistic evaluation of linguistic and communicative abilities in relation to the child's social and cultural environment and operate within ecological models of development (De Lamo White & Jin, 2011). Collection of information from the child and their parents, caregivers, and teachers through observation, conversation, and interview techniques enables a well-rounded understanding of the child's real-world functioning. Examples of procedures for sociocultural assessment approaches are outlined in Cheng (1990,

1997) and Westby (1990). While sociocultural assessment approaches offer a comprehensive view of children in their environment, they are time-, energy-, and financially intensive undertakings that are logistically impossible for many professionals working with D/HH children. However, some information key to a sociocultural approach can be gathered through the use of questionnaires and structured interviews that prompt professionals to ask the right questions. A range of parent interview questionnaires that could be used for linguistically diverse and multilingual D/HH children is available. Such measures include the Alberta Language and Development Questionnaire (Paradis et al., 2010), the Alberta Language Environment Questionnaire (Paradis, 2011), the COST IS0804 Questionnaire (Tuller, 2015), and the Language Experience and Proficiency Questionnaire (Marian et al., 2007).

FUTURE DIRECTIONS

Assessment involves gathering and interpreting data for a variety of reasons, including identification of strengths and weaknesses, diagnosis of disorder, determining service eligibility, developing education or intervention plans, and monitoring progress. The assessment process and interpretation of assessment results is more challenging for bilingual D/HH children but no less important. The future direction of assessments for these children lies in the development and use of reliable and valid assessment approaches that are sensitive to the unique needs of this group. Professionals working with bilingual D/HH children need to continually update their skills and knowledge of these assessments and be alert to emerging evidence for assessment approached within the field of deafness and in the related fields of speech-language pathology, linguistics, education, language education, and special education. Furthermore, future research is needed into the intervention approaches, as well as the fidelity, intensity, and frequency of intervention necessary for successful outcomes, which is currently an area of unmet need (Crowe & Guiberson, 2019; Guiberson & Crowe, 2018). As the linguistic (and cultural) diversity of D/HH children in our clinics and schools continues to grow (also see Chapter 1.1), appropriate assessment of these children will more often become a key part of daily practice for all professionals.

REFERENCES

Baker, A. E., & van den Bogaerde, B. (2014). KODAs: A special form of bilingualism. In D. Quinto-Pozos (Ed.), *Multilingual aspects of signed language communication and disorder* (pp. 211–234). Multilingual Matters.

Ball, M. J., Esling, J. H., & Dickson, B. C. (2018). Revisions to the VoQS system for the transcription of voice quality. *Journal of the International Phonetic Association*, *48*(2), 165–171. https://doi.org/10.1017/S0025100317000159

Ball, M. J., Howard, S. J., & Miller, K. (2018). Revisions to the extIPA chart. *Journal of the International Phonetic Association, 48*(2), 155–164. https://doi.org/10.1017/S0025100317000147

Ball, M. J., Muller, N., Klopfenstein, M., & Rutter, B. (2009). The importance of narrow phonetic transcription for highly unintelligible speech: Some examples. *Logopedics Phoniatrics Vocology, 34*(2), 84–90. https://doi.org/10.1080/14015430902913535

Ball, M. J., Muller, N., Rutter, B., & Klopfenstein, M. (2009). My client is using non-English sounds! A tutorial in advanced phonetic transcription part I: Consonants. *Contemporary Issues in Communication Science Disorders, 36*, 133–141.

Bedore, L. M., & Peña, E. D. (2008). Assessment of bilingual children for identification of language impairment: Current findings and implications for practice. *International Journal of Bilingual Education and Bilingualism, 11*(1), 1–29. https://doi.org/10.2167/beb392.0

Bedore, L. M., Peña, E. D., Garcia, M., & Cortez, C. (2005). Conceptual versus monolingual scoring: When does it make a difference? *Language, Speech, and Hearing Services in Schools, 36*(3), 188–200. https://doi.org/10.1044/0161-1461(2005/020)

Cheng, L.-R. L. (1990). The identification of communicative disorders in Asian-Pacific students. *Journal of Childhood Communication Disorders, 13*(1), 113–119. https://doi.org/10.1177/152574019001300112

Cheng, L.-R. L. (1997). Diversity: Challenges and implications for assessment. *Journal of Children's Communication Development, 19*(1), 55–62. https://doi.org/10.1177/152574019701900107

Chiat, S. (2015). Nonword repetition. In S. Armon-Lotem, J. de Jong, & N. Meir (Eds.), *Methods for assessing multilingual children: Disentangling bilingualism from language impairment* (pp. 125–150). Multilingual Matters.

Crowe, K., & Guiberson, M. (2019). Evidence-based interventions for learners who are deaf and/or multilingual: A systematic quality review. *American Journal of Speech-Language Pathology, 28*, 964–983. https://doi.org/10.1044/2019_AJSLP-IDLL-19-0003

Crowe, K., Marschark, M., & McLeod, S. (2019). Measuring intelligibility in signed languages. *Clinical Linguistics and Phonetics, 33*(10–11), 991–1008. https://doi.org/10.1080/02699206.2019.1600169

Cruz-Ferreira, M. (2018). Assessment of communication abilities in multilingual children: Language rights or human rights? *International Journal of Speech-Language Pathology, 20*(1), 166–169. https://doi.org/10.1080/17549507.2018.1392607

De Lamo White, C., & Jin, L. (2011). Evaluation of speech and language assessment approaches with bilingual children. *International Journal of Language and Communication Disorders, 46*(6), 613–627. https://doi.org/10.1111/j.1460-6984.2011.00049.x

Eddington, D. (2007). Flaps and other variants of /t/ in American English: Allophonic distribution without constraints, rules, or abstractions. *Cognitive Linguistics, 18*(1), 23–46. https://doi.org/10.1515/COG.2007.002

Enns, C. J., Haug, T., Herman, R., Hoffmeister, R., Mann, W., & McQuarrie, L. (2016). Exploring signed language assessment tools in Europe and North America. In M. Marschark, V. Lampropoulou, & E. K. Skordilis (Eds.), *Diversity in deaf education* (pp. 171–218). Oxford University Press.

Fenson, L., Marchman, V. A., Thal, D. J., Dale, P. S., Reznick, J. S., & Bates, E. A. (2007). *MacArthur-Bates Communicative Development Inventories* (2nd ed.). Paul H. Brookes.

Firchow, I., & Firchow, J. (1969). An abbreviated phoneme inventory. *Anthropological Linguistics, 11*(9), 271–276.

Grosjean, F. (1989, Jan). Neurolinguists, beware! The bilingual is not two monolinguals in one person. *Brain and Language, 36*(1), 3–15.

Guiberson, M., & Atkins, J. (2012). Speech-language pathologists' preparation, practices, and perspectives on serving culturally and linguistically diverse children. *Communication Disorders Quarterly, 33*(3), 169–180. https://doi.org/10.1177/1525740110384132

Guiberson, M., & Crowe, K. (2018). Interventions for children with hearing loss from bilingual backgrounds: A scoping review. *Topics in Language Disorders, 38*(3), 225–241. https://doi.org/10.1097/TLD.0000000000000155

Guzman-Orth, D., Lopez, A. A., & Tolentino, F. (2017). *A framework for the dual language assessment of young dual language learners in the United States*. Educational Testing Service. https://doi.org/10.1002/ets2.12165

Hambly, H., Wren, Y., McLeod, S., & Roulstone, S. (2013). The influence of bilingualism on speech production: A systematic review. *International Journal of Language and Communication Disorders, 48*(1), 1–24. https://doi.org/10.1111/j.1460-6984.2012.00178.x

Hapsburg, D. v., & Peña, E. D. (2002). Understanding bilingualism and its impact on speech audiometry. *Journal of Speech Language and Hearing Research, 45*(1), 202–213. https://doi.org/10.1044/1092-4388(2002/015)

Howard, S. J., & Heselwood, B. C. (2002). Learning and teaching phonetic transcription for clinical purposes. *Clinical Linguistics and Phonetics, 16*(5), 371–401. https://doi.org/10.1080/02699200210135893

Hua, Z., & Dodd, B. (2000). The phonological acquisition of Putonghua (Modern Standard Chinese). *Journal of Child Language, 27*(1), 3–42. https://doi.org/10.1017/S030500099900402X

International Phonetic Association. (2015). The international phonetic alphabet. http://www.internationalphoneticassociation.org/content/ipa-chart

Kohnert, K. (2010). Bilingual children with primary language impairment: Issues, evidence and implications for clinical actions. *Journal of Communication Disorders, 43*(6), 456–473. https://doi.org/10.1016/j.jcomdis.2010.02.002

Kohnert, K., & Medina, A. (2009). Bilingual children and communication disorders: A 30-year research retrospective. *Seminars in Speech and Language, 30*(4), 219–223. https://doi.org/10.1055/s-0029-1241721

Lee, K. Y. S., Lam, J. H. S., Chan, K. T. Y., Van Hasselt, C. A., & Tong, M. C. F. (2017). Applying Rasch model analysis in the development of the Cantonese tone identification test (CANTIT). *International Journal of Audiology, 56*(Supplement 2), 60–73. https://doi.org/10.1080/14992027.2017.1294766

Ling, D. (1989). *Foundations of spoken language for the hearing-impaired child*. Alexander Graham Bell Association for the Deaf.

Lockart, R., & McLeod, S. (2013). Factors that enhance English-speaking speech-language pathologists' transcription of Cantonese-speaking children's consonants. *American Journal of Speech-Language Pathology, 22*(3), 523–539. https://doi.org/10.1044/1058-0360(2012/12-0009)

Maller, S. J., Singleton, J. L., Supalla, S. J., & Wix, T. (1999). The development and psychometric properties of the American Sign Language Proficiency Assessment (ASL-PA). *Journal of Deaf Studies and Deaf Education, 4*(4), 249–269. https://doi.org/10.1093/deafed/4.4.249

Mann, W., Peña, E. D., & Morgan, G. (2015). Child modifiability as a predictor of language abilities in deaf children who use American Sign Language. *American Journal of Speech-Language Pathology, 24*(3), 374–385. https://doi.org/10.1044/2015_AJSLP-14-0072

Marian, V., Blumenfeld, H. K., & Kaushanskaya, M. (2007). The Language Experience and Proficiency Questionnaire (LEAP-Q): Assessing language profiles in bilinguals and multilinguals. *Journal of Speech, Language, and Hearing Research, 50*(4), 940–967. https://doi.org/10.1044/1092-4388(2007/067)

Marshall, C. R., Jones, A., Fastelli, A., Atkinson, J., Botting, N., & Morgan, G. (2018). Semantic fluency in deaf children who use spoken and signed language in comparison with hearing peers. *International Journal of Language and Communication Disorders, 53*(1), 157–170. https://doi.org/10.1111/1460-6984.12333

McLeod, S. (2007). *The international guide to speech acquisition*. Thomson Delmar Learning.

McLeod, S. (2018). Multilingual children's speech. http://www.csu.edu.au/research/multilingual-speech

McLeod, S., & Crowe, K. (2018). Children's consonant acquisition in 27 languages: A cross-linguistic review. *American Journal of Speech-Language Pathology, 27*(4), 1546–1571. https://doi.org/10.1044/2018_AJSLP-17-0100

McLeod, S., Crowe, K., & Shahaeian, A. (2015). Intelligibility in Context Scale: Normative and validation data for English-speaking preschoolers. *Language, Speech, and Hearing Services in Schools, 46*(3), 266–276. https://doi.org/10.1044/2015_LSHSS-14-0120

McLeod, S., Harrison, L. J., & McCormack, J. (2012). *Intelligibility in context scale*. Charles Sturt University. http://www.csu.edu.au/research/multilingual-speech/ics

McLeod, S., Verdon, S., & International Expert Panel on Multilingual Children's Speech. (2017). Tutorial: Speech assessment for multilingual children who do not speak the same language(s) as the speech-language pathologist. *American Journal of Speech-Language Pathology, 26*, 691–708. https://doi.org/10.1044/2017_AJSLP-15-0161

Montebello Unified School District Instructional Division. (1978). *Student Oral Language Observation Matrix (SOLOM)*. Author. http://www.cal.org/twi/EvalToolkit/appendix/solom.pdf

Naumann, C. (2016). The phoneme inventory of Taa (West!Xoon Dialect). In R. Vossen & W. H. G. Haacke (Eds.), *Lone tree: Scholarship in the service of the Koon: Essay in the memory of Anthony T Traill* (pp. 311–351). Köppe.

Pascoe, M., & Norman, V. (2011). Contextually relevant resources in speech-language therapy and audiology in South Africa: Are there any? *South African Journal of Communication Disorders, 58*(1), 2–5. https://doi.org/10.4102/sajcd.v58i1.35

Paradis, J. (2011). Individual differences in child English second language acquisition: Comparing child-internal and child-external factors. *Linguistic Approaches to Bilingualism, 1*(3), 213–237. https://doi.org/10.1075/lab.1.3.01par

Paradis, J., Emmerzael, K., & Duncan, T. S. (2010). Assessment of English language learners: Using parent report on first language development. *Journal of Communication Disorders, 43*(6), 474–497. https://doi.org/10.1016/j.jcomdis.2010.01.002

Phạm, B., McLeod, S., & Harrison, L. J. (2017). Validation and norming of the Intelligibility in Context Scale in Northern Viet Nam. *Clinical Linguistics and Phonetics, 31*(7–9), 665–681. https://doi.org/10.1080/02699206.2017.1306110

Singh, L., & Fu, C. S. L. (2016). A new view of language development: The acquisition of lexical tone. *Child Development, 87*(3), 834–854. https://doi.org/10.1111/cdev.12512

Teoh, A. P., & Chin, S. B. (2009). Transcribing the speech of children with cochlear implants: Clinical application of narrow phonetic transcriptions. *American Journal of Speech-Language Pathology, 18*(4), 388–401. https://doi.org/10.1044/1058-0360(2009/08-0076)

Thordardottir, E., Rothenberg, A., Rivard, M., & Naves, R. (2006). Bilingual assessment: Can overall proficiency be estimated from separate measurement of two languages. *Journal of Multilingual Communication Disorders, 4*(1), 1–21. https://doi.org/10.1080/14769670500215647

Tuller, L. (2015). Clinical use of parental questionnaires in multilingual contexts. In S. Armon-Lotem, J. de Jong, & N. Meir (Eds.), *Methods for assessing multilingual children: Disentangling bilingualism from language impairment* (pp. 301–330). Multilingual Matters.

Washington, K. N., Fritz, K., Crowe, K., Shaw, B., & Wright, R. (2019). Bilingual preschoolers' spontaneous productions: Considering Jamaican Creole and English. *Language, Speech, and Hearing Services in Schools, 50*(2), 179–195. https://doi.org/10.1044/2018_LSHSS-18-0072

Westby, C. E. (1990). Ethnographic interviewing: Asking the right questions to the right people in the right ways. *Journal of Childhood Communication Disorders, 13*(1), 101–111. https://doi.org/10.1177/152574019001300111

Williams, C. J., & McLeod, S. (2012). Speech-language pathologists' assessment and intervention practices with multilingual children. *International Journal of Speech-Language Pathology, 14*(3), 292–305. https://doi.org/10.3109/17549507.2011.636071

Xu, L., Chen, X., Lu, H., Zhou, N., Wang, S., Liu, Q., Li, Y., Zhao, X., & Han, D. (2011). Tone perception and production in pediatric cochlear implants users. *Acta Oto-Laryngologica, 131*(4), 395–398. https://doi.org/10.3109/00016489.2010.536993

Yip, M. J. W. (2002). *Tone.* Cambridge University Press.

6.3

Discussion of Issues Related to Assessing the Signed and Spoken Language Skills of Bi/Multilingual Children

Lisa M. Bedore, Kathryn Crowe, Elizabeth D. Peña, Kathleen Durant, and Stephanie McMillen

While there is a growing body of evidence describing best practice in the assessment of bilingual children who use spoken languages, there is currently scant evidence or recommendations available regarding the assessment of bilingual children who use signed languages. In this discussion, we therefore outline how knowledge from the assessment of spoken languages can be used to inform practice in assessing signed languages for bilingual deaf and hard-of-hearing (D/HH) children. Recommendations will be made for applying knowledge about assessment in hearing bilingual children to assessment of bilingual D/HH children, particularly those who use more than one signed language. Consideration will also be given to emerging assessment methods for signed languages that could inform assessment practices with bilingual hearing children.

USING KNOWLEDGE OF THE ASSESSMENT OF BI-/MULTILINGUAL CHILDREN IN SPOKEN LANGUAGE TO INFORM SIGNED LANGUAGE ASSESSMENT

The current lack of knowledge regarding best practice in the assessment of signed languages in bi-/multilingual children means that much can be learned from advances in knowledge of appropriate assessment of spoken languages in bi-/multilingual children. There are four interrelated issues that are both critical and timely to discuss in reference to the assessment of children who use more than one spoken language and that can inform assessment of bi-/multilingual children who use one or more signed languages: (1) differential

Lisa M. Bedore, Kathryn Crowe, Elizabeth D. Peña, Kathleen Durant, and Stephanie McMillen, *Discussion of Issues related to Assessing the Signed and Spoken Language Skills of Bi/Multilingual Children* In: *The Handbook of Language Assessment Across Modalities.* Edited by: Tobias Haug, Wolfgang Mann, and Ute Knoch, Oxford University Press.
 DOI: 10.1093/oso/9780190885052.003.0019

diagnosis, (2) appropriate assessment materials, (3) linguistic bias, and (4) language environment. These issues are highly entwined and will be discussed in relation to the challenges and opportunities that they pose and how they are being addressed in research and practice.

Differential Diagnosis

Diagnosis of speech and/or language impairment in bilingual children is an issue with a long history. Differential diagnosis of a speech or language disorder, as opposed to a delay, requires evidence that the impairment lies in the linguistic system and impacts all languages a child uses. If language difficulties are not evident in the language in which the child has the most knowledge (based on their cumulative experiences), then this is evidence that the linguistic system is intact, and the difficulty relates to inadequate exposure to or experience with the delayed language. As yet there are no satisfactory solutions to differential diagnosis that encompasses all bilingual populations for either hearing or D/HH children. However, considerable progress has been made toward accurate differential diagnosis of bilingual children without hearing loss who use spoken languages when specific diagnoses (e.g., developmental language disorder [DLD]) and/or combinations of languages (e.g., Spanish-English) are considered. Such emerging research provides guidance for those seeking to examine speech and/or language impairment in bilingual children who use signed languages.

Appropriate Assessment Materials

There are many recommendations on what constitutes best practice in assessment for bilingual users of spoken languages. For example, Speech Pathology Australia specified in its clinical guidelines for working in a culturally and linguistically diverse society that clinicians must consider the linguistic features of children's first language(s) and assess both languages used by a child (Speech Pathology Australia, 2016). Guidelines for assessment of bilingual children who use spoken languages are usually general, and their implementation is frequently impeded by practical issues such as a shortage of appropriate assessment tools, appropriate assessment tools being inaccessible, and practitioners lacking of knowledge and experience in the assessment of bilingual children (Caesar & Kohler, 2007; Kritikos, 2003; Williams & McLeod, 2012). Furthermore, time constraints and caseload demands can limit the possibility of thorough evaluation of bilingual children even when the tools, knowledge, and expertise are in place (McLeod et al., 2013). In the United States, recently graduated speech-language pathologists (SLPs) report that while they are aware that languages spoken by children should be taken into account in clinical decision-making, they are often unaware of the home languages of children on their caseload (ASHA, 2014). SLPs frequently report that assessing children from bilingual backgrounds is one of the most challenging clinical tasks they face. SLPs also often report delaying any assessment of bilinguals until the child has acquired enough skills in the community language to complete an assessment. They may also apply their knowledge of monolingual spoken language assessment and development to bilingual children (ASHA, 2010; Thordardottir, 2010; Williams & McLeod, 2012). All these issues similarly exist in the assessment of bilingual children who use signed languages and may even be magnified due to lack of awareness, skills, and resources. Those seeking to assess signed language bilinguals should closely attend to solutions in terms of practices and resources for the assessment of spoken language bilinguals as they continue to emerge.

Specifically considering bilingual D/HH children, there are currently no clear guidelines as to what constitutes appropriate assessment for differential diagnosis of speech and language disorders. Generally, at least by definition, D/HH children are excluded from the possibility of having speech sound disorder or DLD due to the presence of a hearing loss being a complicating factor. However, there is clear evidence that D/HH children may experience speech and language difficulties that may be unrelated to their hearing loss and that are not due to inadequate language exposure or experience (Mason et al., 2010; Quinto-Pozos, 2014; Quinto-Pozos et al., 2017). With that being said, professional organizations are continuing to refine and expand documentation regarding best practices with culturally and linguistically diverse (CLD) children. The American Speech Language and Hearing Association (ASHA, n.d.) recently updated its Practice Portal with guidelines around current definitions, ethical and professional responsibilities, and recommendations for evidence practices to be used with bilingual clients and their families. While there are no guidelines that deal specifically with diagnosis of language disorders in signed languages at this stage, attending to the guidelines for spoken languages and spoken language bilinguals is a good starting point.

The availability of appropriate assessment materials is a constant struggle for practitioners who aim to conduct appropriate assessments of bilingual children's speech and language skills in spoken languages. This is not a struggle unique to bilingual children; it is also true for the majority of languages used in the world today. For the vast majority of languages, there is a lack of norm-referenced standardized measures, criterion-referenced measures, language processing measures, and evaluated dynamic assessment approaches for assessing monolingual children who use spoken languages. For example, McLeod maintains a comprehensive list of speech sound tests in languages other than English in which 125 tests are identified, but these tests represent only 39 languages (https://www.csu.edu.au/research/multilingual-speech/speech-assessments). Of these only 11 are designed or normed with bilingual children in mind. Even when the language pairing of Spanish-English is considered, which is the largest group of bilinguals in the United States, there is a small set of high-quality assessment tools appropriate for assessing the skills of bilingual children and making a diagnosis of speech and/or language disorder, but these need to be expanded for other language groups. Contributing to misdiagnosis and delay is the lack of normative data on the linguistic development of monolingual children in the majority of languages used in the world and for a range of language pairings. This issue is heightened for assessments of signed languages for both monolinguals and especially bilinguals. Knowledge and practices for the development of assessments of spoken languages for bilingual children can inform the development of assessments of signed languages.

Linguistic Bias

The shortage of knowledge concerning typical monolingual language acquisition in most languages hinders the development of assessment practices and materials appropriate for bilingual children who use spoken languages. However, there is growing research interest in the identification of cross-linguistic features, structures, and processes in language acquisition which can give practical insights into the language development of typically and atypically developing bilingual children. Ongoing research seeks to identify robust indicators of speech and language learning difficulties based on this new data, and researchers and clinicians work to develop these into indicators that can be used in assessment to facilitate the diagnosis of speech and language disorders in bilingual populations. These indicators, called *clinical markers*, represent areas of special difficulty that are notable relative to general delays and, in the case of bilinguals, in the face of divided linguistic experience. Assessments built around clinical markers and challenging item types effectively differentiate children with and without DLD (Bedore et al., 2018; Paradis, 2017; Paradis et al., 2010). Examples of robust clinical markers in spoken languages are past tense *-ed* in English and case marking in German. Such research methods provide promise for future research considering signed languages. To date, identifying such clinical markers is much more challenging for signed languages given factors such as the incredible heterogeneity of language exposure, experiences, and skills which are considered typical within populations of signed language users and the relatively scant literature that currently exists on typical and atypical development. However, this is an area of promising future research in signed languages, with approaches to assessment such as semantic and phonological fluency tasks and non-sign repetition tasks potentially leading the way in examining underlying language skills through signed languages.

Language Environment

One further critical issue that affects both language acquisition and interpreting the meaning of assessment results is environmental in nature. This is the quality and quantity of language input and how it impacts on the growth trajectory of speech and language skills in bilingual children. This is of particular importance to D/HH children who may not be immersed in a rich language learning environment due to reduced access to spoken language through audition. For children without hearing loss who are Spanish-English bilinguals, there is converging evidence that the quantity of language that children hear and use is important for getting started and making gains using the language (Bohman et al., 2010). This accounts for concurrent language knowledge (Bedore et al., 2012) and the role it plays in how much language content children know in the early school years (Bedore et al., 2018). The richness in the language environment—indexed by factors such as mother's vocabulary size, parent education level, and numbers of interlocuters—all contribute to the child's language outcomes, particularly in the domain of vocabulary (Bedore et al., 2016; Paradis et al., 2010). This is important not only in terms of which language they are exposed to, but also the quality and quantity of their exposure to each language.

The issue of language environment in assessment is particularly pertinent in the assessment of signed languages, although not considered enough. Reduced access to rich and varied models in the signed languages that a child is acquiring will necessarily impact on his or her rate and quality of acquisition and therefore his or her performance on assessments. For example, bilingual D/HH learners may have little to no access to high-quality language models of the signed language/s they are acquiring in their home as few D/HH children are born into families where the parents are signed language users (Mitchell & Karchmer, 2004) and parents cannot be expected to develop high levels of skills in a new language (i.e., a signed language) in the child's early years of language exposure (Knoors & Marschark, 2012). In addition, children acquiring a signed language outside of the home, such as in their school environment, may also have limited access to a rich language environment. A consequence of the practice of mainstreaming D/HH children means that often there may only be one child using a signed language in a class or even a school, and the only language model for the child may be an interpreter (qualified or unqualified) and/or a visiting teacher of the deaf. For a child relying on education as the source of a model for language acquisition, this poses a particularly deprived and atypical context for language acquisition that will necessarily be reflected in assessments of a child's signed language skills. This issue is intensified if the child is accessing a different signed language in their home environment. Access to signed language is known to be key in language acquisition for D/HH children, yet assessment of children's language environment rarely plays a significant role in language assessments. There is much that can be learned from the language environment of spoken language bilinguals in the assessment of children in a bilingual signed language environment.

USING KNOWLEDGE OF THE ASSESSMENT OF SIGNED LANGUAGES TO INFORM SPOKEN LANGUAGE ASSESSMENT

One area of signed language test development that is particularly challenging is related to vocabulary assessment given that many signs are highly visually motivated (Östling et al., 2018). As an example, the Carolina Picture Vocabulary Test (CPVT; Layton & Holmes, 1985) is a receptive vocabulary test in ASL. In this task a child is presented with a sign and much choose the meaning of the sign from an array of four pictures, meaning there is a 25% chance that they can select the correct answer by guessing. In a study by White and Tischler (1999), the CPVT was administered to 30 children in first, fourth, or ninth grade who had no exposure ASL. On average they scored 73%, at a rate far higher than chance. This demonstrated the incompatibility of signed language vocabulary knowledge with assessment methods traditionally used to assess spoken languages. This is an assessment difficulty that exists, albeit to lesser extent, in some spoken languages. In languages such as Icelandic, words can be built by compounding free morphemes, which makes the meaning of complex words more transparent. For example, in Iceland *risaeðla* (dinosaur) is a compound of giant + lizard and *sóttvarnalæknir* (epidemiologist) is a compound of infection + prevention + doctor. Thus, traditional receptive vocabulary tests based on picture selection have difficulty in accurately assessing knowledge of vocabulary in the same way that the CPVT does.

One solution to this methodological difficulty with assessment can be seen in the framework used by the British Sign Language Vocabulary Test (BSL-VT; see Mann & Marshall, 2012) and its adapted versions for ASL (ASL-VT; see Mann et al., 2015) and Finnish Sign Language (FinSL-VT; see Kanto et al., 2021). These tests use a four-level approach for assessing the relationship between word forms and meanings, originally developed for spoken language (Laufer et al., 2004; Laufer & Goldstein, 2004) and adapted for signed language (Mann & Marshall, 2012): "meaning recognition (matching a sign to four pictures), form recognition (matching a picture to signs), form recall (picture naming), and meaning recall (sign association)" (p. 1033). The original model was developed within the context of adult second language acquisition but, to our knowledge, has never been used with children. By reapplying the adapted signed language model back to spoken language assessment, a meaningful examination of children's vocabulary knowledge in a greater range of languages may be possible. Such a paradigm could be particularly informative for assessing linguistically diverse children to gain a better understanding of the depth as well as the breadth of their vocabulary knowledge. Standardized assessments of vocabulary knowledge typically allow children one attempt at demonstrating knowledge of each word in a pass/fail context. However, the model utilized in the BSL-VT, ASL-VT, and the FinSL-VT recognizes the different degrees of strength that exist between word form and word meaning and uses the four tasks to assess the strength of this relationship, rather than determining if it is present or absent.

SUGGESTIONS FROM SIGNED LANGUAGE RESEARCH FOR SPOKEN LANGUAGE RESEARCH

There is no easy solution to the challenges that practitioners encounter in assessing the speech and spoken language skills of bilingual children. The best possible practices in assessment of bilingual children, whether hearing or D/HH, use evidence-based, nonstandardized testing practices derived from research. Gold standard assessment practices beyond norm-referenced tests include dynamic assessment (DA) and converging concerns from interviews collected from parents and teachers. DA, which is a pretest-teach-posttest method, uses a mediated leaning experience to evaluate children's language learning ability. It can be used to evaluate skills in domains such as vocabulary, macrostructure and microstructures in narratives, classifier use, and grammatical structures. Where possible, this should be conducted in all languages used by a child to examine whether any difficulties observed are language-specific or language-independent. This approach has been shown to accurately differentiates bilingual children with a language impairment from their typically developing peers while reducing testing biases pertinent to CLD populations (Peña et al., 2001, 2006, 2014). Parent and teacher questionnaires focusing on observable behaviors and real-time judgments best provide reliable information about children's language knowledge in the language that they share with the child. In fact, parent questionnaires, in particular, were highly reliable in determining their children's language ability across both Spanish and English in pre-kindergarten or kindergarten (Bedore et al., 2011).

SUGGESTIONS FOR SIGNED LANGUAGE ASSESSMENT

As for spoken languages, there is no easy solution to the challenges that practitioners encounter in assessing the signed language skills of bilingual D/HH children. The suggestions outlined for assessment of spoken languages in bilingual D/HH children are all equally valid for assessment of signed languages in this group. Of particular note is that there is now a growing body of evidence for the use of DA methods with signed language users (Mann & Haug, 2014; Mann et al., 2015; also see Chapter 3.2).

CONCLUSION

In conclusion, the current lack of research concerning reliable and valid assessments of bilingual users of spoken languages is amplified for D/HH children. Where best practices for assessment of hearing bilingual children exist, although knowledge and resources are lacking, for bilingual D/HH children evidence on best practices is still in the early stages of development. This is more so for D/HH children who use two or more signed languages or more than two languages divided across different modalities. There is much existing evidence concerning the assessment of bilingual hearing children that can inform both the research agenda and practices of those working to improve the possibilities, standards, and accuracy of assessments used with bilingual D/HH learners.

REFERENCES

ASHA. (n.d.). *Bilingual service delivery (Practice Portal)*. Retrieved August 7, 2019, from https://www.asha.org/Practice-Portal/Professional-Issues/Bilingual-Service-Delivery/Bilingual-Service--Delivery-Content-Development/

ASHA. (2010). *2010 schools survey*. American Speech Language & Hearing Association.

ASHA. (2014). *2014 school surveys*. American Speech Language & Hearing Association.

Bedore, L. M., Peña, E. D., Anaya, J. B., Nieto, R., Lugo-Neris, M. J., & Baron, A. (2018). Understanding disorder within variation: Production of English grammatical forms by English language learners. *Language, Speech, and Hearing Services in Schools, 49*(2), 277–291. https://doi.org/10.1044/2017_LSHSS-17-0027

Bedore, L. M., Peña, E. D., Griffin, Z. M., & Hixon, J. G. (2016). Effects of age of English exposure, current input/output, and grade on bilingual language performance. *Journal of Child Language, 43*(3), 687–706. https://doi.org/10.1017/S0305000915000811

Bedore, L. M., Peña, E. D., Joyner, D., & Macken, C. (2011). Parent and teacher rating of bilingual language proficiency and language development concerns. *International Journal of Bilingual Education and Bilingualism, 14*(5), 489–511. https://doi.org/10.1080/13670050.2010.529102

Bedore, L. M., Peña, E. D., Summers, C., Boerger, K., Greene, K., Resendiz, M., & Gillam, R. B. (2012). The measure matters: Language dominance profiles across measures in Spanish English bilingual prekindergarten students. *Bilingualism: Language and Cognition, 15*(3), 616–629. https://doi.org/10.1017/S1366728912000090

Bohman, T. M., Bedore, L. M., Peña, E. D., Mendez-Perez, A., & Gillam, R. B. (2010). What you hear and what you say: Language performance in Spanish

English bilinguals. *International Journal of Bilingual Education and Bilingualism, 13*(3), 325–344. https://doi.org/10.1080/13670050903342019

Caesar, L. G., & Kohler, P. D. (2007). The state of school-based bilingual assessment: Actual practice versus recommended guidelines. *Language, Speech, and Hearing Services in Schools, 38*(3), 190–200. https://doi.org/10.1044/0161-1461(2007/020)

Kanto, L., Syrjälä, H., & Mann, W. (2021). Assessing vocabulary knowledge in deaf and hearing children using Finnish Sign Language. *Journal of Deaf Studies and Deaf Education*, 147–158. doi:10.1093/deafed/enaa032

Knoors, H., & Marschark, M. (2012). Language planning for the 21st century: Revisiting bilingual language policy for deaf children. *Journal of Deaf Studies and Deaf Education, 17*(3), 291–305. https://doi.org/10.1093/deafed/ens018

Kritikos, E. P. (2003). Speech-language pathologists' beliefs about language assessment of bilingual/bicultural individuals. *American Journal of Speech-Language Pathology/American Speech-Language-Hearing Association, 12*(1), 73–91. https://doi.org/10.1044/1058-0360(2003/054)

Laufer, B., Elder, C., Hill, K., & Congdon, P. (2004). Size and strength: Do we need both to measure vocabulary knowledge? *Language Testing, 21*, 202–226. https://doi.org/10.1191/0265532204lt277oa

Laufer, B., & Goldstein, Z. (2004). Testing vocabulary knowledge: Size, strength, and computeradaptiveness. *Language Learning, 54*, 399–436. https://doi.org/10.1111/j.0023-8333.2004.00260.x

Layton, T. L., & Holmes, D. W. (1985). *Carolina picture vocabulary test*. Modern Education.

Mann, W., & Haug, T. (2014). Mapping out guidelines for the development and use of sign language assessments: Some critical issues, comments, and suggestions. In D. Quinto-Pozos (Ed.), *Multilingual aspects of signed language communication and disorder* (pp. 123–139). Multilingual Matters.

Mann, W., & Marshall, C. (2012). Investigating deaf children's vocabulary knowledge in British Sign Language. *Language Learning, 62*(4), 1024–1051. https://doi.org/10.1111/j.1467-9922.2011.00670.x

Mann, W., Peña, E. D., & Morgan, G. (2015). Child modifiability as a predictor of language abilities in deaf children who use American Sign Language. *American Journal of Speech-Language Pathology/American Speech-Language-Hearing Association, 24*(3), 374–385. https://doi.org/10.1044/2015_AJSLP-14-0072

Mann, W., Roy, P., & Morgan G. (2015). Adaptation of a vocabulary test from British Sign Language to American Sign Language. *Language Testing*, 33, 3–22. https://doi.org/10.1177/0265532215575627

Mason, K., Rowley, K., Marshall, C. R., Atkinson, J. R., Herman, R., Woll, B., & Morgan, G. (2010). Identifying specific language impairment in deaf children acquiring British Sign Language: Implications for theory and practice. *British Journal of Developmental Psychology, 28*(1), 33–49. https://doi.org/10.1348/026151009X484190

McLeod, S., Verdon, S., Bowen, C., & International Expert Panel on Multilingual Children's Speech. (2013). International aspirations for speech-language pathologists' practice with multilingual children with speech sound disorders: Development of a position paper. *Journal of Communication Disorders, 46*(4), 375–387. https://doi.org/10.1016/j.jcomdis.2013.04.003

Mitchell, R. E., & Karchmer, M. A. (2004). Chasing the mythical ten percent: Parental hearing status of deaf and hard of hearing students in the United States. *Sign Language Studies*, *4*(2), 138–163. https://doi.org/10.1353/sls.2004.0005

Östling, R., Börstell, C., & Courtaux, S. (2018). Visual iconicity across sign languages: Large-scale automated video analysis of iconic articulators and locations. *Frontiers in Psychology*, *9*(725). https://doi.org/10.3389/fpsyg.2018.00725

Paradis, J. (2017). Parent report data on input and experience reliably predict bilingual development and this is not trivial. *Bilingualism: Language and Cognition*, *20*(01), 27–28. https://doi.org/10.1017/S136672891600033X

Paradis, J., Emmerzael, K., & Duncan, T. S. (2010). Assessment of English language learners: Using parent report on first language development. *Journal of Communication Disorders*, *43*(6), 474–497. https://doi.org/10.1016/j.jcomdis.2010.01.002

Peña, E. D., Gillam, R. B., & Bedore, L. M. (2014). Dynamic assessment of narrative ability in English accurately identifies language impairment in English language learners. *Journal of Speech, Language, and Hearing Research*, *57*(6), 2208–2220. https://doi.org/10.1044/2014_JSLHR-L-13-0151

Peña, E. D., Gillam, R. B., Malek, M., Ruiz-Felter, R., Resendiz, M., Fiestas, C., & Sabel, T. (2006). Dynamic assessment of school-age children's narrative ability: An experimental investigation of classification accuracy. *Journal of Speech, Language, and Hearing Research*, *49*(5), 1037–1057. https://doi.org/10.1044/1092-4388(2006/074)

Peña, E. D., Iglesias, A., & Lidz, C. S. (2001). Reducing test bias through dynamic assessment of children's word learning ability. *American Journal of Speech-Language Pathology/American Speech-Language-Hearing Association*, *10*(2), 138. https://doi.org/10.1044/1058-0360(2001/014)

Quinto-Pozos, D. (2014). *Multilingual aspects of signed language communication and disorder*. Multilingual Matters.

Quinto-Pozos, D., Singleton, J. L., & Hauser, P. C. (2017). A case of specific language impairment in a deaf signer of American Sign Language. *Journal of Deaf Studies and Deaf Education*, *22*(2), 204–218. https://doi.org/10.1093/deafed/enw074

Speech Pathology Australia. (2016). *Clinical guidelines: Working in a culturally and linguistically diverse society*. Speech Pathology Australia.

Thordardottir, E. (2010). Towards evidence-based practice in language intervention for bilingual children. *Journal of Communication Disorders*, *43*(6), 523–537. https://doi.org/10.1016/j.jcomdis.2010.06.001

White, A., & Tischler, S. (1999). Receptive sign vocabulary tests: Tests of single-word vocabulary or iconicity? *American Annals of the Deaf*, *144*(4), 334–338. https://doi.org/10.1353/aad.2012.0324

Williams, C. J., & McLeod, S. (2012). Speech-language pathologists' assessment and intervention practices with multilingual children. *International Journal of Speech-Language Pathology*, *14*(3), 292–305. https://doi.org/10.3109/17549507.2011.636071

Topic 7

Construct Issues in Second Language Assessments

7.1

Construct in Assessments of Spoken Language

Susy Macqueen

A *construct* can be considered two things: whatever an assessment is designed to find out about and whatever it actually finds out about. It is hoped, and often presumed, that these two things are the same; for example, if a test is designed to assess speaking ability, then it actually does find out about the test-taker's speaking ability. Thus, when we understand that a score is an indication of speaking ability, we do so by trusting that the assessment did actually find out about speaking ability. Moreover, we trust that the assessment found out about aspects of speaking ability that are relevant to the decisions the score is used for.

These aspects of language assessments—purpose, design, interpretation, and use—all depend fundamentally on the assessment construct.[1] They also concern different groups of stakeholders in different ways. The *design* might predominantly involve the actions of test developers with a technical view of construct or teachers working with specific stipulations about language ability from a curriculum. The *use* of a test construct might involve the actions of policy-makers or employers who have to interpret very general statements about constructs; for example, "spoken Standard Mandarin (Putonghua) proficiency" in the *Putonghua Shuiping Ceshi* (Zhang, 2013). Thus, an assessment construct is not a "black box" or a singular static entity. Rather, constructs comprise "spheres of activity" which involve different parties with various relationships to the assessment instrument. This chapter explores spoken language assessment constructs in terms of their theoretical, practical, and social dimensions and their associated spheres of activity. First, key concepts and issues relating to constructs in the assessment of speaking ability are set out. Theories of language ability as they apply to the assessment of spoken language are then discussed. Finally, the ways constructs are operationalized, communicated to, and understood by users, assessees, and other actors in assessment processes are offered as a multidimensional and holistic view of constructs across diverse stakeholder worlds.

Susy Macqueen, *Construct in Assessments of Spoken Language* In: *The Handbook of Language Assessment Across Modalities.* Edited by: Tobias Haug, Wolfgang Mann, and Ute Knoch, Oxford University Press. © Oxford University Press 2022. DOI: 10.1093/oso/9780190885052.003.0020

THE NOTION OF "CONSTRUCT" IN SPOKEN LANGUAGE ASSESSMENTS

Broadly speaking, language assessments are designed to find about "language ability" in a particular language variety or code (e.g., Standard Mandarin Chinese, American Sign Language). This means that there are two phenomena of interest inherent in any language assessment construct. One, *language ability*, is complex social, psychological, and cognitive phenomenon: "the capacity for creating and interpreting discourse" (Bachman & Palmer, 2010, p. 209). Language ability cannot simply be measured in the same way that, say, physical length can because length doesn't have to be elicited by a test method. The other phenomenon, *language variety*, refers to linguistic patterns (e.g., morphosyntactic, lexical, phonological, discoursal) which have resulted from social, historical, political, economic, cognitive, and physiological processes. People's linguistic patterns are complex and dynamic (Beckner et al., 2009), and assessment constructs prioritize some usage patterns over others. Thus, language assessment constructs are imbued with social values (Shohamy, 2001). Because language assessment constructs comprise these two, highly complex phenomena, they are especially vulnerable to unfairness and method effects.

Assessing speaking ability poses particular challenges. Spoken language is by nature more prone to variability than written language, which has a much more restricted range of signs and symbols and is more constrained formally in terms of correctness. Just considering one aspect of spoken language, pronunciation, we find that even within one named language variety, it is exquisitely patterned across geographical space, age, and social strata, to name a few of the well-researched variables (e.g., Labov, 1966; Trudgill, 1974). Spoken language can also be very fluid in the use of linguistic resources across named language boundaries, such as in code-switching and other multilingual practices. Although spoken language is usually less bound by prescribed notions of correctness than written language, in "standard language cultures," where an idealization of a particular language variety has gained a high-status role across social, educational, and political domains, the written form is so entrenched in the social psyche that there is a general tendency "to evaluate spoken usage on the model of written usage" (Milroy, 1999; Milroy & Milroy, 1999, p. 47).

Assessment constructs are often identified in very broad terms, such as "Japanese language speaking ability." Over the years, language assessment developers and researchers have come up with various methods of observing evaluable behaviors which are considered indicative of some aspect of the theoretical construct that is understood to underlie the performance. For example, within the construct of "[Language] speaking ability," assessment designers often include *construct components* such as grammatical accuracy, fluency, vocabulary, pronunciation, and coherence/cohesion. Construct components are hypothesized to relate to one another and to the broader construct (Bachman, 1990, p. 257). Each construct component is operationalized through a method which elicits something observable and measurable. Thus, we have a theoretical construct level (e.g., spoken language competence and specified components or subconstructs) and an operational construct level (e.g., role-play and rating scale) (Bachman, 1990). Relationships are hypothesized at both a *theoretical level* (i.e., abstract, unobservable conceptualizations arising from theory/research) and an *operational level* (i.e., observable samples of performance constructed in assessment practices). Each of these will be elaborated in the following sections.

THEORETICAL CONSTRUCT

In any assessment situation, a method is used to find out about an ability that is theorized to exist. These processes occur regardless of whether the theory and method are explicit and conscious or not. Even in language assessment situations where no construct has been articulated or even consciously thought about, something (usually a sample of language use) is evaluated through some method. Imagine, for example, a situation in which a doctor needs to decide whether or not to request an interpreter to assist with a consultation (i.e., a future performance). The doctor would attempt to elicit some indication of the speaking ability of the patient, for example, through simple questions or conversation openings (i.e., a method), in order to gauge how likely it is that the consultation will be able to proceed so that all parties are able to deliver, comprehend, and negotiate the necessary information and, as a result, the patient's health concern can be appropriately treated (i.e., an assessment purpose). The "construct" in this situation would be something like "health-related language proficiency," which would be likely to include such things as the ability to understand and respond comprehensibly to questions about pain and symptoms in Language X. Although this assessment is purely practice-based, highly specific, and not linked to any articulation of theory or formal method, the doctor is engaging in the business of sampling in order to predict about an unobservable language ability in the unfolding consultation. The difference between this informal assessment event and an established language test with a strong validation agenda lies in the degree to which the ability of interest is explicitly theorized and the test method is systematized and standardized. As McNamara observes, "even practical approaches which try to eschew theory imply a theoretical position" (1995, p. 164). Thus, in most assessment situations, the reason that scores vary is presumed to be because of a *theoretical construct*, which may arise intuitively from experience—an unarticulated, "pre-theoretical" construct as in the medical consultation—or it may be extensively elaborated as a model of language ability. No matter what the state of its development, the theoretical construct is assumed to explain the variation in what is observed or sampled and is, therefore, always and only an assumption once it has taken on an operationalized form. Let us now consider some key models and approaches that have shaped understandings of theoretical constructs.

Theoretical Construct Models and Approaches

Theoretical models of language ability have been developed for the purposes of understanding what the capacity for communication is and how it occurs. Dell Hymes (1971/1972) aligned language ability with language use in social contexts, rather than the ideal forms of internal syntactic knowledge prioritized by Chomsky at the time (1965). Following Hymes's emphasis on language use in social context, several theorists developed proposals for how the capacity for language use might be analyzed for the purposes of language learning, teaching, and assessment (Bachman, 1990; Bachman & Palmer, 2010; Canale & Swain, 1980; Celce-Murcia, 2008; Douglas, 2000). Most of these proposals separate the capacity to use language into the *what* or knowledge components and the *how* or execution components, which relate to how language knowledge is mobilized in context (see comparative analysis in McNamara, 1995). All models encapsulate a view of language which (1) separates linguistic units into various, relatively basic elements such as grammar, vocabulary, and components of phonology and (2) includes some mobilization of these elements in broader discourse, represented in terms of intradiscoursal relationships such as cohesion and/or contextual relations such as appropriateness.

The well-established model proposed by Bachman (1990) and Bachman and Palmer (2010) of communicative language ability divides language knowledge (the "what" of language use) into *organizational knowledge* (including grammar, vocabulary, phonology, cohesion) and *pragmatic knowledge* (including the use of language for effect, such as delivering an insult or creating an imaginary world). The "how" of language use in this model is a set of metacognitive strategies which are mobilized to manage language use: setting goals, appraising a situation for the linguistic resources needed, and selecting content and language knowledge. While this and most models of communicative competence tend to emphasize the appropriate use of linguistic phenomena in context, Levelt's model of speaking (Levelt, 1993) is more concerned with "how" through modeling psycholinguistic processes. Models that derive from the communicative competence tradition tend to underpin assessment procedures that rely on human comprehension processes for scoring tasks which elicit episodes of relatively spontaneous speech (e.g., May, 2009; Wang et al., 2018). On the other hand, tests which elicit more constrained speaking samples (e.g., sentence repetition) and rely exclusively on computational scoring methods based on theories of human comprehension processes tend to refer to psycholinguistic processes, such as those described by Levelt (e.g., Van Moere, 2012).

The dynamic nature of spoken interaction poses a challenge for both theoretical models of language ability and their operationalization in test methods. The main issue is that the very activity of testing is based on an assumption that there is some degree of stability across an individual's ability elicited for evaluation in the assessment situation and the (future) manifestation of that ability in the relevant criterion or target domain. Much research and theory has pointed to the fact that there are a great many forces at work in oral assessment contexts which make it difficult to generalize about individual abilities beyond the test sample. These include the influence of interviewer behavior (Brown, 2003) and that of other interactants (Lazaraton & Davis, 2008) as well as the co-constructed nature of spoken performance (McNamara, 1997; Swain, 2001). The central point has been that models of language ability have not adequately attended to the social nature of talk, instead presuming spoken language to be sufficiently represented and judged as an individual cognitive ability that is portable across contexts. McNamara (1997) points to the multiple interactions which occur in the assessment context, not just between the humans involved, but the artifacts as well, such as the task, the rating scale, indeed, the whole process of interpretation. Chalhoub-Deville argues for the inseparability of ability from assessment context, termed: "ability—in language user—in context" (2003, p. 373). She suggests a rigorous embedding of context in theoretical models that underpin test design through a greater understanding of "the complex interaction of linguistic and nonlinguistic knowledge, cognitive, affective, and conative attributes engaged in particular situations" (p. 380).

Empirical work relevant to this challenge includes consideration of interactional behaviors such as turn-taking ability, listener backchannels, and eye contact (Al-Gahtani & Roever, 2011; Ross, 2018). Focusing on choice of language code, Kramsch and Whiteside's (2008) notion of "symbolic competence" is more far-reaching than the ability to "approximate or appropriate for oneself someone else's language": it denotes the ability to "shape the very context in which the language is learned and used" (p. 664). In their conceptualization, the language object is also dynamically construed. An individual's decisions about which language variety to use is "not dictated by some pre-existing and permanent value" of the variety, but rather emerges meaningfully from "subjective perceptions of shifting power dynamics within the interaction" (p. 664).

Also in the vein of a more dynamic communicative competence, Harding (2014) proposes the subconstruct component of "adaptability": "how a candidate copes in a novel or challenging language situation in real time" (p. 192), including the ability to move between different varieties of language, different domains of use, and changes in language use via technological innovation (p. 194). Similarly, Fulcher and Davidson propose "adaptivity," which occurs "as human beings engage in complex conversational mechanisms to make themselves understood to one another" (2007, p. 50). In this subconstruct, they include the ability to accommodate one's utterances to the language proficiency of an interlocutor by, for example, using simpler words or slowing down. This implies that being adaptive includes the capacity to assess the proficiency of an interlocutor within the dynamics of spoken interaction: an assessment within an assessment.

While theory and research are rising to the challenge of interaction between agents and artifacts in the assessment event, the theory of language that underpins the test construct lies fairly dormant. Identifying and distinguishing between construct components is difficult since language use is a complex phenomenon which does not reduce to simple component parts without losing its communicative quality (Beckner et al., 2009; Larsen-Freeman & Cameron, 2008). Despite this, reduction to language units is inherent in some way in most models and arguably even more so in assessment methods, both those based on theoretical models of language ability and those that have an unarticulated theoretical basis. Even distinctions that are well-entrenched in language assessment practice across receptive and productive skills have fuzzy and contestable boundaries. The constructs of grammar and vocabulary, for example, are often treated as separable and distinct, as evidenced in subconstructs such as "grammatical range and accuracy" and "lexical resource" (IELTS, 2018). However, determining whether a test item targets a feature of either grammar or vocabulary is not always possible, and some errors are difficult to analyze as distinctly lexical or grammatical (Alderson & Kremmel, 2013). Furthermore, much theory and research now attests to the existence of *formulaic language*, an amalgam of syntactic and lexical patterning, not merely as memorized chunks that appear at the early stages of language learning (evident in some rubric descriptors), but as a phenomenon which occurs at all levels of development (Macqueen & Knoch, 2020; Wray, 2008).

Finally, social values are embedded in constructs as much as in the uses and consequences of test use (Messick, 1989). *Grammatical accuracy* is a construct component in many speaking assessments, and the basic method is quantity of errors. The norms which serve as the ideal against which errors are determined are typically those of particular groups of native speakers (Housen & Kuiken, 2009). This points to the broader issue of societal power relations in the use of language assessments, including whose norms are used for judgment purposes and whose norms inhabit the high-status level of the target language domain (Davies et al., 2003; Knoch & Macqueen, 2020).

OPERATIONALIZED CONSTRUCT

A distinction is usually made between what is assessed (the theoretical construct) and how it is assessed (the operationalized construct). Bachman (1990) describes the process of defining constructs operationally as "determining how to isolate the construct and make it observable" (p. 43). Most theoretical speaking constructs are operationalized through tasks which elicit spoken language, the quality of which is judged in relation to a purpose or a prescribed standard. This involves two systematic procedures which play critical construct-determining roles: (1) the elicitation of a sample and (2) a judgment about its quality. Both of these are often broken down further, although the different components of the speaking ability might be unevenly distributed in tasks and scoring. For example, a test which contains a read-aloud task and a monologue on a familiar topic may prioritize (through task, scoring, or both), the construct component of *intelligibility* in the read-aloud task and *grammatical accuracy* in the monologue. The operationalization of construct through scoring procedures ranges from qualitative methods that use criteria and level descriptions to quantitative scores for predetermined units such as test items or countable language features. For example, the number and length of pauses, something that is both observable and quantifiable, might be hypothesized to relate to the construct component of "fluency" (Fulcher & Davidson, 2007).

As discussed earlier, recent theoretical discussions have argued for a greater awareness of the role and impact of the assessment context on the test construct. In this vein, it is useful to think of the context as being embedded in the *operationalized construct*, rather than the other way around. There are three layers of context: societal, infrastructural, and simulation (for a more detailed discussion, see Knoch & Macqueen, 2020). First, the broader societal context is embedded through the social value indexed by the language variety whose patterns are considered representative of subconstructs such as "grammatical accuracy." Second, the test infrastructure, for example, the task, the criteria, and rating scale, is the built environment in which a theoretical language ability can be made observable (Stern & Harley, 1992). Third, the operationalized construct emerges in the assessment moment from an individual's current linguistic and sociocognitive capacity in interaction with the specific assessment task and conditions (e.g., a question on the topic of "traditions" posed by an automated interlocutor) and the individual's state and circumstances (e.g., nervousness). This final layer of context is called the *simulation layer* since it is the moment in which a person takes on the identity and role of an assessee. Simulation occurs irrespective of how contextualized the assessment task is, provided that the assessee understands they are engaging in the act of being assessed. Construct operationalization is often considered at the infrastructural layer only, in the work of assessment designers. However, the operationalized construct (1) emerges from and regenerates in a societal layer, (2) is built in an infrastructural layer, and (3) is realized in a simulation layer. Thus, it is relevant to policy, design, impact, and validation.

Although there has been considerable scholarship on theoretical constructs, when a judgment is made about someone's language ability, some sort of construct operationalization happens irrespective of the explicitness or elaborateness of construct theorization. If there is an articulated theoretical construct, the operationalized construct is, ideally, congruent with it. While this is the intended relationship, it should not be assumed. The degree of congruence between theoretical and operationalized construct is the focus of test design and validation research. If something other than the intended theoretical construct is operationalized, then we have something interfering with the measurement which shouldn't be or something significant missing from it, respectively known as *construct irrelevant variance* and *construct under representation* (Messick, 1994).

CONSTRUCT DIMENSIONS AND SPHERES OF ACTIVITY

The discussion so far has focused on construct dimensions that are familiar in the assessment literature, which has long grappled with the problem of how to make unobservable abilities observable in order to measure them. However, language assessments have social lives, sometimes quite high-profile ones, where the social sorting job they do influences societal structure, as in the case of language tests in migration processes. As mechanisms which underpin social sorting, test constructs are boundary objects that communicate between social worlds in an understandable code (Macqueen et al., 2016). For example, the familiar scoring system of a recognized test communicates about an applicant's language ability to migration officials. As well as being mechanisms of communication in this way, assessments are also subject to interpretation by stakeholders (McNamara, 2012).

Stated and Perceived Constructs

Assessment practices are driven by educational and sociopolitical needs or mandates (Fulcher, 2010). As with any standard means of doing something, certain assessment methods and products become entrenched and trusted the more they are used. Commercial tests might be repurposed for new uses which are not necessarily in line with their theoretical constructs or intended purpose. Therefore, in policy-making, what the test provider says the test is testing—the *stated construct*—and whatever policy-makers understand the test to be testing—the *perceived construct*—are two highly consequential aspects of the discourse of test use (see Table 7.1.1).

The *stated construct* is the description of what is being measured by the assessment that is articulated to the range of stakeholders (test-takers, students, policy-makers, raters, teachers, etc.). The stated constructs of commercial tests are often vague and brief; for example, the *Test of Chinese as a Foreign Language: Speaking* (TOCFL Speaking) assesses "Chinese learners' non-academic speaking ability" (Steering Committee [SC-TOP], 2007), and stated constructs may be accompanied by an indication of the intended domain of relevance (e.g., "everyday life" in the case of TOCFL Speaking). Depending on the type of assessment, the stated construct and its elaborations can be found in explicit statements on test websites, in sample materials, in curriculum documents, in rating scale descriptions, and in teachers' communications to students.

The *perceived construct* refers to interpretations of a test construct. Stakeholders' interpretations of construct are filtered through a dynamic constellation of beliefs, experiences, knowledge, and attitudes about the nature of language/languages, language acquisition, and language assessments (Knoch & Macqueen, 2020). A distinction between stated and perceived constructs is necessary because beliefs about language and language tests are powerful and can override test providers' statements about construct and intended purpose.

Perceived constructs are relevant to many assessment spheres of activity (see Table 7.1.1). For instance, perceived constructs may be the focus of political debates (Macqueen & Ryan, 2019) and public consultations about test use (Pill & Harding, 2013). They are also demonstrable in institutional understandings of the meaning of the test scores (O'Loughlin, 2011), in raters' interpretations of rating scales (Zhang & Elder, 2011), and in raters' perceptions of how samples align to scales (Carey et al., 2011). Perceived constructs are also relevant to assessees' activity, behavior, and strategies. For instance, test-takers' motivation to prepare for a test can be affected by whether a test construct is perceived as relevant or not (Kim & Elder, 2015), and performance in a test might demonstrate perceptions of construct ideologies, such as monolingual norms (Rydell, 2015). Finally, test preparation may be based on teachers' perceptions of the "rules of the game," as separate from "language development" or the domain beyond the test (Saif et al., 2019, p. 13).

Spoken language assessments are especially vulnerable to bias resulting from perceived constructs due to the fact that listeners are highly sensitive to phonological differences, a sensitivity which persists

Table 7.1.1 Dimensions of constructs and their spheres of activity

Construct dimension	Definition	Spheres of activity
Stated construct	Description of what the assessment claims to assess and its intended interpretation and use/s	• Test descriptions and other available information (e.g., sample tests) • Curriculum documents, course descriptions • Teacher/institutional communication • Sanctioned assessment preparation activities (e.g., classroom activities explicitly aimed at preparation and official test preparation guides or texts) • Policy documents stipulating assessment focus, construct or framework • Rating scale or framework descriptors
Operationalized construct	What is actually elicited by the assessment method and experienced by an individual assessee in particular assessment circumstances at the time of assessment	• Actual performance of an individual assessee elicited by specific assessment form that emerges in relation to aspects of the immediate and broader context • Test specifications, assessment design, tasks, topics, test version, and other elements of assessment infrastructure in interaction with the assessee
Theoretical construct	Theoretical, underlying, unobservable ability which is assumed to explain differences in assessee responses and their classification (e.g., score) differences	• An ability (or ability component) theorized in academic literature and research (e.g., communicative competence) • An ability (or ability component) theorized through experience (e.g., specific language proficiency needed for understanding medical treatment risks) • An ability (or ability component) assumed to exist due to the fact that it is routinely assessed • Expectations of classification (e.g., score) differences
Perceived construct	What users understand is being assessed, the purpose the assessment is understood to be serving and beliefs and attitudes to language, language acquisition, language proficiency and (language) assessment which affect the perception of what is being assessed	• Discourse of stakeholders (e.g., political debate, media representations, institutional policies, talk about test use, descriptions and explanations about test, score meanings and uses) • Washback practices • Users' (e.g., raters', assessees') interpretations of scales and descriptors

Adapted from "Dimensions of constructs and their spheres of activity," Table 2.2, p. 49, *Assessing English for Professional Purposes*, Ute Knoch & Susy Macqueen, Routledge, 2020. Reproduced with permission.

even when other aspects of language (e.g., morphology) are native-like (Isaacs, 2018). Research in this area often focuses on the effects of perceived constructs (e.g., the effect of rater familiarity with the speech patterns of particular first language backgrounds). In fact, spoken language assessments are always affected by perceived constructs to some extent since all raters have their own "language lens" of attitudes, beliefs, and experiences (Knoch & Macqueen, 2020, p. 47), something that rater training aims to mitigate. There is also evidence to suggest that raters evaluate samples agentively, with conscious knowledge of their perceived constructs. For example, in a study of test raters who had Indian language backgrounds, Xi and Mollaun (2011) found that the raters were conscious of their familiarity with the Indian accent characteristics of the assessees and appeared to take a more analytic approach to rating these candidates' English in order to "correct" for their perceived constructs (p. 1244). In automated testing practices, perceived constructs may be embedded through processes such as the composition of corpora used to generate rating algorithms and machine training on human scoring (Bejar, 2012). They may also be limited by the "perception" of linguistic features that is possible by computational means. For example, segmental features of pronunciation may be more amenable to automated scoring (Isaacs, 2018), even though suprasegmental features such as prosody and word stress may be key in the subconstruct of intelligibility (Harding, 2017; Moyer, 1999). It is important to note that the perceptions embedded in machine scoring are not dynamic in the way that human raters' perceived constructs are. It is therefore essential that automated scoring methods have inbuilt safeguards such as monitoring and appeals processes that involve human raters.

The construct dimensions set out in Table 7.1.1 show the spheres of activity of each dimension. These spheres of activity (third column), while not exhaustive, give a sense of how far-reaching "construct activity" is. The spheres are also overlapping and messy: a dynamic network of activities by invested agents. A teacher's communication about an upcoming assessment, for instance, is activity related to both perceived and stated construct dimensions. However, separating the dimensions is a useful way of ensuring that important aspects of construct activity are not forgotten in assessment design, use, and validation. The nature and activities of each dimension and the congruence between them are ongoing questions for language assessment users, developers, and researchers.

IMPLICATIONS FOR PRACTICE

The theoretical configurations of language ability described here pose challenges for assessment designers and users in terms of the two objects of assessment we began with: *ability* and *language*. For ability, the challenge is to understand and evaluate situated ability where context is embedded in construct, rather than a separate variable (Larsen-Freeman & Cameron, 2008). For the language object, the challenge is to systematically elicit and evaluate linguistic repertoires relevant to the test purpose, rather than a contained, 'standard' language system. For example, a language test for doctors for skilled migration purposes might include code-switching ability, where a patient population would be best served by doctors who could use more than one language in consultations (Knoch & Macqueen, 2020). However, efforts toward the assessment of situated, dynamic, and emergent constructs of language ability have practical, theoretical, and sociopolitical challenges—the attraction of cheaper and faster but less social, automated test methods not least among them.

It might appear from the discussion so far that, in test development, elaborate theorizing lays the foundations for test method and development. In reality, few assessments have highly theorized constructs, and those that do tend to become more developed theoretically *after* the construct has emerged in operationalized form and validation efforts have begun. Most assessments are tethered intuitively to other proficiency structures such as established tests and frameworks in the case of standardized instruments and to prior assessment practice, curriculum documents, and state standards or benchmarks in the case of classroom-based methods. These established practices may or may not arise from articulated or tested models of ability. An analysis of construct dimensions shown in Table 7.1.1 can identify gaps in construct activity or its problematic aspects and enable congruent understandings across stakeholder groups.

FUTURE DIRECTIONS

The onward march of computational methods that recognize and analyze spoken data is an obvious direction in the assessment of speaking. Developments such as automated scoring, are sociotechnical: that is, they are an integration of social phenomena (e.g., language status, policy imperatives, market forces) and technical tools (e.g., audio recorder, bandwidth) (see Bijker, 1997). Sociotechnical developments give rise to new or different kinds of concerns relating to test fairness and impact. For example, test washback may be unproductive in terms of language learning if technical constraints result in relatively superficial aspects of spoken production as the primary score-bearing matter.

A rising challenge for operationalizing speaking constructs is the nature of "intelligibility" and its relationship to native speaker norms. Discussions on this topic highlight that *intelligibility* is often a more appropriate construct than *nativelikeness* (e.g., Harding, 2017; Levis, 2005). This is for two reasons: first, many assessments are taken for the purposes of communication in lingua franca contexts where native varieties are not necessarily the most intelligible, and, second, research in second language acquisition has shown that learners are unlikely to sound like first language speakers of a variety even in ideal learning circumstances (e.g., Moyer, 1999). The distinction between intelligibility and nativelikeness is troublesome because a perceived construct (i.e., the "language lenses" of raters and automated scoring algorithms) inhabits the space of a robust theoretical one (see discussions in Harding, 2013; Isaacs, 2018). To address this gap, the comprehension competence of the "listener" that lurks within existing assessment infrastructures such as rating scale descriptions, rater training, and automated scoring needs to be made explicit and then evaluated in relation to a generalized comprehension competence of the target domain.

A further challenge for theoretical constructs of speaking is the inclusion of formulaic language (or "formulaicity"). While research and linguistic theory have attested to the pervasiveness of lexicogrammatical formulae in fluent speech (e.g., Read & Nation, 2006; Wood, 2010; Wray, 2002), grammar and the lexicon are entrenched as separate phenomena in speaking assessments through the theoretical bias present in much second language acquisition research (discussed in Wray, 2002). Although formulaic language is difficult to operationalize due to its formal complexity and variability, there is scope in both human and automated rating methods for much greater attention to this phenomenon (e.g., Xu, 2018). Furthermore, explorations into the interaction between *intelligibility* and *formulaicity* offer the potential to reconfigure comprehension and production in a sociocognitive, usage-based perspective that is more congruent with the language variation found in domains of use.

Finally, there is a need to monitor and investigate the proliferation of stated constructs in the forms of frameworks and categorizations of standardized tests. There is a danger that radically simplified stated constructs obscure the specific nature of the operationalized constructs. Attention to the relationship between the stated, theoretical, operationalized, and perceived construct dimensions can provide a counterpoint to the increasing tendency to lump diverse assessment instruments and contexts together in alignment with "parent standards," such as the Common European Framework of Reference (CEFR; Council of Europe, 2001). A constructive direction for research is examining the discourse surrounding test use decisions and the adequacy of stated constructs for policy-making audiences.

CONCLUSION

This chapter has examined the notion of an assessment construct by first considering the nature of speaking as a means of communication and the main ways it is represented in assessments. We explored theories that guide assessment practices, even ad hoc ones, and we charted key approaches to competence and ability. From theory we turned to assessment practices. First, we encountered the societal, infrastructural, and simulation mechanisms through which an operationalized construct emerges. The conceptualization of an assessment construct was then broken into four dimensions: theoretical, operationalized, stated, and perceived. Seeing constructs in terms of the spheres of activity around four dimensions allows us to take a more holistic view of the building, selection, and impact of assessment constructs across diverse stakeholder worlds. By theorizing these activities as a dynamic network of construct-related activity, there may be a potential for more congruence between how people understand and use language assessments and the operationalized constructs that are experienced by assessees.

NOTE

1. In this chapter, "assessment" is used as the superordinate term for all types of assessment. "Test" refers to an instrument administered in secure, timed conditions, typically with different versions. Someone who is assessed is referred to as an "assessee" (a general term) or a "test-taker" for tests.

REFERENCES

Al-Gahtani, S., & Roever, C. (2011). Proficiency and sequential organization of L2 requests. *Applied Linguistics, 33*(1), 42–65. https://doi.org/10.1093/applin/amr031

Alderson, J. C., & Kremmel, B. (2013). Re–examining the content validation of a grammar test: The (im) possibility of distinguishing vocabulary and structural knowledge. *Language Testing, 30*(4), 535–556. https://doi.org/10.1177/0265532213489568

Bachman, L. F. (1990). *Fundamental considerations in language testing*. Oxford University Press.

Bachman, L. F., & Palmer, A. S. (2010). *Language assessment in practice*. Oxford University Press.

Beckner, C., Blythe, R., Bybee, J., Christiansen, M. H., Croft, W., Ellis, N. C., Holland, J., Ke, J., Larsen-Freeman, D., & Schoenemann, T. (2009). Language is a complex adaptive system: Position paper. *Language Learning, 59*(Supplement 1), 1–26. https://doi.org/10.1111/j.1467-9922.2009.00533.x

Bejar, I. I. (2012). Rater cognition: Implications for validity. *Educational Measurement: Issues and Practice, 31*(3), 2–9. https://doi.org/10.1111/j.1745-3992.2012.00238.x

Bijker, W. E. (1997). *Of bicycles, bakelites, and bulbs: Toward a theory of sociotechnical change*. Cambridge, Mass.: MIT Press.

Brown, A. (2003). Interviewer variation and the co–construction of speaking proficiency. *Language Testing, 20*(1), 1–25. https://doi.org/10.1191/0265532203lt242oa

Canale, M., & Swain, M. (1980). Theoretical bases of communicative approaches to second language teaching and testing. *Applied Linguistics, 1*(1), 1–47. https://doi.org/10.1093/applin/I.1.1

Carey, M. D., Mannell, R. H., & Dunn, P. K. (2011). Does a rater's familiarity with a candidate's pronunciation affect the rating in oral proficiency interviews? *Language Testing, 28*(2), 201–219. https://doi.org/10.1177/0265532210393704
Celce-Murcia, M. (2008). Rethinking the role of communicative competence in language teaching. In E. A. Soler & M. P. S. Jordà (Eds.), *Intercultural language use and language learning* (pp. 41–57). Springer.
Chalhoub-Deville, M. (2003). Second language interaction: Current perspectives and future trends. *Language Testing, 20*(4), 369–383. https://doi.org/10.1191/0265532203lt264oa
Chomsky, N. (1965). *Aspects of the theory of syntax*. MIT Press.
Council of Europe. (2001). *Common European Framework of Reference for Languages: Learning, Teaching, Assessment (CEFR)*. Modern Languages Division, Strasbourg. Cambridge University Press. https://rm.coe.int/1680459f97
Davies, A., Hamp–Lyons, L., & Kemp, C. (2003). Whose norms? International proficiency tests in English. *World Englishes, 22*(4), 571–584. https://doi.org/10.1111/j.1467-971X.2003.00324.x
Douglas, D. (2000). *Assessing languages for specific purposes*. Cambridge University Press.
Fulcher, G. (2010). *Practical language testing*. Hodder Education.
Fulcher, G., & Davidson, F. (2007). *Language testing and assessment: An advanced resource book*. Routledge.
Harding, L. (2013). Pronunciation assessment. In C. A. Chapelle (Ed.), *The encyclopedia of applied linguistics*. Wiley-Blackwell.
Harding, L. (2014). Communicative language testing: Current issues and future research. *Language Assessment Quarterly, 11*(2), 186–197. https://doi.org/10.1080/15434303.2014.895829
Harding, L. (2017). Validity in pronunciation assessment. In O. Kang & A. Ginther (Eds.), *Assessment in second language pronunciation* (pp. 30–48). Routledge.
Housen, A., & Kuiken, F. (2009). Complexity, accuracy, and fluency in second language acquisition. *Applied Linguistics, 30*(4), 461–473. https://doi.org/10.1093/applin/amp048
Hymes, D. H. (1971/1972). On communicative competence. In J. B. Pride & J. Holmes (Eds.), *Sociolinguistics: Selected readings* (pp. 269–293). Penguin.
IELTS. (2018). IELTS Speaking Band Descriptors. https://www.ielts.org/-/media/pdfs/speaking–band–descriptors.ashx?la=en
Isaacs, T. (2018). Shifting sands in second language pronunciation teaching and assessment research and practice. *Language Assessment Quarterly, 15*(3), 273–293. https://doi.org/10.1080/15434303.2018.1472264
Kim, H., & Elder, C. (2015). Interrogating the construct of aviation English: Feedback from test takers in Korea. *Language Testing, 32*(2), 129–149. https://doi.org/10.1177/0265532214544394
Knoch, U., & Macqueen, S. (2020). *Assessing English for professional purposes*. Routledge.
Kramsch, C., & Whiteside, A. (2008). Language ecology in multilingual settings. Towards a theory of symbolic competence. *Applied Linguistics, 29*(4), 645–671. https://doi.org/10.1093/applin/amn022
Labov, W. (1966). *The social stratification of English in New York City*. Center for Applied Linguistics.

Larsen-Freeman, D., & Cameron, L. (2008). *Complex systems and applied linguistics*. Oxford University Press.

Lazaraton, A., & Davis, L. (2008). A microanalytic perspective on discourse, proficiency, and identity in paired oral assessment. *Language Assessment Quarterly, 5*(4), 313–335. https://doi.org/10.1080/15434300802457513

Levelt, W. J. M. (1993). *Speaking: From intention to articulation*. MIT Press.

Levis, J. M. (2005). Changing contexts and shifting paradigms in pronunciation teaching. *TESOL Quarterly, 39*(3), 369–377. https://doi.org/10.2307/3588485

Macqueen, S., & Knoch, U. (2020). Adaptive imitation: Formulaicity and the words of others in L2 English academic writing. In G. G. Fogal & M. H. Verspoor (Eds.), *Complex dynamic systems theory and L2 writing development* (pp. 81–108). John Benjamins.

Macqueen, S., Pill, J., & Knoch, U. (2016). Language test as boundary object: Perspectives from test users in the healthcare domain. *Language Testing, 33*(2), 271–288. https://doi.org/10.1177/0265532215607401

Macqueen, S., & Ryan, K. (2019). Test mandate discourse: Debating the role of language tests in citizenship. In C. Roever & G. Wigglesworth (Eds.), *Social perspectives on language testing: Papers in honour of Tim McNamara* (pp. 55–71). Peter Lang.

May, L. (2009). Co–constructed interaction in a paired speaking test: The rater's perspective. *Language Testing, 26*(3), 397–421. https://doi.org/10.1177/0265532209104668

McNamara, T. (1995). Modelling performance: Opening Pandora's box. *Applied Linguistics, 16*(2), 159–179. https://doi.org/10.1093/applin/16.2.159

McNamara, T. (1997). 'Interaction' in second language performance assessment: Whose performance? *Applied Linguistics, 18*(4), 446–466. https://doi.org/10.1093/applin/18.4.446

McNamara, T. (2012). Language assessments as shibboleths: A poststructuralist perspective. *Applied Linguistics, 33*(5), 564–581. http://doi.org/10.1093/applin/ams052

Messick, S. (1989). Validity. In R. L. Linn (Ed.), *Educational measurement* (3rd ed., pp. 13–103). American Council on Education and Macmillan.

Messick, S. (1994). The interplay of evidence and consequences in the validation of performance assessments. *Educational Researcher, 23*(2), 13–23. https://doi.org/10.3102/0013189X023002013

Milroy, J. (1999). The consequences of standardisation in descriptive linguistics. In T. Bex & R. J. Watts (Eds.), *Standard English: The widening debate* (pp. 16–39). Routledge.

Milroy, J., & Milroy, L. (1999). *Authority in language: Investigating standard English* (4th ed.). Routledge.

Moyer, A. (1999). Ultimate attainment in L2 phonology: The critical factors of age, motivation, and instruction. *Studies in Second Language Acquisition, 21*(1), 81–108. https://doi.org/10.1017/S0272263199001035

O'Loughlin, K. (2011). The interpretation and use of proficiency test scores in university selection: How valid and ethical are they? *Language Assessment Quarterly, 8*(2), 146–160. https://doi.org/10.1080/15434303.2011.564698

Pill, J., & Harding, L. (2013). Defining the language assessment literacy gap: Evidence from a parliamentary inquiry. *Language Testing, 30*(3), 381–402. https://doi.org/10.1177/0265532213480337

Read, J., & Nation, I. S. P. (2006). *An investigation of the lexical dimension of the IELTS Speaking Test by measuring lexical output, variation and sophistication, and the use of formulaic language* (vol. 6). IELTS Australia and British Council Research Report Series.
Ross, S. (2018). Listener response as a facet of interactional competence. *Language Testing*, *35*(3), 357–375. https://doi.org/10.1177/0265532218758125
Rydell, M. (2015). Performance and ideology in speaking tests for adult migrants. *Journal of Sociolinguistics*, *19*(4), 535–558.
Saif, S., Ma, J., May, L., & Cheng, L. (2019). Complexity of test preparation across three contexts: Case studies from Australia, Iran and China. *Assessment in Education: Principles, Policy & Practice*, 1–18. https://doi.org/10.1080/0969594X.2019.1700211
Shohamy, E. (2001). *The power of tests: A critical perspective on the uses of language tests*. Longman.
Steering Committee for the Test of Proficiency–Huayu. (2007). TOCFL Speaking: About the test. https://www.sc–top.org.tw/english/SP/test1.php
Stern, H. H., & Harley, B. (1992). *Issues and options in language teaching*. Oxford University Press.
Swain, M. (2001). Examining dialogue: Another approach to content specification and to validating inferences drawn from test scores. *Language Testing*, *18*(3), 275–302. https://doi.org/10.1177/026553220101800302
Trudgill, P. (1974). *The social differentiation of English in Norwich*. Cambridge University Press.
Van Moere, A. (2012). A psycholinguistic approach to oral language assessment. *Language Testing*, *29*(3), 325–344. https://doi.org/10.1177/0265532211424478
Wang, Z., Zechner, K., & Sun, Y. (2018). Monitoring the performance of human and automated scores for spoken responses. *Language Testing*, *35*(1), 101–120. https://doi.org/10.1177/0265532216679451
Wood, D. (2010). *Formulaic language and second language speech fluency: Background, evidence and classroom applications*. Continuum.
Wray, A. (2002). *Formulaic language and the lexicon*. Cambridge University Press.
Wray, A. (2008). *Formulaic language: Pushing the boundaries*. Oxford University Press.
Xi, X., & Mollaun, P. (2011). Using raters from India to score a large-scale speaking test. *Language Learning*, *61*(4), 1222–1255. https://doi.org/10.1111/j.1467-9922.2011.00667.x
Xu, J. (2018). Measuring "spoken collocational competence" in communicative speaking assessment. *Language Assessment Quarterly*, *15*(3), 255–272. https://doi.org/10.1080/15434303.2018.1482900
Zhang, Q. (2013). Language policy and ideology: Greater China. In R. Bayley, R. Cameron, & C. Lucas (Eds.), *The Oxford handbook of sociolinguistics*. (pp. 563–586). Oxford University Press.
Zhang, Y., & Elder, C. (2011). Judgments of oral proficiency by non–native and native English speaking teacher raters: Competing or complementary constructs? *Language Testing*, *28*(1), 31–50. https://doi.org/10.1177/0265532209360671

7.2

Construct in Assessments of Signed Language

Tobias Haug

Descriptions of test constructs in second signed language assessment, such as vocabulary knowledge, are rare and far from receiving the attention by the field of signed language test research that they deserves. Detailing the construct in second signed language assessment poses a challenge for obvious reasons: only very few published studies on signed language tests for adult learners are available, and none of them focuses on construct-related issues. Equally, there is a shortage of operationally used test instruments that are accessible for review.

A small number of available signed language tests and assessment procedures are used in tertiary education, for example, to evaluate the signing skills of students in signed language interpreter training programs. However, these tests are often used exclusively by the specific program (usually offered by a university), with limited or no access from outside the university. Such assessment instruments have not always been validated in a systematic way. In the field of signed language teaching and learning in tertiary education in Europe, there is an ongoing process to implement the Common European Framework of Reference (CEFR) (Council of Europe, 2001) and, consequently, the CEFR is used as a model to define signed language proficiency (and thus contributes to the construct of a test) (see Chapter 7.1).

In the following sections, I (1) review published studies on second signed language assessment, focusing specifically on construct representation; (2) discuss tests that are used for hiring and promotion; (3) provide an example of how to define the construct for a signed language test; and (4) present future directions in this field.

CONSTRUCT REPRESENTATION IN SECOND SIGNED LANGUAGE ASSESSMENT SERVING DIFFERENT (GENERAL) PURPOSES

Anecdotally, we know that, in the planning stage of test development, the construct is often defined rather vaguely as part of the targeted

Tobias Haug, *Construct in Assessments of Signed Language* In: *The Handbook of Language Assessment Across Modalities*. Edited by: Tobias Haug, Wolfgang Mann, and Ute Knoch, Oxford University Press. © Oxford University Press 2022. DOI: 10.1093/oso/9780190885052.003.0021 linguistic structure (e.g., vocabulary), modality (comprehension, production, or interaction), or test method (e.g., a Yes/No vocabulary test which focuses on vocabulary size). Instead of being addressed explicitly in published documentation on signed language assessment, it tends to be "implied." By "implied" I mean that either the name of a test also represents the tested construct (e.g., "vocabulary size test" for Swiss German Sign Language/*Deutschschweizerische Gebärdensprache* [DSGS]; Haug et al., 2019) or the targeted, linguistic structures of the test (e.g., aspect of morphology and syntax, as in the American Sign Language [ASL] Comprehension Test; Hauser et al., 2015).

Since most test discussed in this chapter are primarily used within the context of research projects (e.g., Sentence Repetition Test for ASL) or as part of training programs in institutions of tertiary education, no public information is available about these tests for test-takers. Instead, such information may be shared exclusively within the program (i.e., prior to an exam of signed language proficiency). An exception is the Sign Language Proficiency Interview (SLPI), which has public information available at the website of the National Technical Institute of the Deaf (NTID), a college of the Rochester Institute of Technology (RIT) (see Chapter 9.2 for more information on the SLPI).

In what follows, I review published studies of second signed language assessment to investigate how the construct representation is addressed in these tests. For example, Bochner and colleagues (Bochner et al., 2016) while discussing validity evidence of the ASL Discrimination Test (ASL-DT) address the issue of the construct. The ASL-DT targets receptive skills to discriminate phonological and morphophonological contrasts in ASL. Bochner et al. argue that a test of (morpho)phonological contrasts can serve as a proxy for overall ASL proficiency and is not focusing on subcomponents that make up ASL proficiency, such as vocabulary knowledge or grammar. They build their argument on a review of second (spoken) language studies addressing various aspects and their relations to spoken language proficiency (the term "spoken language" is not used in the sense of the subskill "speaking" but as contrast to the different modality of signed languages). Even though the construct of the ASL-DT is not derived from signed language studies (because of the lack of such studies), it frames and defines the construct based on empirical studies of spoken language proficiency. There are plans to include the ASL-DT in a larger ASL test battery to be used to assess the ASL proficiency of staff and faculty of the NTID (J. Bochner, personal communication, May 13, 2019).

Another example of a test for assessing a signed language as second language (L2) is the ASL Comprehension Test (ASL-CT) by Hauser and colleagues (Hauser et al., 2015). This test is primarily used for research purposes. The target group(s) of the ASL-CT are adult users of ASL with varying signing skills. The ASL-CT can be used, for example, in studies where ASL skills are an important variable for the inclusion in studies that, for example, look at the age of access to ASL and ASL skills or for neuroimaging studies (Hauser et al., 2015). While Hauser and colleagues do not mention the construct of the ASL-CT explicitly, it is implied through their discussion of the target linguistic structures of ASL that are represented in items of receptive ASL skills (i.e., morphology and syntax).

The same is true for another signed language test, the ASL Sentence Repetition Test (ASL-SRT; Hauser et al., 2008). The ASL-SRT is used as an instrument to assess ASL proficiency, targeting different groups of ASL users. The test represents specific aspects of (manual and nonmanual) morphology and syntax that are represented in the stimuli sentences. The developers state that the ASL-SRT can be used as an instrument to test global ASL proficiency. This could be understood as the construct of the ASL-SRT even though the authors do not explicitly frame "ASL proficiency" within a model of communicative language ability (CLA; e.g., Bachman, 1990) as the basis that defines the construct theoretically.

While the three tests discussed so far are more indirect measures of signed language proficiency, the SLPI is a more direct measure of signed language proficiency (Newell et al., 1983) that assesses the communicative competence or functional competence of an adult learner of ASL (cf. Chapter 9.2 for a more detailed description of the instrument). As with the other signed language assessments, the construct of the SLPI is not discussed explicitly but rather implied in the instrument's name and description. Different functional language descriptors on a rating scale define different ASL skills at 11 levels. This rating scale and documentation on how to use the rating scale is publicly available. Because the rating scale usually serves as an operationalization of the test construct, it provides a starting point for investigating the test construct more broadly. An adapted version of the SLPI also exists for Sign Language of the Netherlands (*Nederlandse Gebarentaal* [NGT]; Van den Broek-Laven et al., 2014). This adapted version, the NGT-Functional Assessment (NGT-FA), is aligned to the six levels of the CEFR (Council of Europe, 2001) and also could be interpreted as the construct, described in the "regular" can-do descriptors of the CEFR scale used (Scale for Fluency).

A test instrument similar to the SLPI is the ASL Proficiency Interview (ASLPI), which was developed at Gallaudet University (2020) (cf. Chapter 9.2 for more information about the instrument). In contrast to the previously mentioned assessments, the ASLPI is included in the Praxis Program of the Educational Testing Service (ETS) as a requirement for "candidates who plan to teach American Sign Language (ASL) as a language other than English [and for] candidates who plan to teach students who are deaf and hard of hearing" (Educational Testing Service, 2019) in the state of Connecticut. The ASLPI is delivered and scored by trained test administrators and raters from Gallaudet University. On the ASLPI's website (Educational Testing Service, 2019), the test-takers (or other interested parties) are informed that the test is "a holistic language evaluation used to determine global ASL proficiency." This can be interpreted as the construct of the ASLPI. The ASLPI operates on 11 different levels, ranging from "0," "0+," "1," "1+," to "5" (there is no "5+"). For each level a detailed description is provided at the Gallaudet University website (see Gallaudet University, 2020).

Finally, Haug (2017) developed two vocabulary size tests for DSGS, an L1/L2 translation test, and a yes/no test. He defines the construct as the "size of vocabulary knowledge of beginning adult learners of DSGS at the level of A1 [according to the CEFR]" (p. 21). Even though the construct is defined explicitly, it is not framed within a model of CLA nor does it use scales and descriptors of a language framework like the CEFR.

Two things become clear from this description: (1) explicit construct descriptions are rarely available for signed language assessments, and (2) many signed language assessments (with the exception of the SLPI) often draw on more indirect measures of language proficiency (i.e., are more cognitive).

CONSTRUCT REPRESENTATION IN TESTS OF SECOND SIGNED LANGUAGE ASSESSMENT FOR SPECIFIC PURPOSES

In the field of testing languages for specific purposes, "the test content and test method are derived from an analysis of a specific language use situation" (Douglas, 2000, p. 1). "Language for specific purposes" refers to a specific language use domain, such as air traffic controllers or the business domain (Douglas, 2000). This notion should equally apply for specific purposes in signed language assessment.

Transferring the idea of language for specific purposes to signed language assessment, persons who are planning to become teachers of the deaf and who will be using ASL at work should be assessed with an instrument that serves this specific purpose. For example, a prospective teacher of the deaf should not only have general high ASL proficiency, but he or she should be able to, for example, use the appropriate ASL register to communicate with deaf students in the school context effectively or use ASL signs that are appropriate for deaf students.

Linking this notion to the previously presented ASLPI, it is apparent that the ASLPI is an assessment instrument for more general purposes (i.e., assessing a global ASL proficiency) and thus does not test the specific ASL skills of prospective teachers of the deaf. The general construct of ASL proficiency, as stated at the ETS website, is represented in the testing method and the scoring instrument of the ASLPI.

ETS also provides within its Praxis Program the ASL Assessments for prospective teachers of the deaf in the state of Georgia (GACE, 2017). This assessment includes two test formats: the first is a computer-delivered test that contains mostly multiple-choice questions, the second one is the ASLPI. As for the first test format (Test 1), it is clearly defined into different content subareas, all of which represent objectives specific for teachers of deaf children: "Objective 2: Demonstrates knowledge of language as a means to transmitting culture and demonstrates knowledge of theories of second–language learning" (GACE, 2017, p. 3). Based on the provided information on the ETS website, it is not clear, but it can be assumed, that Test 1 is rather a knowledge test specifically for the field of teaching deaf children and that Test 2 assesses globally ASL skills using the ASLPI. Based on the available information about Test 1, it is not entirely clear if the construct of this test assesses content knowledge of becoming a teacher for the deaf (which would not be a language for specific purpose testing) and/or a language for specific purpose test (e.g., "Objective 4B: Demonstrates knowledge of the phonological structure of American Sign Language, including phonological parameters; i.e., handshape, movement, location, palm orientation, and nonmanual signals"; GACE, 2017, p. 5).

Revisiting the SLPI, at the NTID's Academic Affairs website[1] are guidelines available that clearly describe the need for faculty to be able to communicate in ASL for both "work and social topics" (NTID, 2018, p. 10–11), assessed by the SLPI. The NTID defines a level of "advanced" skills as the minimum level of ASL proficiency for this purpose (i.e., the 8th level out of 11 proficiency levels, the 11th level being the highest). The SLPI is used here, for example, for promotion to the rank of tenured faculty. As such, the SLPI's purpose is clearly that of an instrument to assess ASL skills for more general purposes. The documents of the NTID's Academic Affairs website define the necessary skills also in more global terms (i.e., work and social topics).

Two observations can be made related to the notion of specific purpose testing: (1) while the ASLPI is a global measure of ASL proficiency, it is used to assess the specific ASL skills required to work as a teacher of the deaf (i.e., the construct and purpose do not match); and (2) the SLPI, as used at the NTID, is a global assessment as well, but is also used as a more global assessment. Here the purpose and construct match.

AN EXAMPLE OF CONSTRUCT DEFINITION FOR A SIGNED LANGUAGE TEST

In this section, I define the construct of vocabulary knowledge within CLA (Bachman, 1990), but also define what the lexicon of a signed language might look like in order to describe the construct in more concrete terms.

Bachman (1990) and Bachman and Palmer (1996) define CLA along two interacting components (and subcomponents): *language knowledge* and *strategic competence* (see also Chapter 7.1). Bachman and Palmer further divide language knowledge into *organizational knowledge* and *pragmatic knowledge*. Both components are further subdivided; the subcomponents of organizational knowledge are *grammatical knowledge* and *textual knowledge*. Grammatical knowledge is further subdivided into *vocabulary*, *morphology* (only in Bachman, 1990), *syntax*, and *phonology/graphology*. Textual knowledge is subdivided into *cohesion* and *rhetorical organization*. The focus here is on defining the construct of vocabulary knowledge within this model of CLA as one component of grammatical knowledge. To do so, empirical studies on the signed language lexicon will be reviewed as the basis to investigate if the CLA model's component of vocabulary is also applicable to signed languages. In theory, the whole model could be applied to signed languages, but it was decided to focus here on vocabulary knowledge only. Bachman's CLA has been chosen because it is known to be one of the state-of-the-art models of CLA (Alderson & Banerjee, 2002). The construct definition was defined during the development of two vocabulary size tests for DSGS (Haug, 2017).

Signed Language Vocabulary

With regard to the signed language lexicon, Johnston and Schembri (2007) proposed a model for the organization of the mental lexicon in signed languages based on their research on Australian Sign Language (Auslan). This model divides the mental lexicon into a *native* and a *non–native* signed language lexicon. The native lexicon is further divided into a *conventional* and a *productive lexicon.* The conventional (or *established*) lexicon consists of signs (lexical types) that have a stable form–meaning relationship; for example, the German Sign Language (*Deutsche Gebärdensprache*, DGS) sign AUTO ("car"), which can be used in different contexts without a change in meaning (König et al., 2012).

The productive lexicon is considerably different and does not consist of an easy-to-determine number of signs. Sign forms that can be labeled as "productive" are realized and understood in a given context to convey a specific meaning. The signs themselves are not conventionalized, although their sublexical units (especially the handshapes) are. The sublexical units of productive signs are combined in a context-specific way to convey, for example, the meaning of "a person is approaching me." To represent the concept of *person*, the signer needs to select a specific handshape (often a single upright index finger) and the location, movement, and orientation of the hand, then transmit the meaning of how and from where the person is approaching and with what kind of path (straight, wavy, etc.). Accordingly, when the sign is produced in a different location with a different direction and manner, the meaning can change from "a person comes straight at me" to "meandering slowly away." Because of the multiple possibilities for choosing the parameters of the form, no citation entry in the mental lexicon is possible. That is, no base form exists for productive signs. This is why productive forms, while used extensively in actual signing, often do not appear in (printed or electronic) signed language lexicons.

The number of conventional sign types of a signed language is difficult to determine: estimates range from 2,500 to 5,000 signs for Auslan and DGS, respectively (Ebbinghaus & Heßmann, 2000; Johnston & Schembri, 1999). Since there is a potentially large number of context-specific meanings, the size of the productive lexicon cannot be determined.

The non-native lexicon describes the parts of a signed language where, for example, loan signs from other signed languages are conceptualized, which (through the process of lexicalization) may eventually become part of the native conventional lexicon.

Summarizing this short literature review and applying it to the CLA model, it can be said that within the domain of grammatical knowledge, the subcomponent of vocabulary used in spoken languages can be equally applied to signed languages, considering the conventional lexicon only. This has been applied in the aforementioned vocabulary tests for DSGS. It becomes even more complex when the construct of a vocabulary test is broadened to include also signs from the productive lexicon, which also touches on signed language morphology.

In this chapter, I reviewed existing signed language tests and raised the issue of how the construct is represented in these tests—mostly implicitly. Additionally, I presented an example how the construct of a vocabulary size test for DSGS could be defined.

FUTURE DIRECTIONS

One important issue for future research related to the construct of second signed language assessment is that the construct of signed language tests needs to be addressed in the test specifications or other available information of the test. Additionally, future research should also address how "signed language proficiency" can be defined on theoretical grounds. One possibility could be to define signed language proficiency by applying a model of CLA (Bachman, 1990) or derive the construct from scales of the CEFR that have been aligned to signed languages (Leeson et al., 2016). It has become a more common practice to develop signed language tests with CEFR descriptors serving as constructs. The lack of a defined construct might have a direct impact on the validity of a test; that is, "construct validity concerns the extent to which performance on tests is consistent with predictions that we make on the basis of a theory of abilities, or construct" (Bachman, 1990, pp. 254–255).

NOTE

1. https://www.rit.edu/ntid/president/academic–affairs

REFERENCES

Alderson, J. C., & Banerjee, J. (2002). Language testing and assessment (Part 2). *Language Teaching*, *35*(2), 79–113. https://doi.org/10.1017/S0261444802001751

Bachman, L. F. (1990). *Fundamental considerations in language testing*. Oxford University Press.

Bachman, L. F., & Palmer, A. (1996). *Language testing in practice*. Oxford University Press.

Bochner, J. H., Samar, V. J., Hauser, P. C., Garrison, W. M., Searls, J. M., & Sanders, C. A. (2016). Validity of the American Sign Language discrimination test. *Language Testing*, *33*(4), 473–495. https://doi.org/10.1177/0265532215590849

Council of Europe. (2001). *Common European Framework of Reference for languages: Learning, teaching, assessment*. Cambridge University Press; Council of Europe.

Douglas, D. (2000). *Assessing language for specific purposes*. Cambridge University Press.

Ebbinghaus, H., & Heßmann, J. (2000). Leben im Kommunikationskonflikt: Zur Ungleichsprachigkeit Hörender und Gehörloser [Livening in a conflict of communication: Differences in the languages between deaf and hearing people]. In E. Hess–Lüttich & H. W. Schmitz (Eds.), *Botschaften verstehen: Kommunikationstheorie und Zeichenpraxis. Festschrift für Helmut Richter* (pp. 47–66). Peter Lang.

Educational Testing Service. (2019). About the American Sign Language proficiency interview. https://www.ets.org/praxis/ct/aslpi/

GACE. (2017). GACE American Sign Language Assessment Test at a Glance. http://gace.ets.org/s/pdf/gace_taag_american_sign_language.pdf

Gallaudet University. (2020). The American Sign Language proficiency interview. https://www.gallaudet.edu/the-american-sign-language-proficiency-interview

Haug, T. (2017). *Development and evaluation of two vocabulary tests for Swiss German Sign Language*. Master thesis, Lancaster University. https://doi.org/10.13140/RG.2.2.25397.17129

Haug, T., Ebling, S., Boyes Braem, P., Tissi, K., & Sidler–Miserez, S. (2019). Sign language learning and assessment in German Switzerland: Exploring the potential of vocabulary size tests for Swiss German Sign Language. *Language Education & Assessment*, *2*(1), 20–40. https://doi.org/10.29140/lea.v2n1.85

Hauser, P. C., Paludneviciene, R., Riddle, W., Kurz, K. B., Emmorey, K., & Contreras, J. (2015). American Sign Language comprehension test: A tool for sign language researchers. *Journal of Deaf Studies and Deaf Education*, *21*(1), 64–69. https://doi.org/10.1093/deafed/env051

Hauser, P., Supalla, T., & Bavelier, D. (2008). American Sign Language sentence reproduction test: Development and implications. In R. Müller de Quadros (Ed.), *Sign languages: Spinning and unraveling the past, present and future.*

TISLR9, forty five papers and three posters from the 9th. Theoretical Issues in Sign Language Research Conference (pp. 160–172). Editora Arara Azul.

Johnston, T., & Schembri, A. (1999). On defining lexeme in a signed language. *Sign Language & Linguistics, 2*(2), 115–185. https://doi.org/10.1075/sll.2.2.03joh

Johnston, T., & Schembri, A. (2007). *Australian Sign Language: An introduction to sign language linguistics*. Cambridge University Press.

König, S., Konrad, R., & Langer, G. (2012). Lexikon: Der Wortschatz der DGS [Lexicon: The vocabulary of German Sign Language]. In H. Eichmann, M. Hansen, & J. Heßmann (Eds.), *Handbuch Deutsche Gebärdensprache: Sprachwissenschaftliche und anwendungsbezogene Perspektiven* (pp. 111–164). Signum.

Leeson, L., Van den Bogaerde, B., Rathmann, C., & Haug, T. (2016). *Sign languages and the Common European Framework of Reference for Languages common reference level descriptors*. Council of Europe.

Newell, W., Caccamise, F., Boardman, K., & Ray Holcomb, B. (1983). Adaptation of the Language Proficiency Interview (LPI) for assessing sign communicative competence. *Sign Language Studies, 41*, 311–347.

NTID. (2018). NTID policy on promotion in rank of tenured faculty. https://www.rit.edu/ntid/sites/rit.edu.ntid/files/acadaffairs/ntid_policy_on_promotion_in_rank_of_tenured_faculty_march_2018_revised_9_10_18_1.pdf

Van den Broek–Laven, A., Boers–Visker, E., & Van den Bogaerde, B. (2014). Determining aspects of text difficulty for the Sign Language of the Netherlands (NGT) Functional Assessment instrument. *Papers in Language Testing and Assessment—Special Issue, 1*, 53–75.

7.3

Discussion of Issues Related to Assessment Constructs in Spoken and Signed Languages

Susy Macqueen and Tobias Haug

Spoken language assessments have had a relatively long incubation in educational and other domains. This has allowed common understandings to develop about what spoken communication is and how it can be assessed. In contrast, signed language assessment constructs have been emerging as the demand for assessment instruments has grown in research and educational contexts. Assessing signed languages draws attention to assessment practices and understandings that are entrenched and taken-for-granted in the assessment of spoken languages. In this discussion, we highlight some of the theoretical, ideological, and practical challenges for assessing signed and spoken language abilities.

CHALLENGES FOR SPOKEN ASSESSMENT CONSTRUCTS: IDEOLOGIES, THEORIES, AND MINDSETS

Underpinning the assessment of standard spoken languages is a "literacy mindset" which has well-formed sentences at its core. As minority languages that do not have a widely used written forms (Boyes Braem, 2012), the assessment of signed language offers insights into the assumptions that underlie many spoken language assessments. "Standard" spoken languages, such as *Pǔtōnghuà* (Standard Chinese) or British English, are varieties of language which have become codes of education and government and are strongly tied to written forms (Haugen, 1966). It is their high social status and economic value which tend to make them popular choices for second language (L2) learning and hence L2 assessment. The anchoring of standard languages in their written forms creates a sense that a standard language is uniform, logical, and correct (Milroy & Milroy, 2012). The commonly used speaking criterion of *grammatical accuracy*, therefore, arises from an understanding of acceptable morphosyntactic regularities in target language usage, as well as the notion of a written sentence as the fundamental

Susy Macqueen and Tobias Haug, *Discussion of Issues Related to Assessment Constructs in Spoken and Signed Languages* In: *The Handbook of Language Assessment Across Modalities.* Edited by: Tobias Haug, Wolfgang Mann, and Ute Knoch, Oxford University Press. © Oxford University Press 2022. DOI: 10.1093/oso/9780190885052.003.0022 unit. Thus, we encounter descriptions such as: "produces basic sentence forms and some correct simple sentences but subordinate structures are rare" for Band 4 of the Grammatical Range and Accuracy criterion in the International English Language Testing System (IELTS) speaking scale (IELTS, 2018). Similarly, tasks that are designed around the notion of "complete sentences," such as read-aloud or sentence completion tasks have a writing-to-speak premise rather than a spoken one. Furthermore, the anchoring of spoken assessment in its written form is evident in the fact that spoken language is presumed to be assessable through both auditory and written modes. In auditory modes, a human rater listens to a test recording, and, in written ones, test scores are based on the analysis of transcripts that have been generated through automated speech recognition. Unlike 'standard' spoken languages, signed languages are not tethered to written notions of correctness. Therefore, signed language constructs can model how the modes of speaking and writing might be disassociated so that spoken language can be assessed in its own terms.

A challenge for L2 spoken language assessment is to determine gradations of accuracy that are not beholden to written forms. At one end of a comprehensibility scale are spoken patterns that are incomprehensible to the proficient mass of target language speakers (regardless of whether it is their first language [L1] or L2). At the other end are spoken patterns that are completely comprehensible but different from the target (standard) language variety, either in the patterns of groups who speak a close variety as an L1 or in the variation of groups of L2 users. Although many theorists have interrogated the ownership of spoken norms that are accorded the highest value in rating scales and scoring algorithms, truly decoupling spoken language assessment from standard written forms requires us to "think outside the sentence."

There are several fruitful lines of inquiry which can help reconfigure spoken language theoretical constructs. Auer (2009) has pointed out that structuralism has resulted in the conceptualization of any syntactic structure as a "finished product," rather than an "emerging syntactic gestalt," and he offers an analysis of how syntax evolves in a time-bound manner in interaction (p. 1, 6). McCarthy and Carter (2002) argue for greater use of spoken corpus evidence to create a "socially embedded grammar, one with criteria for acceptability based on adequate communicability in real contexts among real participants" (p. 56). They point to the interpersonal effects on grammar and flexibility in positioning of clause elements as characteristics of a distinctly spoken grammar.

Beyond grammar, much work on spoken languages in the past 20 years attests to the important contribution of formulaic language to fluent speech (e.g., McCarthy, 2006; Wood, 2010; Wray, 2000). *Formulaic language* refers to lexicogrammatical patterning of many kinds (e.g., "a true friend," "Let me just check when/what/whether . . . ," "it all depends") which has varying degrees of predictability, semantic transparency, and flexibility. While formulaicity is also pervasive in written language, its instantiation in spoken language is made more complex by the involvement of a range of suprasegmental and segmental semiotic resources. Despite the abundance of research and the inclusion of "formulaic competence" in Celce-Murcia's theoretical model of communicative competence (2008), its incorporation in the assessment infrastructures (e.g., rating scales) which elicit the operationalized constructs of either spoken or written language assessment has been minimal. Typically, formulaic language appears in rating scales as a characteristic of early L2 learning in the form of an overreliance on phrasebook chunks. Although obvious formulae are observable in early L2 learning stages, predictable lexicogrammatical patterning is actually a pervasive feature of fluent speech. Reorienting both human and machine rating to this phenomenon would help shift emphasis from the confines of the written grammatical sentence. Theoretical constructs underpinning such a shift in operationalized constructs would constitute a move from a more structuralist orientation to a more usage-based one (e.g., as set out in Bybee, 2010; Ellis, 2019).

CHALLENGES FOR SIGNED LANGUAGES: STATED AND THEORETICAL CONSTRUCTS

Language assessment occurs within a broader system in which a language code or variety (e.g., Standard Spoken Tamil or British Sign Language) and certain patterns of use (e.g., those present in formal interviews) are prioritized at societal/institutional levels as worth teaching and learning and, hence, worth assessing. Thus, the very existence of an assessment is usually an indication that standardization is under way. At the very least, decisions about assessable patterns of language use or models of ideal test performance are likely to have been established, subconsciously or otherwise, by the test developers as part of the process of test development. Thus, in striving to develop signed language assessments, questions of "status" and "community" arise. Adam (2015) describes several situations in which signed language standardization projects have been driven by different agendas, both from within Deaf communities or associations and from outside. He points to the fact that standardization efforts have the potential to accord status and recognition to a signed language variety, which may be empowering for users of the variety and disempowering for those who do not use that variety. This is, of course, no different to the effects of standardization for any language, but, in the case of signed languages, which are minority languages, Adam notes that it is important to consider who is doing the standardization and whether language ownership has been considered in the process. In a study of the views of Deaf signed language teachers in the United Kingdom and Germany, Eichmann (2009) observed that standardization efforts were seen as attempting to "fix" the language, driven by the needs of hearing L2 learners and hearing teachers of Deaf children. The teachers expressed concern that language standardization would create "double minorities" when the selected variety renders other varieties "incorrect" (p. 301). Language assessment is a byproduct of standardization that is driven by institutional language learning, and it powerfully entrenches correctness. Thus, there may be cause to interrogate the discourse (i.e., the *perceived construct* in Macqueen, Chapter 7.1) surrounding signed language tests and their uses.

Some signed language tests have been developed for research purposes and are only used within the context of a specific research project (see Chapter 7.2). The stated construct for these tests may be mentioned in associated publications, but these tests are less likely to generate much social impact when compared to tests used in educational contexts (where standard language ideologies are typically nurtured) or commercial tests. However, given the contribution of such tests to knowledge-building and replication research, developers and users of research instruments of any modality should be clear about the nature and limits of the construct they are operationalizing in research. They should also report the information provided to participants about the test so readers can get some sense of the perceived constructs the test might have generated; that is, what kind of test the participants thought they were doing and why they thought they were doing it.

FUTURE DIRECTIONS

So far, we have discussed theoretical and ideological challenges for the assessment of signed and spoken language abilities. In this section, we consider practical and empirical directions that may address these challenges, offering insights into the nature of operationalized assessment constructs across modalities and their underpinning theoretical models.

As discussed earlier, the development of theoretical models of signed language acquisition would enable greater explicitness (of descriptions of language use) and robustness (of the explanatory model causing score variance) of signed language assessment constructs. As described in Chapter 7.1, there are two theoretical focuses in language assessment: language variety and language ability. Learner corpora that are carefully built from authentic interactions in clearly specified acquisitional contexts and a range of domains are the best sources for construct description and explanation. The creation of well-specified corpora is especially important given the diversity of circumstances in which L1 and L2 signed languages are learned (Meier, 2016). Learner corpora can provide empirical insight in the developmental patterns of child adult learners of an L2 and thus could inform the theoretical definition of a language assessment construct. For signed languages, there are only two existing learner corpora: one for Irish Sign Language and another for Swedish Sign Language (Schönström et al., 2015). A third learner corpus is in planning for Swiss German Sign Language.

Corpora can also inform the theory of language that underpins assessment constructs, particularly linguistic phenomena which are idiosyncratic and improvisatory rather than rule-governed and regularized. In his discussion of signed language vocabulary (see Chapter 7.2), Haug mentions Johnston and Schembri's model of the signed language lexicon (2007), which distinguishes between stable lexemes that consistently mean the same thing (and are therefore listable in a dictionary) and "productive" lexemes which are complex, context-dependent composites. This phenomenon of conventionalized, context-dependent composites is examined in Schembri, Cormier, and Fenlon's analysis of "indicating verbs" in Australian Sign Language and British Sign Language (2018) based on the construction grammar approach (Goldberg, 1995). Their analysis demonstrates that indicating verbs are a holistic composite of phonological, semantic, morphosyntactic, discourse, and pragmatic features (in the form of dietic gestures). Capturing a learner's facility with such diverse semiotic combinations in an assessment context is a challenge for signed language assessments, just as formulaic language is for spoken language assessments.

Both spoken "formulaic language" and the signed holistic composites just discussed have been associated with the cognitive mechanism of "chunking" (Miller 1956). Chunks are combinations that are "retrieved whole from memory" (Wray, 2000, p. 465). Lepic (2019) proposes that chunking is common to oral/aural formulaic language and visual/gestural complexes, both of which "exhibit an analyzable internal structure and holistic properties simultaneously" (p. 1). Chunking enables automatic retrieval of semiotic complexes (Ellis, 1996). It economizes on the effort needed to assemble and comprehend complex utterances such as "I don't really mind whether we eat out or not," which comprise interlocking formulae. However, for learners of an L2, internalizing target lexicogrammatical patterns and gaining control of their degrees of flexibility is a gradual process (see, e.g., Macqueen & Knoch 2020). This developmental process could be tapped in operationalized constructs. For example, a spoken language assessment might incorporate the extent to which words and formulaic fragments are communicatively combined and manipulated (Read & Nation, 2006; Wood, 2010; Xu, 2018). Future developments in operationalized constructs in both signed and spoken languages, therefore, should strive to encompass meaningful combinations of traditionally separated components (e.g., morphosyntax, lexis, gesture) so that more of the complexity of speech, sign, and modality is represented in the construct.

Studies of acquisition and language use are necessary for the development of robust, well-articulated *theoretical constructs*, which are assumed to cause score variance (see Chapter 7.1). However, theory development typically moves much more slowly than is useful for practitioners and researchers who are seeking to use and improve assessment practices. Assessment infrastructures, such as tasks, raters, and rating scales, are the built environment in which a theoretical language ability is made observable and measurable (see Chapter 7.1). Thus, another way to develop the theoretical dimensions of constructs is by interrogating and elaborating existing assessment infrastructures. In this kind of practice-based approach, existing assessment instruments (e.g., a rating scale) and practices (e.g., rating behavior) are examined to shed light on the nature of the construct being operationalized in relation to theorized developmental trajectories. One example of practice-based development is described in a study by Isaacs, Trofimovich, and Foote (2018) who set out to elaborate the use of an existing L2 English comprehensibility scale. The scale development procedure was teacher-oriented since teachers were the target users of the scale and therefore the intended audience whose "listener effort in processing the speech" was fundamental in the operationalization of the comprehensibility construct (p. 208). While the original scale was developed through a combination of methods including statistical analysis of ratings, discourse features, and naïve rater introspection, this later elaboration systematically collected and incorporated a large number of teachers' perceived constructs into the rating scale. This practice-based approach resulted in a better alignment between a mass of domain insiders' *perceived constructs* and the elaborated scale descriptors.

Such a process of development and elaboration could also be applied to existing signed language assessments. Increasingly, existing assessment instruments are adapted for use in different contexts with different language varieties, as, for example, the adaptation of the BSL Receptive Skills Test (Herman et al., 1999) into various languages (Haug & Mann, 2008), including to test the progress of adult learners of L2 New Zealand Sign Language (Powell et al., 2019). While test adaptions are a practical solution in the absence of research on developmental trajectories on which to base new assessment instruments (Kotowicz et al., 2020), these adaptation processes for use with both L1 and L2 populations are good opportunities for construct exploration, development, and elaboration work.

Technological developments are in constant interaction with assessment constructs, giving rise to a continuous stream of possibilities and caveats (see also Chapters 12.1–12.3). One significant technological challenge in the assessment of spoken language has been the simulation of face-to-face interaction, as, for example, through a task that requires an assessee to respond verbally to automated prompts. While such methods enable a highly standardized delivery, they severely restrict the representation of interactional competence, with limited representation of the sequential, organizational features of communication such as turn-taking (Young, 2000). Spoken and signed interactions are intricately co-constructed in real life (e.g., Baker & Van den Bogaerde, 2020; Sacks et al., 1974), and capturing this phenomenon in automated delivery is work-in-progress for the field. At the same time, communication in many domains is increasingly mediated through computers and various forms of communication technology. This rapid naturalization of technology in human communication means that assessment developers will need to grapple with the representation of both videotelephonic and face-to-face interactional competence in assessment constructs. Future developments may include the expansion of operationalized constructs to include phenomena such as managing discourse in computer-mediated interactions, turn-taking with computers as co-interactants (Herijgers et al., 2019), adapting three-dimensional signs to a two-dimensional space, and adapting manual and nonmanual signs for increased clarity in the virtual context (Keating & Mirus, 2003; Keating et al., 2008).

Thinking about what is assessed—the construct—in any language assessment inevitably raises big questions about the nature of language use, the nature of developmental trajectories, and whose language patterns determine the standards. It is, however, relatively easy to gloss over these substantial considerations when defining and operationalizing constructs within the practical, financial, and time constraints typical of test development projects and policy decision-making. Deliberate attention paid to the relationship between what is actually operationalized as an assessment construct and what is theorized, claimed, and understood to be assessed by various stakeholders, from assessees to policy-makers, will go some way to ensuring that the big questions continue to be asked.

REFERENCES

Adam, R. (2015). Standardization of sign languages. *Sign Language Studies, 15*(4), 432–445. https://doi.org/10.1353/sls.2015.0015

Auer, P. (2009). On-line syntax: Thoughts on the temporality of spoken language. *Language Sciences, 31*(1), 1–13. https://doi.org/10.1016/j.langsci.2007.10.004

Baker, A., & Van den Bogaerde, B. (2020). Overlap in turn–taking in signed mother–child dyadic and triadic interactions. In G. Morgan (Ed.), *Understanding deafness, language and cognitive Development: Essays in honour of Bencie Woll.* (pp. 33–52). John Benjamins.

Boyes Braem, P. (2012). Evolving methods for written representations of signed languages of the deaf. In A. Ender, A. Leemann, & B. Waelchli (Eds.), *Methods in contemporary linguistics* (pp. 411–438). De Gruyter Mouton.
Bybee, J. (2010). *Language, usage and cognition*. Cambridge University Press.
Celce-Murcia, M. (2008). Rethinking the role of communicative competence in language teaching. In E. A. Soler & M. P. S. Jordà (Eds.), *Intercultural language use and language learning* (pp. 41–57). Springer.
Eichmann, H. (2009). Planning sign languages: Promoting hearing hegemony? Conceptualizing sign language standardization. *Current Issues in Language Planning, 10*(3), 293–307. https://doi.org/10.1080/14664200903116287
Ellis, N. C. (1996). Sequencing in SLA: Phonological memory, chunking, and points of order. *Studies in Second Language Acquisition, 18*(1), 91–126. https://doi.org/10.1017/S0272263100014698
Ellis, N. C. (2019). Essentials of a theory of language cognition. *Modern Language Journal, 103*, 39–60. https://doi.org/10.1111/modl.12532
Goldberg, A. (1995). *Constructions: A construction grammar approach to argument structure*. University of Chicago Press.
Haug, T., & Mann, W. (2008). Adapting tests of sign language assessment for other sign languages: A review of linguistic, cultural, and psychometric problems. *Journal of Deaf Studies and Deaf Education, 13*(1), 138–147. https://doi.org/10.1093/deafed/enm027
Haugen, E. (1966). Dialect, language, nation 1. *American Anthropologist, 68*(4), 922–935.
Herijgers, M. M., van Charldorp, T. T., & Maat, H. H. P. (2019). Human-human-computer triads in institutional encounters. *Journal of Pragmatics, 150*, 1–16. https://doi.org/10.1016/j.pragma.2019.06.010
Herman, R., Holmes, S., & Woll, B. (1999). *Assessing BSL development: Receptive Skills Test*. Forest Books.
IELTS. (2018). IELTS Speaking Band Descriptors. https://www.ielts.org/-/media/pdfs/speaking-band-descriptors.ashx?la=en
Isaacs, T., Trofimovich, P., & Foote, J. A. (2018). Developing a user-oriented second language comprehensibility scale for English-medium universities. *Language Testing, 35*(2), 193–216. https://doi.org/10.1177/0265532217703433
Johnston, T., & Schembri, A. (2007). *Australian Sign Language (Auslan): An introduction to sign language linguistics*. Cambridge University Press.
Keating, E., Edwards, T., & Mirus, G. (2008). Cybersign and new proximities: Impacts of new communication technologies on space and language. *Journal of Pragmatics, 40*(6), 1067–1081. https://doi.org/10.1016/j.pragma.2008.02.009
Keating, E., & Mirus, G. (2003). American Sign Language in virtual space: Interactions between deaf users of computer-mediated video communication and the impact of technology on language practices. *Language in Society, 32*(5), 693–714. https://doi.org/10.1017/S0047404503325047
Kotowicz, J., Woll, B., & Herman, R. (2021). Adaptation of the British sign language receptive skills test into Polish Sign Language. *Language Testing, 38*(1), 132–153. https://doi.org/10.1177/0265532220924598
Lepic, R. (2019). A usage-based alternative to "lexicalization" in sign language linguistics. *Glossa: A Journal of General Linguistics, 4*(1), 1–30. https://doi.org/10.5334/gjgl.840

Macqueen, S., & Knoch, U. (2020). Adaptive imitation: Formulaicity and the words of others in L2 English academic writing. In G. G. Fogal & M. H. Verspoor (Eds.), *Complex dynamic systems theory and L2 writing development* (pp. 81–108). John Benjamins.

McCarthy, M. (2006). *Fluency and confluence: What fluent speakers do*. Explorations in Corpus Linguistics. Cambridge University Press.

McCarthy, M., & Carter, R. (2002). Ten criteria for a spoken grammar. E. Hinkel & S. Fotos (Eds.), *New perspectives on grammar teaching in second language classrooms* (pp. 53–78). Lawrence Erlbaum.

Meier, R. P. (2016). Sign language acquisition. Oxford Handbooks Online. Oxford University Press. https://doi.org/10.1093/oxfordhb/9780199935345.013.19

Miller, G. A. (1956). The magical number seven, plus or minus two: Some limits on our capacity for processing information. *Psychological review*, *63*(2), 81–97.

Milroy, J., & Milroy, L. (2012). *Authority in language: Investigating standard English* (4th ed.). Routledge.

Powell, D., Boon, A., & Luckner, J. (2019). Improving the New Zealand Sign Language skills of educators. *Deafness & Education International*, *21*(4), 227–239. https://doi.org/10.1080/14643154.2019.1589974

Read, J., & Nation, I. S. P. (2006). *An investigation of the lexical dimension of the IELTS Speaking Test by measuring lexical output, variation and sophistication, and the use of formulaic language* (vol. 6): IELTS Australia and British Council Research Report Series.

Sacks, H., Schegloff, E. A., & Jefferson, G. (1974). The simplest systematics for the organization of turn–taking for conversations. *Language*, *50*(4), 696–735.

Schembri, A., Cormier, K., & Fenlon, J. (2018). Indicating verbs as typologically unique constructions: Reconsidering verb 'agreement' in sign languages. *Glossa: A Journal of General Linguistics*, *3*(1), 1–40. https://doi.org/10.5334/gjgl.468

Schönström, K., Dye, M., Leeson, L., & Mesch, J. (2015, July). *Building up L2 corpora in different signed languages: SSL, ISL and ASL* [Poster]. 2nd International Conference on Sign Language Acquisition, Amsterdam.

Wood, D. (2010). *Formulaic language and second language speech fluency: Background, evidence and classroom applications*. Continuum.

Wray, A. (2000). Formulaic sequences in second language teaching: Principle and practice. *Applied Linguistics*, *21*(4), 463–489. https://doi.org/10.1093/applin/21.4.463

Xu, J. (2018). Measuring "spoken collocational competence" in communicative speaking assessment. *Language Assessment Quarterly*, *15*(3), 255–272. https://doi.org/10.1080/15434303.2018.1482900

Young, R. F. (2000). *Interactional competence: Challenges for validity*. Paper presented at the Annual Meeting of the American Association for Applied Linguistics: Vancouver, BC, Canada.

Topic 8

Validation of Second Language Assessments

8.1

Validation of Spoken Language Assessments for Adult L2 Learners

Carol A. Chapelle and Hye-won Lee

WHAT IS VALIDATION?

Validation refers to the process of undertaking research to investigate whether test scores are appropriate for their intended uses. Such research yields findings that serve as evidence in justifying test score use in important decisions, such as admitting an applicant to a university, certifying the adequacy of a candidate's speaking ability for performing a particular job, placing a student at a certain level in a sequence of language courses, or planning the specifics of their future instruction. Speaking test scores are also used in some countries as part of the applications made for citizenship. Moreover, researchers use scores from speaking tests as data in research on language acquisition. The uses of tests are sometimes referenced on a continuum from high-stakes (meaning that test results have important implications) to low-stakes (meaning that test results have little impact). Some argue that low-stakes tests require less validation. However, any time that people are spending their time taking tests, the tests should be worthy of the time spent and the test results should be informative for their intended purpose. All test use has some form of impact on test-takers and test users; the job of testers is to investigate the extent to which the proposed uses of tests are valid. They do so by conducting validation research.

Validation research for a test is rarely if ever completed in a single study, and researchers investigating speaking tests have identified the many critical points in need of investigation in validity studies (Knoch & Chapelle, 2018; McNamara, 1996). Validation research requires use of multiple types of data that must be interpreted to result in an "integrated evaluation of the test" (Cronbach, 1971, p. 445). In other words, Cronbach wanted to emphasize that validation research should result in an overall evidence-based judgment of the adequacy of the test scores for a particular purpose. This perspective is reflected in the influential academic presentations in language testing by Bachman (1990) and Bachman and Palmer (1996, 2010), even if not in all books

Carol A. Chapelle and Hye-won Lee, *Validation of Spoken Language Assessments for Adult L2 Learners* In: *The Handbook of Language Assessment Across Modalities.* Edited by: Tobias Haug, Wolfgang Mann, and Ute Knoch, Oxford University Press. DOI: 10.1093/oso/9780190885052.003.0023 for language teacher education. The key figures in educational and psychological testing since Cronbach have agreed on the need to integrate various types of evidence from research (e.g., Kane, 2006, 2013; Messick, 1989) to make a judgment about test interpretation and use.

For any test, a judgment is based on more than a single claim so validation is never complete with a single investigation of one claim. Instead, multiple claims, each with its own inference, are structured together into what Cronbach (1988) called a "validity argument" (p. 4), which was explicated and formalized by Kane (2013).

Kane explicated the concept of the validity argument in part by demonstrating that certain types of claims are dependent on the credibility of other types of claims. For example, any claims about the construct (see Chapter 7.1) that a test assesses are credible only to the extent that claims about the quality of the test development process are warranted. Such relationships among the claims are expressed in a validity argument by the way that they are structured to demonstrate how they depend on one another. Figure 8.1.1 illustrates the basic outline of the claims and inferences in a validity argument, with seven claims that account for five aspects of score meaning. The structuring

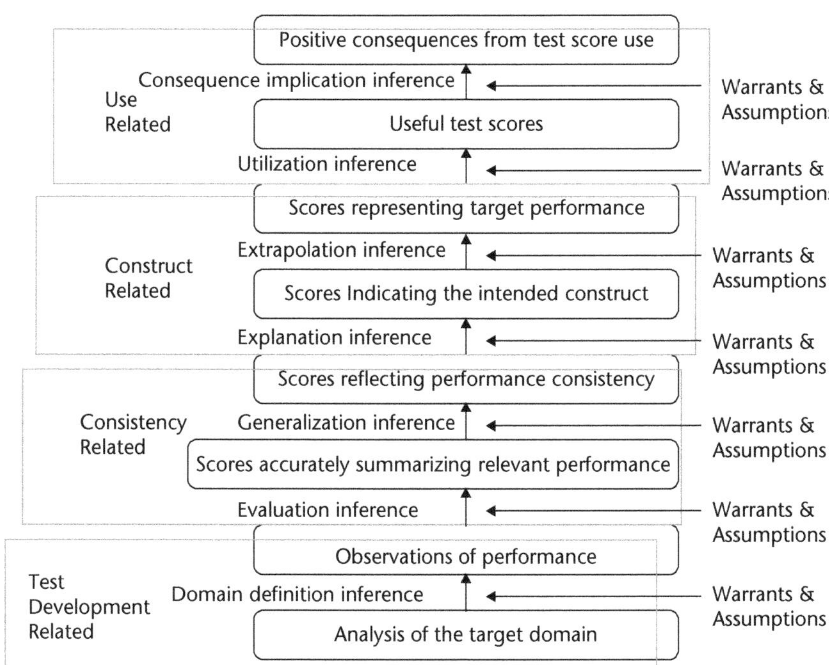

Figure 8.1.1 Schematic diagram of four types of inferences structured in an interpretation/use argument, which provides the basis of a validity argument. From Chapelle (2021).

of claims based on their relationships to one another—rather than listing claims, types of evidence, or types of validities—distinguishes argument-based validity from other approaches that have appeared in language testing research (Chapelle, 2012).

Figure 8.1.1 is read by starting at the bottom and following the chain of inferences to those at the top, which indicate the use-based claims. These claims about test use, utilization, and consequences serve as the conclusion for the integrated validity argument. In this way the diagram reflects that the use of the test is the bottom line, so to speak, as indicated by the definition of validity that appears in the *Standards for Educational and Psychological Testing*: "the degree to which evidence and theory support the interpretations of test scores for proposed uses of test scores" (American Education Research Association, American Psychological Association, & the National Council on Measurement in Education, 2014, p. 1). This definition states that justifying the test score use is the ultimate goal of validation, but doing so also involves other issues in need of investigation.

Figure 8.1.1 depicts the other issues, with inferences used to refer to the process of coming to a logical conclusion that is supported by evidence. The conclusion from each inference is a claim, and the evidence needed to support each inference is identified by the warrants and assumptions identified as critical for making the inference. Setting up such an argument and then using it to create a validity argument requires an understanding of the inferences underlying test score use.

HOW IS VALIDATION DONE?

The claims that testers make about the interpretation and use of test scores need to be justified by appropriate evidence. The credibility of each claim depends on the degree of support the tester presents for the corresponding inference. Therefore, the validation process typically focuses on investigating the inferences. Investigations are focused on specific statements called *warrants* that express in greater detail what must be accepted as plausible to authorize their respective inference. Even more detail is presented in assumptions that underlie the warrants. *Assumptions* make explicit the types of evidence required to make a warrant plausible. Examples of such validation research appear in the professional journals such as *Language Testing* and *Language Assessment Quarterly* as well as in other professional literature and documentation about tests even though testers are just beginning to use the language of argument-based validation with claims, inferences, warrants, and assumptions. Examples of how each of the four types of inferences has been investigated for speaking tests are provided here with reference to Figure 8.1.1.

Inference About the Quality of Test Development Processes.

Starting at the bottom of Figure 8.1.1, the inference about test development processes—domain definition—leads to a conclusion (claim) that the assessment has been designed and administered appropriately. Its place at the bottom of the diagram indicates that domain definition is the most fundamental inference to be justified in a validity argument. The inference connects language performance in the target domain—a specific real-life setting identified based on the test purpose—to observed performances in the test domain. It is necessary to verify this inferential link if a test developer wants to claim that the observation of test performances demonstrates relevant language abilities. To achieve such a goal, the tester first analyzes the target domain.

An example of this type of analysis was conducted by Youn (2013), who developed a classroom-based English for Academic Purposes (EAP) speaking assessment. A test was needed to assess second language (L2) pragmatics in interaction in academic tasks so she surveyed stakeholders in an EAP context about their needs for learning L2 pragmatics. She then identified a range of situations that students may encounter with interlocutors in the target domain, such as making an appropriate request to a professor and disagreeing politely with classmates during discussion. Based on the needs analysis findings, she developed two types of open role-play tasks (ORPTs) that can simulate the identified target situations: one with a professor interlocutor and the other involving two students. This test development supported the domain definition inference, leading to the conclusion that the test development process was done appropriately.

INFERENCES ABOUT THE CONSISTENCY OF TEST SCORES

Two types of inferences are made about the consistency of the test scores. The *evaluation* inference allows for a claim to be made about the accuracy of the scores as summaries of speaking performance. This inference has as its premise the observations of performance on test tasks. To be able to make an evaluation inference, evidence is needed to support warrants about task administration for obtaining accurate samples of performance, the appropriateness of scoring rubrics, and the consistency of rating procedures. Investigations and monitoring of task administration is an ongoing concern in operational testing but is rarely reported as research in the professional journals. In contrast, many validation studies of speaking tests illustrate the issues involved in creating and implementing a rating scale that will result in accurate ratings for tasks.

Youn's (2013) test development research, described earlier, also included a method of linguistic analysis, *conversation analysis*, to create rating criteria (Youn, 2015). To assess students' varying degrees of pragmatic competence in interaction, the scoring rubric needed to be sensitive to emerging features of the students' interaction. The process of developing the rating scale as well as the follow-up quantitative analysis of its consistent use by raters served as backing for the evaluation inference. Rather than a linguistically based analysis, Elder and McNamara (2016) sought support for evaluation by investigating test score users' perspectives of their rating scale. The test was the Occupational English Test (OET) for assessing English proficiency for healthcare professionals. The speaking part of the test consists mainly of two role-plays where a test-taker plays the role of a doctor, nurse, or physiotherapist, and an interlocutor plays the patient role. In an attempt to learn what criteria are valued in communication in the target domain, the researchers conducted a qualitative analysis of feedback given by some healthcare educators and supervisors on trainees' communication with patients in various (simulated) clinical settings and were able to identify, to some degree, some language-related criteria that they incorporated into their rubric. Such domain-related studies have multiple purposes, but the focus of the study highlighted here is that the researchers were attempting to maximize the accuracy and relevance of the response evaluation process to create an effective rubric for raters to use.

A critical area of investigation for making evaluation inferences is the process of *rater training*. Davis (2016) investigated the role of rater training and experience on scoring patterns in the Test of English as a Foreign Language (TOEFL) iBT Speaking Test. Twenty teachers, experienced in teaching English learners but inexperienced in scoring TOEFL speaking tasks, participated in the study. They scored four batches of 100 spoken responses over a few days. The first individual scoring after a brief orientation was followed by a rater training session providing exemplars with scoring rationales and scoring calibration exercises. The findings revealed that training contributed to a slight improvement in consistency of scoring patterns within the raters themselves but had little effect on interrater consistency. Gained experience over scoring sessions (relatively short, approximately 2 weeks) did not make much change, either; however, it did improve scoring accuracy, defined as agreement with pre-established reference scores. It was also found that more accurate raters tended to review exemplars more frequently than did less accurate ones. It was concluded that training with some form of scoring aids would help to sustain quality of scores assigned by raters and possibly provide support for the evaluation inference in the speaking part of the TOEFL iBT validity argument.

The *generalization* inference allows for a claim to be made about the consistency of the test scores across parallel versions of tasks within and across test forms, raters, and occasions of testing. This inference has as its premise the accurate ratings on the test tasks. To make a generalization inference, evidence is needed to support warrants about consistency of ratings for the whole test. This is a challenge for speaking assessments because, even if raters can consistently rate individual speaking tasks, obtaining a consistent test score requires a sufficient number of tasks on the test. Strictly in terms of reliability, it would be ideal to include as many tasks as possible, but there are limits to the numbers of tasks a test-taker can complete from a logistical and economic perspective.

The research on the TOEFL iBT speaking test provides a good example of how generalizability (G) theory was used to evaluate the impact of the aforementioned issues on reliability. Lee (2006) carried out G studies in the prototyping phase of the test to decide the optimal number of speaking tasks and check whether justification could be found for combining scores on different task types in one composite score. Increasing the number of tasks, up to five or six, had a fairly large effect on the score dependability[1]; reporting a single composite score for the whole speaking section appeared to be justified. These results guided test configuration and score reporting in the subsequent prototyping and finalizing phases and served as essential pieces of evidence supporting the generalization inference of the validity argument for the TOEFL iBT (Chapelle et al., 2008).

CONSTRUCT-RELATED INFERENCES

Construct-related inferences are made when test users conclude that the intended speaking construct has been assessed. Speaking can be defined in a number of different ways depending on how much emphasis is to be given to particular aspects (e.g., pronunciation vs. coherence) and on the genre and registers of speaking (e.g., dialogic client interviews conducted in a healthcare setting vs. monologic oral research presentations at an international conference). The speaking construct should be defined as appropriate for a certain intended test use.

The *explanation* inference allows for a claim to be made about the speaking construct assessed by the test. This inference has as its premise that the test scores are consistent, as concluded from the generalization inference. To make an explanation inference, evidence is needed to support warrants about the internal structure of the construct, the components and processes that make up the construct, the hypothesized relationships of the construct to other related and unrelated constructs, or any combination of the three. These types of warrants about the construct serve as hypotheses to be tested by validation research using a range of quantitative and qualitative methods, including discourse analyses, cognitive processing techniques, and some statistical analyses such as correlation, factor analysis, and group difference tests.

An example of a study that investigated the internal structure of test scores intended to reflect an oral proficiency construct was conducted by Yan, Cheng, and Ginther (2018). They investigated the Oral English Proficiency Test (OEPT), a local speaking test for prospective international teaching assistants (ITAs) in a US university. The test consists of 10 main items in three task types: text-based, graph-involved, and listening-integrated. The researchers used a confirmatory factor analysis to examine whether the test scores were consistent with the construct as they had theorized it. Three models were tested: one with a single speaking factor and the other two each with two factors. The two-factor models were configured differently, one with a speaking factor and a factor for all the task types, and the other with separate speaking and listening factors. The third model demonstrated the best fit to the data, which they interpreted to mean that the OEPT measures a largely unidimensional construct of oral English proficiency even though listening comprehension is also accounted for in the two-factor model. The researchers interpret the finding as consistent with their understanding of the construct and therefore a piece of supporting evidence for the explanation inference.

The warrants supporting explanation refer to a theoretical construct hypothesized to affect performance regardless of context (e.g., fluency). The *extrapolation* inference allows for conclusions about the degree to which the test construct reflects the aspects of the theoretical construct related to the language use domain of interest to test users (i.e., the genre and register of the speaking situations of interest to the score users). Extrapolation inferences can be supported by two types of warrants, both stating a relationship between test performance and performance in the context of interest. One type of warrant states the degree of relationship between speaking test scores and scores from another test that is supposed to measure speaking in the same context of interest. Using such a concurrent correlational analysis as an approach for supporting extrapolation has the obvious limitation that it assumes the criterion test reliability assesses the same thing that the test under investigation does. Other indicators, such as evaluations conducted by the test-takers' supervisor, teacher, or colleagues, are also used in such analyses to attempt to supply data on how well the test scores assess the construct of interest. Such research needs to be theorized appropriately to state the expected relationships between the test scores and the other indicators, taking into account the degree of similarity and difference between what the test measures and what is assessed by the criterion observations, as well as the reliability of both.

A second type of warrant states a comparison between test performance and performance in the domain of interest to test users. Such studies examine language use. For example, Brooks and Swain (2014) collected speaking samples from 30 international graduate students in both the TOEFL speaking test setting and the target domain—students' in- and out-of-class settings in their real life. Grammatical and discourse features and vocabulary use of the samples from these different contexts were compared. Speech samples from the test setting were more complex but less accurate in grammar, and performances in both the test and the class demonstrated more use of conjunctions, connectives, and content words. Speech from the out-of-class context used questions and informal language more than those in the other contexts. The researchers concluded that, despite overlapping linguistic features, the number and type of features that were dissimilar between the performances across the contexts "expose a potential weak link" in the validity argument by failing to provide strong support for the extrapolation inference (p. 371) and point to areas to consider as test tasks are revised in the future.

LaFlair and Staples (2017) conducted a similarly motivated investigation of extrapolation by comparing student speaking performances on the Michigan English Language Assessment Battery with those from relevant subdomains of existing corpora. They conducted a quantitative corpus-based register analysis, which allowed them to identify patterns of co-occurring linguistic features. Although identifying some similarities across the two sources of language samples—the test performances and the corpora—the researchers interpreted the linguistic analysis as underscoring the fundamentally different communicative purposes between the test and the target domain. The detailed findings produced through the use of linguistic analysis present new opportunities for appraisal of extrapolation, on the one hand, and integration of linguistic analysis in validation practices, on the other.

INFERENCES ABOUT TEST USE

Inferences about test score use are made when test users accept that the scores are appropriate and useful for making certain decisions resulting in the intended consequences. A *utilization* inference leads to claims about test use such as the following:

- Scores are useful for making decisions about admission of applicants to universities in the United States.
- Scores are useful for certifying a candidate's expertise to perform a particular job.
- Scores are useful for placing a student at a certain level in a program of study.
- Scores are useful for planning a student's future instruction.

Such claims also serve as the grounds for a *consequence implication* inference, which would lead to claims about the intended consequences of each of these test score uses that may seem apparent to testers. Such positive consequences would include admitting the best prepared applicants, certifying candidates with appropriate experience, achieving an appropriately homogeneous class of students, and providing well-targeted instruction.

An example of a study investigating the utilization inference for a speaking test evaluated use of the score on the TOEFL iBT speaking test for decisions about teaching assignments for ITAs. The primary use of the TOEFL iBT is for admission decisions in English-medium universities, so the validation study was needed to investigate the validity of a different claim about usefulness of the test (Xi, 2008). Four North American universities where decision-making procedures for teaching assignments already existed participated. The study design focused on the correspondence between existing practices and the decisions that would result from the use of the TOEFL iBT Speaking test. Several analyses suggested that the use of the TOEFL iBT speaking scores would result in similar teaching assignments as the existing methods. Analyses included correlations between scores on the TOEFL speaking test and local ITA screening tests, with logistic regression analyses showing that the TOEFL speaking scores were significant predictors of TA assignments. These findings were interpreted as warranting the use of the TOEFL speaking test for an additional purpose.

The claims resulting from the consequence implication inference are supported by the study of the effects, including washback on teaching, of the test score use. For instance, Hirai and Koizumi (2009) developed a semi-direct classroom speaking assessment called the Story Retelling Speaking Test (SRST) and administered a questionnaire to learn about students' perceptions of test qualities, including impacts on their learning. Questions related to positive impacts were responded to positively; students commented that they could improve their speaking ability, summary skills, and/or vocabulary through frequent practice and be motivated to improve further after the test.

With the intent of promoting positive effects on teaching and learning, Muñoz and Álvarez (2010) developed the Oral Assessment System (OAS), consisting of standards, rubrics, tasks, scoring sheets, report cards, and test guidelines, and they investigated its effect on some areas of classroom teaching and learning. Fourteen English as foreign language teachers and 110 college students were surveyed, their classrooms were observed, and external evaluations of students' spoken performance were collected for the analysis. Teachers who participated in the OAS (experimental group) were more aware of class objectives and aligned those with their instructional and assessment tasks. They tended to provide more analytic feedback on student spoken performances with the help of the given rubrics. Students in the experimental group were also clear about what they were to be assessed on, utilized self-assessment more often, and gained higher scores on most of the speaking aspects. In general, the evidence suggested that the OAS brought about the intended positive washback in the classroom.

FUTURE DIRECTIONS

Conceptualizing the process of validation as a multistage argument requires testers to specify the claims that need to be supported for valid test score interpretation and use. Because of the variety of types of claims, validation research is best conceptualized as requiring mixed methods (Creswell & Plano Clark, 2017) to investigate the degree of support that can be obtained (Chapelle, 2020; Moeller et al., 2016). The multiple claims invite examination of the rationale required for each claim, which typically requires testers to engage in a mixed-methods inquiry. The fact that mixed-methods research has become relatively well established in applied linguistics may help to crystalize the idea of a single validity argument in language testing research and practice, where some still conceive of three separate types of validity. Years ago, Cronbach judged, "The 30-year-old idea of three types of validity, separate but maybe equal, is an idea whose time has gone" (Cronbach, 1988, p. 4). Types of validities were anathema for professionals wishing to consolidate professional knowledge around the idea of validity as an "integrated evaluation of the test" (Cronbach, 1971, p. 445). However, as the examples of argument-based validity research increase in language testing, the field may be in a position to move toward Cronbach's idea of validity as an *integrated evaluation* (Cronbach, 1971, p. 445).

NOTE

1. The scoring consistency of criterion-referenced tests, which is a type of test that assesses the performance of test-takers against a set of criteria rather than relatively against each other.

REFERENCES

American Education Research Association, American Psychological Association, & the National Council on Measurement in Education. (2014). *Standards for educational and psychological testing*. American Education Research Association.

Bachman, L. F. (1990). *Fundamental considerations in language testing*. Oxford University Press.

Bachman, L. F., & Palmer, A. (1996). *Language testing in practice: Designing and developing useful language tests*. Oxford University Press.

Bachman, L., & Palmer, A. (2010). *Language assessment in practice: Developing language assessments and justifying their use in the real world*. Oxford University Press.

Brooks, L., & Swain, M. (2014). Contextualizing performances: Comparing performances during TOEFL iBT and real-life academic speaking activities.

Language Assessment Quarterly, 11(4), 353–373. https://doi.org/10.1080/15434303.2014.947532
Chapelle, C. A. (2012). Validity argument for language assessment: The framework is simple. *Language Testing, 29*(1), 19–27. https://doi.org/10.1177/0265532211417211
Chapelle, C. A. (2020). *Argument-based validation in testing and assessment*. Sage Publications.
Chapelle, C. A., Enright, M. K., & Jamieson, J. M. (Eds.). (2008). *Building a validity argument for the Test of English as a Foreign Language*. Routledge.
Creswell, J. W., & Plano Clark, V. L. (2017). *Designing and conducting mixed methods research* (3rd ed.). Sage Publications.
Cronbach, L. J. (1971). Test validation. In R. L. Thorndike (Ed.), *Educational measurement* (2nd ed., pp. 443–507). American Council on Education.
Cronbach, L. J. (1988). Five perspectives on validation argument. In H. Wainer & H. Braun (Eds.), *Test validity* (pp. 34–35). Erlbaum.
Davis, L. (2016). The influence of training and experience on rater performance in scoring spoken language. *Language Testing, 33*(1), 117–135. https://doi.org/10.1177/0265532215582282
Elder, C., & McNamara, T. (2016). The hunt for "indigenous criteria" in assessing communication in the physiotherapy workplace. *Language Testing, 33*(2), 153–174. https://doi.org/10.1177/0265532215607398
Hirai, A., & Koizumi, R. (2009). Development of a practical speaking test with a positive impact on learning using a story retelling technique. *Language Assessment Quarterly, 6*(2), 151–167. https://doi.org/10.1080/15434300902801925
Kane, M. T. (2006). Validation. In R. Brennan (Ed.), *Educational measurement* (4th ed., pp. 17–64). American Council on Education and Praeger.
Kane, M. T. (2013). Validating the interpretations and uses of test scores. *Journal of Educational Measurement, 50*(1), 1–73. https://doi.org/10.1111/jedm.12000
Knoch, U., & Chapelle, C. A. (2018). Validation of rating processes within an argument-based framework. *Language Testing, 35*(4), 477–499. https://doi.org/10.1177/0265532217710049
LaFlair, G. T., & Staples, S. (2017). Using corpus linguistics to examine the extrapolation inference in the validity argument for a high-stakes speaking assessment. *Language Testing, 34*(4), 451–475. https://doi.org/10.1177/0265532217713951
Lee, Y.-W. (2006). Dependability of scores for a new ESL speaking assessment consisting of integrated and independent tasks. *Language Testing, 23*(2), 131–166. https://doi.org/10.1191/0265532206lt325oa
McNamara, T. F. (1996). *Measuring second language performance*. Longman.
Messick, S. (1989). Validity. In R. L. Linn (Ed.), *Educational measurement* (3rd ed., pp. 13–103). Macmillan.
Moeller, A. J., Creswell, J. W., & Saville, N. (Eds.). (2016). *Second language assessment and mixed methods research*, Studies in Language Testing, 43. Cambridge University Press.
Muñoz, A. P., & Álvarez, M. E. (2010). Washback of an oral assessment system in the EFL classroom. *Language Testing, 27*(1), 33–49. https://doi.org/10.1177/0265532209347148

Xi, X. (2008). *Investigating the criterion-related validity of the TOEFL speaking scores for ITA screening and setting standards for ITAs*. (TOEFL iBT Research Report No. TOEFL iBT-03.) Educational Testing Service.

Yan, X., Cheng, L., & Ginther, A. (2018). Factor analysis for fairness: Examining the impact of task type and examinee L1 background on scores of an ITA speaking test. *Language Testing, 36*(2), 207–234. https://doi.org/10.1177/0265532218775764

Youn, S. J. (2013). *Validating task-based assessment of L2 pragmatics in interaction using mixed methods*. Doctoral dissertation, University of Hawai'i, Honolulu. http://hdl.handle.net/10125/100656

Youn, S. J. (2015). Validity argument for assessing L2 pragmatics in interaction using mixed methods. *Language Testing, 32*(2), 199–225. https://doi.org/10.1177/0265532214557113

8.2

Validation of Signed Language Assessments for Adult L2 Learners

Krister Schönström, Peter C. Hauser, and
Christian Rathmann

The evaluation of adult achievement in developing signed language skills is important in signed language research and deaf education yet test developers face challenges when developing measurements that can have an impact on the appropriate use and valid interpretations of test results. Adults learning signed language are not only learning a second language (L2) but one that exploits a new modality, specifically the gestural-visual modality (e.g., Chen-Pichler & Koulidobrova, 2015); hence, signed language L2 tests do not only measure language development but also the ability to process language in a different modality. In contrast with spoken language, where lexical items are primarily expressed sequentially, signed language unfolds both sequentially and simultaneously, with simultaneity achieved through, for example, spatial referencing and inclusion of nonmanual features (Meier, 2002; Padden, 2000). The modality aspect of signed language tests creates the first challenge because there are no spoken language test models. The process of signed language test validation is complicated by the high variation in local signed languages (Schembri & Johnston, 2013) and what we expect from signed language users in a particular setting (see Paludnevičience et al., 2012, for discussion of signed language test development challenges). Despite the challenges, over half a century worth of studies on signed languages around the world has afforded the development of some theory-based signed language assessment instruments.

Most signed language tests have been developed to evaluate deaf students' achievement in learning a local signed language as their first language (L1). A smaller number of tests has been developed for adults learning a local signed language as their second language (L2) (see Landa & Clark, 2019, for review). The evaluation of adult L2 learners' signed language skills is important for the education, health, and quality of life of deaf people. Worldwide, it is rare that teachers,

Krister Schönström, Peter C. Hauser, and Christian Rathmann, *Validation of Signed Language Assessments for Adult L2 Learners* In: *The Handbook of Language Assessment Across Modalities*. Edited by: Tobias Haug, Wolfgang Mann, and Ute Knoch, Oxford University Press. © Oxford University Press 2022. DOI: 10.1093/oso/9780190885052.003.0024 interpreters, and others using signed language professionally have their signed language skill evaluated using instruments with published validity. The need to accurately address signed language skill has driven some teams to explore methods of combining signed language research knowledge with theories of test development. In this chapter, we use the argument-based approach (Kane, 2013; Knoch & Chapelle, 2017; see also Chapter 8.1) to evaluate the validity of a sample of existing L2 signed language tests. The argument-based approach first identifies the test developer's claims, then identifies the grounds (data) that provide backings to support such claims about the test's use and interpretation of results. Theoretical and behavioral research are needed to appropriately support any claim, and, the stronger the claim, the more backings are needed to document validity. In other words, evaluating the plausibility and appropriateness of claims made about test results validates the use of test scores or interpretations. In this sense, validity is a property of the interpretations and use of test scores, not of the test itself.

Although the L2 signed language tests reviewed here were not developed with the argument-based approach in mind, we selected this approach because it provides a framework for evaluating test validity. Ideally, the tests' published validity should clearly and thoroughly articulate claims made about their use and interpretation. This was not the case in our review, so we had to make assumptions about the test developers' claims based on information provided in test publications and the known use of such tests. We did this by exploring the reasoning inherent in the proposed interpretation and use of scores, including assumptions about the conclusions to be drawn based on test performance and decisions made based on those conclusions. For example, Test X's scores on a signed language vocabulary test reflects some level of receptive skill achievement. This achievement may be assumed to be generalizable beyond the test situation (generalization inference), assumed to reflect similar skills in other performance domains (extrapolation inference; e.g., expressive language skills, signed language discourse skills), and/or assumed to contribute to the test-taker's mastery of signed language–based instruction or interpreting for hiring, certification, or promotion (decision inference). These assumptions and inferences may be valid if appropriate backings—theories, empirical research, and test statistics—are provided. Here, we provide examples of a number of well-known signed language tests for adult learners, discuss the validation research of these tests, and account for any gaps in this validation research base.

SIGN LANGUAGE PROFICIENCY INTERVIEW

One of the first widely used adult L2 signed language assessment tests was the Sign Language Proficiency Interview for ASL (SLPI:ASL;

Caccamise & Newell, 1995, see also Chapter 9.2). Caccamise and Newell (1995) claim that the SLPI:ASL results provide an indication of the functional communicative skills of teachers and faculty working with deaf students at schools for the deaf and in universities, respectively. It is used in hiring, tenure and promotion, and program admissions and graduation. The test was created in the 1980s, based on the Oral Proficiency Interview developed by the American Council on the Teaching of Foreign Language. The SLPI is now used, for example, in New Zealand as the SLPI:NZSL, in Kenya as the SLPI:KSL, and in South Africa as the SLPI:SASL, and it inspired the design of InTeck in Sweden.

SLPI test-takers are interviewed for 20 minutes by a fluent signer (often deaf) who has been trained to elicit specific types of utterances, including those that are unique to the visual modality, such as those involving classifiers and the deliberate and meaningful use of the signing space. Inherent in the SLPI's claim to measure functional communication is the notion that the interview successfully elicits evidence of an individual's ability to communicate using the target language. The interview is filmed and later rated by raters using a score sheet with checklist design (see Chapter 9.2, for discussion) to determine whether the test-taker can functionally communicate in a broad sense about different topics. Raters determine the test-taker's level by taking into consideration function and form. In evaluating function, the rater measures the global ability of the candidate to participate in a conversation. Evaluation of form, in contrast, focuses on specific aspects such as (1) vocabulary knowledge, (2) signing rate, (3) fluency, (4) grammar, and (5) comprehension. The test offers 11 ratings, spanning from beginning signed language skill (No Functional Skills) to native-like signed language skills (Superior Plus). Raters are trained on how to distinguish between the constructs entitled at each level. It is important to note here that the use of raters to score test-takers' performance poses a challenge to any test's validity. Knoch (Chapter 9.1) discusses scoring issues when human raters are involved, including measurement error, interviewer effects, and rater effects (sometimes depending on how consistently raters have been trained).

The SLPI:ASL has a procedure to maximize the reliability of ratings and minimize interviewer and rater effects. First, interviews are rated independently by three trained raters then compared by a fourth individual who coordinates the SLPI. If the three ratings are not within one rating level of one another (e.g., if two people assigned a rating of 7 and 8 and the third assigned a rating of 5), the coordinator requests that the raters meet to discuss the test-taker's language use with explicit reference to the construct of each level and negotiate an official rating that is consistent with that construct (negotiation). Then, the raters provide a second set of ratings (post-negotiation). Caccamise and Samar (2009) investigated the interrater reliability of the pre-negotiation ratings, evaluated the degree of deviation of raters' pre-negotiation ratings from their post-negotiation ratings and found that, generally, interrater reliability was high.

Caccamise and Samar (2009) specifically investigated the ratings of 160 adults who took the SLPI at a college that teaches deaf students. They found that eight interviews (5%) required re-ratings, six of which resulted in official ratings and two of which did not because the raters could not agree on the official rating. They demonstrated that 86.6% of the raters provided first independent ratings that were either the same as or within one rating level of those produced by the other members of their rating team, and 13.4% of the raters provided first independent ratings that were not within one rating level of those produced by the other members of their rating team. After second independent ratings (post-negotiation), 96.8% of the raters provided ratings that were either the same as or within one level of those produced by their rating team members, which is an improvement of 10.2%. When comparing the pre-negotiation rating with post-negotiation ratings, 2.5% were not within one level of official ratings; after second independent ratings, this percentage was reduced to 0.6%. Caccamise and Samar's (2009) results support the argument that the SLPI is a good measure of functional communication because the constructs supporting each 11-rating level can be trained and reliably rated.

What is absent from the SLPI validity analysis are the plausibility and appropriateness of the use-related inferences used by the test, as well as an examination of the consequences of the test (i.e., for the employment process). Caccamise and Samar (2009) did not collect any backings for the test's decision inferences. Specifically, they did not make any claims or provide any backings for decisions about who should be hired or promoted versus who should not, although SLPIs are often used for the purpose of such determination. Another criticism of the SLPI is that the generalizability inferences–based ratings might be limited if the trained interviewers and raters do not appropriately handle the natural variations of a local signed language. Arguably, if the interviewers' and raters' training and experience have been based on a specific regional, racial, or ethnic group, and they continue to evaluate the functional communication only within this specific variation of a local signed language, then the need to address how variation is handled to support generalized inferences is not needed. However, if the interviewers and raters are white, middle-class, and have little contact outside their only socioeconomic and/or cultural group, then this could impact validity if the SLPI is used to evaluate, for example, an African American employee's functional communication in a signed environment that mostly includes Black ASL (McCaskill et al., 2011). Similarly, if the same group of interviewers and raters evaluates teachers who work with deaf individuals from diverse backgrounds, generalized inferences made based on the SLPI results would be limited to the test-taker's functional communication with white, middle-class deaf adults.

SENTENCE REPETITION TESTS

One way to further minimize the rater effects often seen in language tests is to control or limit expressive language responses, a tactic taken, for example, by sentence repetition tests (SRTs). SRTs typically involve an examiner reading a sentence and asking the test-taker to repeat it. Repetitions that deviate from the original sentence are scored as incorrect or awarded fewer points, making SRTs easier to score than the SLPI, which involves free responses. SRTs are backed by theoretical and empirical research, making them popular for documenting language fluency and identifying language disorders (e.g., Gaillard & Tremblay, 2016). It is beyond the scope of this chapter to discuss the argument-based validity of spoken language SRTs. Instead, this section discusses the validation of signed language SRTs used with L2 populations.

The ASL Sentence Repetition Test (ASL-SRT, Hauser et al., 2008; Supalla et al., 2014) was developed to measure both child and adult ASL fluency regardless whether participants were deaf or hearing or learned ASL as their L1 or L2. The goal was to develop an ASL fluency test that is brief and easy to score while avoiding floor and ceiling effects. The authors (Hauser et al., 2008) argued that the signed sentences were valid partially because the sentences were created, signed, and evaluated by a team of native deaf signers with doctoral degrees in psychology, thus providing face validity for the items (but see Davies, 2003, for counterarguments on the use of native speakers). When the test was developed, there were no corpus data, existing lists of sign frequencies, or documentations of variation to assist with sentence development. Therefore, the team of native signers used their intuition to decide which signs were most frequent and least varied across the United States. The first version of the ASL-SRT contained 39 video-recorded sentences and was administered to 120 deaf and hearing children and adults, including both native and non-native signers. It demonstrated acceptable interrater reliability (r = .83) and internal consistency (Cronbach alpha = .87 and .88), providing support to the authors' claim that the ASL-SRT items can be appropriately rated and does measure a single construct.

Hauser and colleagues (2008) found that hearing signers evidenced significantly more incorrect repetitions than did deaf signers. Paludnevičience, Hauser, Daggett, and Kurz (2012) describe this as the "24/7 effect"—deaf native signers using ASL as their primary language develop greater ASL skill than do hearing native signers using it less frequently. This effect potentially complicates the development of signed language tests. For this reason, Hauser and colleagues (2008) decided to conduct the remaining psychometric analyses excluding the hearing signers and argued that the ASL-SRT was a good measure of ASL because deaf adults perform better than deaf children, and those who learned ASL earlier in life performed better than those who learned later (sometimes as their L1). The ASL-SRT has been adapted to a number of signed languages, including Swedish Sign Language (*Svenskt teckenspråk* [STS]) (Schönström, 2014) and German Sign Language (*Deutsche Gebärdensprache* [DGS]) (Kubus & Rathmann, 2013).

Schönström and Holmström (2017) modified the STS-SRT (Schönström, 2014), an L1 assessment modeled after the ASL-SRT, to the SignRepL2, designed specifically for adult hearing L2 users of STS. Short sentences were created for hearing STS L2 learners by a team including deaf university lecturers with vast experience teaching STS to this population, thus contributing to the item face validity. The SignRepL2 consists of 40 items—10 sentences each of single-sign, two-sign, three-sign, and four-sign utterances. A 5-point rating scale was developed to capture more variation in fluency among those developing skills in STS. Until now, SignRepL2 validity results are based on 23 adult L2 learners tested before and after 200 hours of STS instruction. The adult learners' ratings had high internal consistency (Cronbach alpha = .904), and the participants' scores were significantly better after 200 hours of STS instruction. Schönström and Holmström (2017) argue that the SignRepL2 is a good measure of nascent STS skills because it was developed with the test population in mind, has good reliability, and has discriminant validity based on STS instruction. The SignRepL2 was not developed for consequence implication inferences but rather to document research participants' L2 competency as a continuous variable or grouping variable (e.g., using median split between high and low performers) in research studies. The validity of the SignRepL2 when used in research would depend on the preliminary analyses to be confirmed with a larger sample and would depend on the inferences made, based on the number of correct repetitions, in studies.

Kubus and Rathmann (2013) adapted the ASL-SRT to German Sign Language (DGS-SRT). They administered the 30-sentence DGS-SRT to 31 L2 students enrolled in two different bachelor degree programs, as well as to 13 native signers. They used a 3-point rating scale to score the repetitions. The preliminary results had high interrater reliability (r = .91). Among the L2 students, they found that the intermediate (2nd-year) students did not perform better than the beginning (1st-year) students, but that the advanced (3rd-year) students performed better than the two less experienced groups. They claimed that the DGS-SRT is a good measure of DGS because of its interrater reliability and discriminant validity between beginning and advanced students. The use and type of interpretations made based on DGS-SRT data, like the SignRepL2, depend how the test is used and how its results are interpreted in research studies.

Each of the SRTs reviewed here was supported by extant linguistic theory and research when developed, thus contributing support to the argument that each is an appropriate language measure. The argument-based validity of the use of the SRTs for L2 learners has been backed by different psychometric analyses, including tests of internal consistency, interrater reliability, face validity, and discriminant validity (L1 outperforms L2; advanced students outperform beginners), though not all analyses were available for all SRTs. The SRT approach to assessing L2 signers' skills appears promising, and the rater effects appear to be better controlled than those observed with the SLPI, though the two have not yet been directly compared. Unlike the SLPI, SRT measures repetition ability but not functional communication skill; therefore, construct-related inferences made based on the number of correct repetitions may be limited. The SRT approach has been challenged by critics who claim that the test is more a memory test than a language test. However, sentence repetition tests have been reported as having a stronger relationship with language skills than with working memory skills (Gaillard & Tremblay, 2016; Klem et al., 2015). Another limitation of the SRT is its use outside of the laboratory because it requires raters who have extensive training on how to code repetitions. Though spoken language SRTs often prove useful to speech-language pathologists and psychologists able to administer and rate them, the use of signed language SRTs by the same professionals often threatens argument-based validity because raters are hard to train and must have native or near-native fluency in the language.

AMERICAN SIGN LANGUAGE COMPREHENSION TEST

Computer-scored assessments are considered objective tests because they do not involve raters, but they are often limited to the measurement of receptive language skills. Such tests are desirable because they can be administered independently on a computer and their results can be available immediately at the conclusion of testing. Hauser, Paludneviciene, Riddle, Kurz, Emmorey, and Contreras (2016) developed an objective receptive test, the ASL Comprehension Test (ASL-CT), for adult L1 and L2 signers. The aim was to create a test to be used in research and, ultimately, in education and other fields, at multiple sites, without raters. They claim that generalized inferences on an individual's receptive and expressive ASL skills can be made based on the test results. The authors claim that it is a good measure of ASL because it was developed by a team of deaf native signers (professors and doctoral students) with linguistic, psychology, and education backgrounds. The team focused on spatial linguistic aspects of ASL that are unique to signed languages and often pose a challenge to L2 signers, such as depicting verbs. The test's 30 items include both phrases and sentences and require understanding of ASL vocabulary, depiction, and syntax. During the test, subjects see either (a) a photo, (b) an action video, or (c) a sign video on a computer screen and are instructed to pick which of four multiple-choice items best matches the stimulus. Choices are in any of the media listed, but, in each item, sign videos are either the stimuli or choices.

The ASL-CT was administered to a sample of 20 deaf native signers, 20 deaf non-native signers, 20 hearing native signers, and 20 hearing non-native signers. Results revealed that the test has an acceptable internal consistency (Cronbach alpha = .83) and good concurrent validity when compared with the ASL-SRT (r = .72). Among the hearing adult L2 signers who took the test, results positively correlated with ASL class level (r = .73). Similar to the ASL-SRT, deaf native signers performed significantly better than deaf non-native signers and hearing native signers, although the deaf non-native signers and hearing native signers' performance was not significantly different. Hauser and colleagues (2016) argue that these findings provide backings for their claim that the percent of correct answers reflects an individual's ability to understand ASL (vocabulary, fingerspelling, and depicting verbs in phrases and sentences), indicating support for consistency-based inferences (i.e., generalization inference), but they did not make claims for more construct-based inferences such as extrapolation inferences or consequence implication inferences.

FUTURE DIRECTIONS

We attempted to evaluate adult L2 sign test publications that describe psychometric properties "of the test" to support its validity without making an overall argument about the validity of the test use and interpretation of results. Professionals who use such tests need to interpret test results with less confidence when the general purpose or use of tests is not described; intended inferences based on test scores are not discussed; and the clarity, coherence, and plausibility of claims are not evaluated. Tests with some psychometric data are still the best option to use over in-house tests without such data, but examiners need to realize that there are limitations to how test results can be appropriately interpreted. The ideal situation would be to have a battery of tests that measure different domains of language use. This is extremely important when test results imply a base for decisions because decisions are better made based on multiple test results rather than on just one.

Future adult L2 signed language competency tests should include unambiguous statements of claims so that it is clear what skills are being evaluated and how data should be interpreted (e.g., Kane, 2006, 2013). Clearly specified claims provide guidance on the kinds of evidence needed for evaluating the inferences and assumptions in the test's use and score interpretation. It is important to make claims and provide theories, empirical research, and data to warrant claims about, for example, the generalization inference of how performance on a sample of language use is related to everyday use of the language. If inferences are to be made from the domain that the test measures to other domains of language use (extrapolation inference), validity must be justified.

Future L2 signed language tests can be better developed and argument-based validity more robustly supported if item development leverages corpus data about actual language use. Psychometric analyses should sample the L2 learning population for whom the test is ultimately intended and should include a representative sample of diverse skills. The different types of language variation that exist within the test-takers' signing community should be carefully considered. The more accurately test items reflect actual language use, the more justified will be generalized inferences of the test's use and interpretations. If test developers claim that test results reflect test-takers' actual language skill outside of the testing situation, then extrapolation inferences will require that developers demonstrate a relationship between test results and actual observed behaviors. And, perhaps most importantly, for tests that are used for making decisions, test developers need to demonstrate that decisions based on tests are justified.

REFERENCES

Caccamise, F., & Newell, W. (1995). Evaluating sign language communication skills: The Sign Communication Proficiency Interview (SCPI). In R. Myers (Ed.), *Standards of care for the delivery of mental health services to deaf and hard of hearing persons* (pp. 33–35). National Association of the Deaf.

Caccamise, F. C., & Samar, V. J. (2009). Sign Language Proficiency Interview (SLPI): Prenegotiation interrater reliability and rater validity. *Contemporary Issues in Communication Science & Disorders, 36*, 36–47.

Chen Pichler, D., & Koulidobrova, H. (2015). Acquisition of a sign language as a second language. In M. Marschark & P. Spencer (Eds.), *Oxford handbook of deaf studies in language* (pp. 218–230). Oxford University Press. https://doi.org/10.1093/oxfordhb/9780190241414.013.14

Davies, A. (2003). *The native speaker: Myth and reality* (vol. 38). Multilingual Matters.

Gaillard, S., & Tremblay, A. (2016). Linguistic proficiency assessment in second language acquisition research: The elicited imitation task. *Language Learning, 66*(2), 419–447. https://doi.org/10.1111/lang.12157

Hauser, P. C., Paludnevicience, R., Riddle, W., Kurz, K. B., Emmorey, K., & Contreras, J. (2016). American Sign Language Comprehension Test: A tool for sign language researchers. *Journal of Deaf Studies and Deaf Education, 21*(1), 64–69. https://doi.org/10.1093/deafed/env051

Hauser, P. C., Paludnevičiene, R., Supalla, T., & Bavelier, D. (2008). American Sign Language-Sentence Reproduction Test: Development and implications. In R. M. de Quadros (Ed.), *Sign language: Spinning and unraveling the past, present and future* (pp. 160–172). Editora Arara Azul.
Kane, M. (2006). Validation. In R. Brennen (Ed.), *Educational measurement* (4th ed., pp. 17–64). Greenwood.
Kane, M. T. (2013). Validating the interpretations and uses of test scores. *Journal of Educational Measurement*, *50*(1), 1–73. https://doi.org/10.1111/jedm.12000
Klem, M., Melby-Lervåg, M., Hagtvet, B., Lyster, S. A. H., Gustafsson, J. E., & Hulme, C. (2015). Sentence repetition is a measure of children's language skills rather than working memory limitations. *Developmental Science*, *18*(1), 146–154. https://doi.org/10.1111/desc.12202
Knoch, U., & Chapelle, C. A. (2017). Validation of rating processes within an argument-based framework. *Language Testing*, *35*(4), 477–499. https://doi.org/10.1177/0265532217710049
Kubus, O., & Rathmann, C. (2013, July). Morphological error analysis in the M2/L2 acquisition of DGS-learners. Paper presented at the *Theoretical Issues in Sign Language Research (TISLR) Conference*, London, UK.
Landa, R., & Clark, M. (2019). L2/Ln sign language tests and assessment procedures and evaluation. *Psychology*, *10*(2), 181–198. https://doi.org/10.4236/psych.2019.102015
McCaskill, C., Lucas, C., Bayley, R., Hill, J. C., Dummet-King, R., Baldwin, P., & Hogue, R. (2011). *The hidden treasure of Black ASL: Its history and structure*. Gallaudet University Press.
Meier, R. (2002). Why different, why the same? Explaining effects and non-effects of modality upon linguistic structure in sign and speech. In R. P. Meier, K. Cormier, & D. Quinto-Pozos (Eds.), *Modality and structure in signed and spoken languages* (pp. 1–16). Cambridge University Press.
Padden, C. A. (2000). Simultaneous interpreting across modalities. *Interpreting*, *5*(2), 169–185. https://doi.org/10.1075/intp.5.2.07pad
Paludnevičience, R., Hauser, P. C., Daggett, D., & Kurz, K. B. (2012). Issues and trends in sign language assessment. In D. Morere & T. Allen (Eds.), *Measuring literacy and its neurocognitive predictors among deaf individuals: An assessment toolkit* (pp. 191–207). Springer.
Schembri, A., & Johnston, T. (2013). Sociolinguistic variation and change in sign languages. In R. Bayley, R. Cameron, & C. Lucas (Eds.), *The Oxford handbook of sociolinguistics*. Oxford University Press. https://doi.org/10.1093/oxfordhb/9780199744084.013.0025
Schönström, K. (2014). *Adaptation of sign language tests*. Presented at the 36th Language Testing Research Colloquium (LTRC), Amsterdam, Netherlands, 4–6 June, 2014. http://urn.kb.se/resolve?urn=urn:nbn:se:su:diva-131831
Schönström, K., & Holmström, I. (2017). *Elicited imitation tasks (EITs) as a tool for measuring sign language proficiency in L1 and L2 signers*. Presented at ALTE 6th Conference, Learning and Assessment: Making the Connections, Bologna, Italy, May 3–5, 2017. http://urn.kb.se/resolve?urn=urn:nbn:se:su:diva-150395
Supalla, T., Hauser, P. C., & Bavelier, D. (2014). Reproducing American Sign Language sentences: Cognitive scaffolding in working memory. *Frontiers in Psychology*, *5*. https://doi.org/10.3389/fpsyg.2014.$1$2

8.3

Discussion of Validation Issues in Signed and Spoken Assessments for Adult L2 Learners

Carol A. Chapelle, Peter C. Hauser, Hye-won Lee, Christian Rathmann, and Krister Schönström

The use of argument-based validity as a framework for discussion of validity issues in spoken and signed second language (L2) assessment reveals many areas of commonality. Common areas include the role of systematic test development practices in the validity argument, the complexity of rating issues, the need to define and assess a construct of functional communication of meaning, and the centrality of test use in the validity argument. By examining these areas of commonality in this chapter, we reveal the fundamental similarities in the basic validity issues faced in spoken and signed language assessment.

The validity of both spoken and signed tests of L2 communication rests on the foundation of systematic and appropriate test design and development procedures. The professional practices of test development are reported elsewhere in this volume (Chapters 1.1–1.3), but what is important for the validity argument is that these practices result in a record of their quality as well as a rationale for their use in creating test tasks that elicit relevant samples of test-takers' performance. In the testing of signed languages, this aspect of the validity argument has been given a lot of weight: The validity argument typically focuses on the quality of test development processes, including data that support claims about domain definition inferences. One element treated as key in this context is the qualifications of the test developers. Schönström, Hauser, and Rathmann (Chapter 8.2) noted, for example, that for the ASL Sentence Repetition, it was considered important that the test content was specified, signed, and evaluated by a team of native deaf signers with research backgrounds. In tests of spoken L2 communication, qualifications are also important but are typically eclipsed by warrants and assumptions about the quality of investigation of the domain of interest for the test. In the example provided by Chapelle and

Carol A. Chapelle, Peter C. Hauser, Hye-won Lee, Christian Rathmann, and Krister Schönström, *Discussion of Validation Issues in Signed and Spoken Assessments for Adult L2 Learners* In: *The Handbook of Language Assessment Across Modalities.* Edited by: Tobias Haug, Wolfgang Mann, and Ute Knoch, Oxford University Press. © Oxford University Press 2022. DOI: 10.1093/oso/9780190885052.003.0025

Lee of the test of spoken L2 pragmatics (Chapter 8.1), the test developer carried out a needs analysis to identify the most important pragmatic functions that should be the focus of the test. In both contexts, the analytic approaches for making decisions about test content will likely benefit from work in corpus linguistics and frameworks for test development. This is especially true for signed languages, which do not have a written mode, and thus signed language corpus research serves as an important source. Through signed language corpora, test developers are in a better position to control linguistic variation and make decisions about test content.

The consistency of scores is a critical concern underlying the validity of both spoken and signed tests of L2 communication, and therefore the inferences of evaluation and generalization are supported for both types of tests. Evaluation inferences require consistency in administration conditions, rating scales with clearly defined and appropriate criteria, and a strong program of rater training and monitoring. Some of these conditions, such as test security, are not typically described in the research literature on spoken L2 assessment even though they are important in operational practice. The research tends to focus on the development of rating scales as well as training raters and monitoring their performance. Generalization inferences are investigated in the research on both spoken and signed communication as testers examine the consistency of test scores across test tasks, test forms, occasions of testing, and raters. In spoken language assessment, consistency across test tasks is investigated using generalizability theory to determine the type and number of test tasks as well as the number of raters needed to achieve the targeted level of consistency in the scores. Consistency of ratings is accomplished through item-response theory, which provides results about the degree of raters' effects on the scores. The use of rating scales and human raters has been found to be essential for assessing the functional communicative success in both signed and oral communication, and therefore the topic of how to create scales and train, monitor, and correct for rater performance is likely to remain critically important. For signed language assessments, recruitment and training of raters can be a challenge due to the limited number of proficient signers with metalinguistic knowledge and training in signed language linguistics. Additionally, as signs often vary widely within the same signed languages depending on region, age, and other demographic factors, raters might only be familiar with their own variations. There is a risk that test developers overestimate the competency of signed language raters, which can lead to unreliable scores. In spoken language assessment, nevertheless, the use of computer-scored testing is used in some testing contexts, the claim being that automated rating processes can provide more reliable scores. The question, of course, for both spoken and signed assessments, is whether the reliable ratings are of interest if they fail to reflect the ability to communicate.

Demonstrating that a test assesses the ability to communicate requires a definition of the construct of communication ability. In a validity argument, the ability to communicate serves as the explanation for the meaning of the scores, if this is defined as the construct for the test. Validation research then needs to investigate the extent to which the theorized construct of communication ability is reflected in the test scores. For tests of spoken language, the construct is variously defined as consisting of a unitary trait, a multicomponential trait, a trait consisting of several areas of language knowledge and strategies, or as performance in certain specific contexts, among others. Because of the range of approaches used for defining communication ability for spoken tests, the methods for investigating construct-related evidence for the validity argument also vary. As for signed languages, because there are no various test approaches for defining communication ability to date, further research on construct-related evidence is needed. Some of the challenges inherent in creating good research designs for investigating explanation inferences are illustrated through the research on signed tests. For example, researchers compare existing groups of test-takers who are known to differ in their signed communication ability, such as deaf adults and deaf children, L1 signers and L2 signers, or deaf signers and hearing signers. Provided the construct theory (cf. Chapters 7.1–7.3) offers a basis for making predictions about test performance, comparisons of test scores between groups can be interpreted in terms of how well the test assesses signed communication ability. Analogies in the design of construct-related research between L2 spoken and signed communication ability are potentially abundant. Equally, the challenges of such research, including how to model and assess important dialect and register variation in observed performance and how to specify the intended scope of extrapolation, are shared by the two areas.

Testers adhering to professional guidelines undertake validation research in view of the intended use(s) of the test. In tests of L2 communication, the attention to test use and consequences has prompted validation studies focusing on specific decisions that are made based on test scores, as well as the effects of making such decisions. The focus on test use in validation studies can, on the one hand, be helpful in limiting the scope of validation research. On the other hand, it can be a challenge for test developers who develop tests that they claim are useful for a range of uses across different contexts. Such a use-free approach to test development creates problems for test users and for advances in the field more broadly. Users need tests that are appropriate for particular purposes; therefore, without necessarily having any knowledge about how to do so, they end up evaluating the validity of a "general purpose" test for their use. For the profession, when test development is not tailored to any particular use, test developers fail to improve testing practice to make testing more informative across a range of uses. Historically, the development of tests without specified uses was a widespread problem, and today this issue still exists among some tests of spoken and signed communication ability.

Tests of L2 signed language have much in common with tests of L2 of spoken languages, and therefore some of the critical issues in the validation of these tests of productive language skills might best be tackled through cross-fertilization. Three fundamental areas would be a good point of departure: (1) achieving a better understanding of the variation in potential uses for tests of communication ability and the implications of the different uses for the particulars of the respective validity arguments, (2) conceptualizing a means of modeling the appropriate range and type of variation in performance to be accepted in test-takers' responses, and (3) systematizing the process of domain analysis in the test development stage to take advantage of existing tools and experience. For both L2 spoken and signed language tests, an argument-based validity framework is useful for analyzing the complex process of validation.

Topic 9

Scoring Issues in Second Spoken and Signed Language Assessment

9.1

Scoring Spoken Second Language Assessment

Ute Knoch

Achieving scores that adequately reflect the test-takers' proficiency level as evidenced in spoken assessment tasks has been the subject of a large body of research in second language (L2) assessment, both in the classroom and in more high-stakes, standardized testing contexts. In fact, this area has attracted more attention than many other important aspects of assessment covered in this book, including score use and interpretation, the test construct, standard-setting, or the use of technology. This chapter summarizes research on scoring L2 spoken assessments, examining issues relating to both rater-mediated and automated scoring. I begin with a brief introduction of scoring carried out by human raters.

SCORING SPOKEN ASSESSMENTS USING HUMAN RATERS

Assessing spoken performances is not a straightforward matter. Many different aspects or facets within an assessment situation may influence the quality of the score reported, with many of these factors being construct-irrelevant and therefore unduly affecting the information that users get from the score and the types of interpretations that they can make (Knoch, Fairbairn & Jin (2021). Figure 9.1.1 presents some of these effects. As can be seen, the raters may be influenced by the training, standardization, and ongoing monitoring they receive. During the rating process, raters interact with a *rating scale* when evaluating performances. These performances have been produced by *test-takers* interacting with the *task* they were presented, as well as the *interlocutor(s)* (if applicable). During scoring, raters may produce possible rater effects while they are generating their scores. Testing agencies then may draw on a variety of methods to adjust scores before reporting them to score users. Based on the scores, feedback and/or retraining may be offered to raters.

Ute Knoch, *Scoring Spoken Second Language Assessment* In: *The Handbook of Language Assessment Across Modalities*. Edited by: Tobias Haug, Wolfgang Mann, and Ute Knoch, Oxford University Press. © Oxford University Press 2022. DOI: 10.1093/oso/9780190885052.003.0026

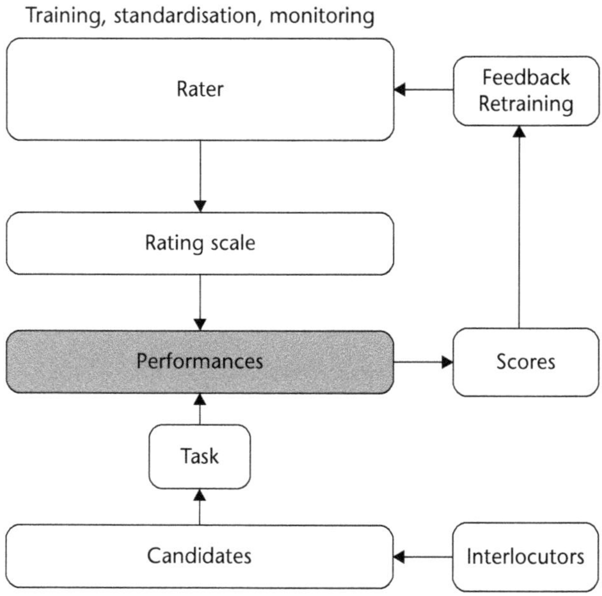

Figure 9.1.1 Aspects influencing test scores in spoken assessment.

Here, I review current research on a selection of these factors (rater effects, rater training, rater feedback, rater characteristics, interlocutor/interviewer effects, rating scales and their development) before describing the alternative to using human raters: automated scoring.

Rater Effects (Rating Quality)

Concerns about the reliability of the rater-mediated assessment of spoken (and written) language have resulted in a substantial amount of research in this area (Fulcher, 2003). This work originated out of unease about the effect of rater differences on test-takers' scores and the consequences on assessment outcomes. Differences in rater severity, for example, can influence a test-takers' final score to such an extent that the candidates' true speaking ability is not fully reflected in their score. While earlier studies mainly relied on correlational techniques to investigate rater reliability, recent work has drawn on more advanced statistical techniques, such as the use of many-faceted Rasch measurement (Linacre, 1989) and Generalizability theory (or G-theory) (Lynch & McNamara, 1998). These techniques are able to model the influence of raters more accurately and, in the case of many-faceted Rasch measurement, a test-taker can be provided with a fair score that is adjusted after taking the rater characteristics into account. These statistical techniques have also made it possible to highlight different areas in which raters may differ (McNamara, 1996; Myford & Wolfe, 2003, 2004).

As mentioned earlier, raters may apply different levels of leniency and harshness and therefore unnecessarily advantage or disadvantage certain candidates. Raters may also differ in their rating consistency, which means that they display an inconsistent picture of leniency and harshness across test-takers. Finally, raters may also display a *rating bias*. This means that they show an interaction effect with certain criteria on the rating scale (in the case of an analytic rating scale[1]), which means that they may rate certain criteria or certain test-taker characteristics more harshly or leniently than others (e.g., when rating test-takers from a certain gender or a particular language background). Such factors have been classified as construct irrelevant variance (Messick, 1989) as they mask the candidates' true ability.

Research into rater reliability in spoken L2 assessment can be broadly divided into studies that set out to investigate overall rating reliability and studies concerned with uncovering one or two particular sources of construct-irrelevant variance. Yan (2014), for example, employed a mixed-method approach to evaluate rater performance on a large-scale oral proficiency tests used to measure the oral proficiency of international teaching assistants. The study uncovered that although the overall rater reliability was acceptable, there was a low rate of exact agreement on scores. The qualitative data (rater verbal protocols) showed that these discrepancies were due to disagreements between raters at lower score levels as well as varied ratings of test-takers from particular backgrounds (e.g., Indian and Chinese examinees), issues that we describe in greater detail later. The authors argue that the use of both quantitative and qualitative data can be used effectively to triangulate different scoring information to gain a more holistic picture of rater reliability.

Rater Training and Rater Feedback

Rater training is usually used to eliminate or at least minimize rater effects. Studies have shown that rater training, which is usually considered a standard procedure in most high-stakes rating contexts, can reduce extreme differences between raters in terms of differences in severity and rater bias (Elder et al., 2005, 2007; Weigle, 1998). Rater training has, however, been criticized for forcing raters to artificially agree and to distract from an authentic listening experience (see, e.g., Charney, 1984) as raters engage with the spoken performances in a different way to a listener in the target language use domain. Despite these criticisms, rater training is considered important to clarify the scoring expectations and procedures to the raters and improve scorers' understanding of the rating criteria.

Some studies have experimented with providing rater training online (Brown & Jaquith, 2007, 2011; Elder et al., 2007; Erlam et al., 2013; Knoch et al., 2007, 2015) to facilitate access to raters working from home in their own time. Others have examined the effectiveness of providing individualized feedback to raters (Elder et al., 2005; Knoch, 2011; Wigglesworth, 1993). In the most recent study with this aim, Knoch (2011) provided longitudinal, individualized feedback to raters based on the output from a many-faceted Rasch analysis. Raters were provided with these reports following each administration of the Occupational English test, a standardized high-stakes test designed to assess the language proficiency of overseas-trained healthcare professionals intending to immigrate to an English-speaking country. The reports provided detailed feedback on each rater's relative leniency and harshness in comparison to the other raters in the group, the raters' consistency, and whether they displayed any biases in relation to any of the scoring criteria. The raters were asked to adjust their rating behavior in their following test administration. Knoch (2011) was able to show that the raters were not able to rate better with the feedback than when not receiving the feedback and that there were also no differences between providing feedback to writing and speaking raters.

Rater Characteristics

Other studies have examined particular sources of construct-irrelevant variance, focusing both on the raters themselves and on the raters' characteristics and their interaction with the ratees (e.g., by examining accent familiarity). Rater characteristics can be divided into (1) rating experience and (2) language and language learning background. Rater experience has been extensively investigated in studies on raters of written assessments/performances (see e.g., Cumming, 1990; Weigle, 1998). Fewer such studies are available in the area of spoken assessment. Isaacs and Thomson (2013), for example, compared the judgments of novice and experienced raters on two scales for comprehensibility, accentedness, and fluency. Although the statistical analysis (many-faceted Rasch analysis) found no significant differences between the ratings of the two groups of raters, verbal reports were able to distinguish different strategies employed by the two groups in dealing with ratings they found difficult. A number of studies have focused on raters' language background to investigate possible interactions between this factor and test-takers' scores (Brown, 1995; Chalhoub-Deville & Wigglesworth, 2005; Kim, 2009; Xi & Mollaun, 2009; Zhang & Elder, 2011). While most quantitative studies found little or negligible interaction effects between raters' first language (L1) and their scoring, studies employing complementary qualitative investigations (usually by employing verbal protocols) were able to uncover some differences in, for example, how the criteria were weighted (Kim, 2009) and in rating behaviors more generally (Zhang & Elder, 2011). More recently, studies have also investigated the influence of raters' language learning background by investigating accent familiarity (Carey et al., 2011;

Winke et al., 2013; Xi & Mollaun, 2006, 2009). Winke et al. (2013), for example, examined whether accent familiarity led to rater bias. In their analysis of 107 ratings of 432 Test of English as a Foreign Language (TOEFL) iBT[2] speech samples, they were able to show that raters who have learned Spanish are more lenient when rating test-takers from a Spanish L1 background and raters who have familiarity with Chinese are more lenient when rating Chinese students. All the studies just listed found some effect for rater familiarity with candidate accents and therefore suggest that this potential issue needs to be specifically addressed in rater training.

Interlocutor/Interviewer Effects

Specific to L2 spoken assessment are interlocutor and interviewer effects which can unduly influence a test-taker's score. For example, *paired speaking tests*, where two or more test-takers interact with each other during a speaking test and are rated based on this interaction, are increasingly becoming popular. May (2011) as well as Ducasse and Brown (2009) conducted verbal protocols with raters and showed how they struggled with awarding individual scores to individual test-takers based on this co-constructed performance, where success of the communication cannot be attributed to just one of the individuals. Studies have also examined how raters deal with judging performances collected with varying interviewers. Brown (2003) was able to show, employing verbal protocols, how some raters compensate for such interviewer variability by assigning different scores than they may have if they would have not found the interviewer to have influenced the communication.

RATING SCALES AND THEIR DEVELOPMENT

Scoring criteria are designed to provide an operational definition of the construct that an assessment is designed to measure (e.g., Davies et al., 1999), and they therefore embody the underlying abilities that test developers are attempting to measure. They are mostly designed for raters (but see Alderson, 1991, for other types of scales) and are aimed at making the rating process as objective as possible (Winke, 2013). Given the importance of rating scales to the assessment process, surprisingly little information is available on how rating scales are developed (e.g., Fulcher, 2003). This is probably because many rating scales are merely adaptations of other rating scales, and development or adaption methods are not well documented.

The quality of a scale, and therefore how well it is able to help raters achieve rating consistency, is directly related to how it was developed (and also how it is incorporated into rater training sessions, as we discussed earlier). When developing a rating scale for spoken performance, test developers need to make a number of decisions. First, they need to decide on the type of rating scale to use. Two main types of scales are generally used in language assessments: holistic and analytic rating scales. *Holistic rating scales* present overall descriptions of spoken performance, while *analytic rating scales* include descriptors for a number of criteria at different score levels. Apart from these two most commonly used scale types, some tests also use detailed diagnostic checklists, where the construct under interest is detailed in even finer details or relies on decision trees (Fulcher et al., 2011; Turner & Upshur, 2002; Upshur & Turner, 1999). The choice of scale is often related to the purpose of the assessment. If an estimation of the overall proficiency level is of interest, a holistic scale may be the most suitable, whereas in a classroom environment, where formative feedback is usually desired, a detailed checklist may be the more appropriate choice.

The next decision relates to how the construct (i.e., the trait of spoken language) is embodied in the set of scales: What criteria are included? Some studies have described in detail how aspects of the speaking construct were translated into rating scale descriptors. Elder et al. (2013) set out to develop professionally relevant speaking scale descriptors for an English screening test for healthcare professionals intending to immigrate to an English-speaking country. In the first stage of the project, they played video performances of medical students interacting with patients to a group of healthcare professionals. In these focus groups, the healthcare professionals commented on any aspects in the spoken performance of the students that they valued. These focus group discussions were recorded, transcribed, and then analyzed. All aspects relevant to language performance, including their ability to actively listen and engage in a patient-centered way, were recorded in detailed checklists. These checklist indicators included aspects not previously included in the speaking descriptors, and the authors argued that the construct of the new scale is more relevant to the domain of assessing languages for specific purposes than the previous, more linguistic criteria.

In another study, May (2011) examined how raters evaluate interactional competence in paired speaking tests. As suggested earlier, raters may have difficulty rating this criterion due to the co-constructed nature of the interactions. May collected verbal protocols from raters when rating this criterion. She also examined rater notes and rater discussions. She discovered a number of features noted by raters, including some that were seen as mutual achievements and were therefore difficult to score individually. She noted that the findings are implications for the construct of interactional competence in speaking tests and the operationalization of the construct in rating scales.

As mentioned earlier, rating scales are often based on intuition or previously designed scales rather than on a theoretical model (Fulcher,

2003). Intuitions may come from one test developer's or researcher's experience or be collated from a group of experts. Often rating scales are changed repeatedly over many years. However, these intuitive development methods have been criticized for lacking theoretical underpinnings and often either under- or misrepresenting the construct they are designed to assess. For this reason, some researchers have suggested that scales should be based on models or theories of language proficiency or language development.

Intuition-based rating scales have been criticized at times for including features which are not actually found in the sample/performance to be rated or for employing vague terminology (e.g., Brindley, 1998; Mickan, 2003; Turner & Upshur, 2002; Upshur & Turner, 1995). For this reason, some researchers have developed rating scales empirically, basing the descriptors on features in real test-takers' performances (see, e.g., Fulcher, 1987, 1996) following discourse analyses of performances at different score levels. Such methods have also been popular in language tests for specific purposes to ensure that the assessment rubrics are closely linked with the domain in question. In a study currently in progress (Knoch, McNamara, et al., 2015), researchers are using a blended approach to rating scale development by first collecting the values of domain experts (in this case healthcare professionals), then developing initial checklist indicators. The next stage involves experienced raters identifying the checklist indicators in test data from the test, resulting in the final revision of the rating rubric, and therefore ensuring that the final rating rubric is both reflective of the professional context in which language is used and empirically grounded.

Regardless of the development method, however, it is important that the scale is theoretically sound and useful to test users. Increasing numbers of scales are developed to be directly linked to assessment or learning frameworks, such as the Common European Framework of Reference (CEFR; Council of Europe, 2001; Deygers & Van Gorp, 2015; Harsch & Martin, 2012). Harsch and Martin (2012) provide a detailed description how they started from the CEFR, which, like most frameworks, was developed for policy purposes and developed for operational rating scales in an iterative process involving trained raters. While their study focused on writing assessment, the same method could be applied to speaking assessment.

SCORE RESOLUTION TECHNIQUES

Despite thorough focus on rater training and ongoing rater standardization techniques, it is generally agreed that raters may not fully agree on scores for performance assessments. To ensure that the scores reported to score users are fair, most large-scale testing agencies employ more than one rater to rate speaking performances because scores from just one rater may not be reflective of the spoken performance if a test-taker is only scored by one harsh or one lenient rater alone. However, this raises the issue of what to do if the two raters do not agree in their ratings. While some agencies routinely employing many-faceted Rasch analysis as part of their test administration, which can easily resolve such differences (Rasch reports a "fair score" that corrects for unduly harsh or lenient raters), researchers have also experimented with other score resolution methods. Studies have, for example, examined whether involving raters in discussions to resolve score differences is more effective compared to simply averaging the scores (Johnson et al., 2000, 2005; Penny & Johnson, 2011). Penny and Johnson (2011) modeled the score accuracy of a variety of such score resolution studies using a Monte Carlo study and varying the factors associated with scoring and resolution. They concluded that more research in this area is necessary but recommended that using an adjudicator with high rater reliability if this is possible.

AUTOMATED SCORING

There is a growing focus on automated scoring of spoken L2 performances on behalf of the language testing industry, with attempts at combining assessments that are administered by machine and machine scored. One of the most well-established and known of these tests is the Versant English Test (Pearson, 2020), a fully automated speaking test. It includes an automated phone response system, a speech recognizer and analyzer, and a score generator (Bernstein et al., 2010; Pearson Education, 2008). The assessment system also includes a digital storage bank for speech samples. Other systems, like the SpeechRater technology developed by the Educational Testing Service, are still restricted to low-stakes contexts where no important decisions are made about test-takers (see, e.g., Zechner et al., 2015). It is important to scrutinize the scoring mechanisms that underlie these systems to gain an understanding of the construct represented in the test. The Versant English Test, for example, targets aspects such as sentence mastery (operationalized in terms of test-takers' syntactic processing of lexical items, phrases and clauses), fluency (operationalized through a range of temporal measures, such as rhythm, phrasing, and timing), pronunciation (operationalized as the ability to produce consonants, vowels, and stress in "native-like manner"), and vocabulary (operationalized as test-takers' ability to produce frequent words in connected speech) (Pearson Education, 2008). It is clear from this list that the construct measured by this test is restricted when compared to the aspects that a human rater can attend to (human raters are able to judge more complicated aspects of speech, such as the content, the communicative effectiveness, discourse structure, and so on). This takes me to the first of two issues that are crucially examined in relation to automated scoring: construct validity. The highly restrictive tasks[3] that are needed in most cases to apply automated scoring systems and the limited types of measures that automated scoring systems rely on (scoring often is highly dependent on fluency and pronunciation) limit the kind of interpretations we can make based on the scores (see, e.g., Bridgeman et al., 2011; Xi, 2012). The second issue is directly related to this issue. The nature of the tasks included in automated spoken assessments is restricted, resulting in constrained tasks that are also highly inauthentic (e.g., Chun, 2008). As one can imagine, there is great controversy regarding the use of automated scoring systems. Proponents of such assessment systems have argued that the context-independent nature of such tasks is a strength of these automated assessments in that the results are generalizable to a wider range of target language use situations (see, e.g., Pearson Education, 2008). Opponents, however, argue against this view, maintaining that tasks should not be decontextualized. Other issues of automated speech scoring relate to the native speaker norms often aspired to by these systems, which focus on accuracy in pronunciation and the similarity to native-speaker norms, rather than how intelligible a speaker is.[4] Similarly, the types of errors assessed as part of the scoring mechanism may not all be equally detrimental to comprehensibility, with those easily detectable by automated scoring machines (such as some grammatical errors) often being classed as less harmful. As can be seen from this discussion, automated scoring systems of L2 speech, while free of the types of scoring errors introduced by raters, are not without their own problems.

FUTURE DIRECTIONS

Future work in spoken L2 performances is inevitably going to focus on improving automated scoring systems, with the aim of broadening the construct they are able to measure. One avenue of further work may be to explore how the different measures used to score can be explored to provide diagnostic information to learners and other stakeholders, in line with automated feedback systems currently being used in written assessment. Work in cognitive diagnosis to L2 testing (Lee & Sawaki, 2009) is promising in this respect, and the greater explication of the target construct needed for such purposes will at the same time deepen our understanding of the theory of L2 speaking.

But future work will not only be limited to automated scoring. Human scoring is here to stay until automated scoring systems become cheaper, more readily available, and able to assess a broader construct. In the meantime, research on human raters will continue. In the near future, an increasing number of research studies will focus on interaction effects between the different facets shown in Figure 9.1.1 (e.g., the interaction between rater training, rater characteristics, and certain candidate characteristics). It is to be expected that more practical implications for rater training will emerge based on these studies. Rater training is likely to be carried out online more frequently, creating different "communities of practice" for raters who tend to work from home and score using computers, rather than listening to live performances.

Irrespective of whether a performance is scored by a human or machine, focus will continue to broaden the construct of what we measure in spoken performances. For example, I anticipate more work concentrating on particular aspects that accompany spoken performances but that have been studied much less frequently, such as the use of body language.

CONCLUSION

The review of the literature on scoring L2 spoken assessments shows that this is an active research area with a solid research base. Studies on human rater scoring have a long history in language assessment. More recently, the focus has shifted to examining automated scoring, but, as the brief review shows, more work is needed in this area. Because of the highly controlled speaking tasks necessary for current automated scoring systems, there are no examples of assessments administered by humans but then machine scored (although the opposite is not uncommon). Automated scoring is attractive because it eliminates many of the factors described earlier in relation to human raters and provides more reliable and objective scores. At the same time, however, scoring technologies still rely on relatively simple features of speech and are therefore only able to measure a more restricted construct compared to human raters.

NOTES

1. An analytic rating scale is a scoring rubric with several categories (e.g., grammar, pronunciation, vocabulary, etc.).
2. The TOEFL is an internet-based test.
3. Tasks used in assessments that rely on automated scoring are usually not reflective of real-life spoken communication. Tasks may draw on test-takers reading back sentences or providing short answers to questions.
4. A further issue is what norms the assessment systems are trained on; that is, whether the system expects speakers to adhere to American English or British English norms or whether other varieties are also acceptable.

REFERENCES

Alderson, C. (1991). Bands and scores. In C. Alderson & B. North (Eds.), *Language testing in the 1990s: The communicative legacy* (pp. 71–86). Modern English Publications/British Council/MacMillan.

Bernstein, J., Van Moere, A., & Cheng, J. (2010). Validating automated speaking tests. *Language Testing, 27*(3), 355–377. https://doi.org/10.1177/0265532210364404

Bridgeman, B., Powers, D., Stone, E., & Mollaun, P. (2011). TOEFL iBT speaking test scores as indicators of communicative language proficiency. *Language Testing, 29*(1), 91–108. https://doi.org/10.1177/0265532211411078

Brindley, G. (1998). Describing language development? Rating scales and SLA. In L. F. Bachman & A. D. Cohen (Eds.), *Interfaces between second language acquisition and language testing research* (pp. 112–140). Cambridge University Press.

Brown, A. (1995). The effect of rater variables in the development of an occupation-specific language performance test. *Language Testing, 12*(1), 1–15. https://doi.org/10.1177/026553229501200101

Brown, A. (2003). Interviewer variation and the co-construction of speaking proficiency. *Language Testing, 20*(1), 1–25. https://doi.org/10.1191/0265532203lt242oa

Brown, A., & Jaquith, P. (2007). *Online rater training: Perceptions and performance.* Paper presented at the Language Testing Research Colloquium, Barcelona, Spain.

Brown, A., & Jaquith, P. (2011). The development and validation of an online rater training and marking system: Promises and pitfalls. In B. O'Sullivan (Ed.), *Language testing: Theories and practices* (pp. 244–261). Palgrave Macmillan.

Carey, M. D., Manell, R. H., & Dunn, P. K. (2011). Does a rater's familiarity with a candidate's pronunciation affect the rating in oral proficiency interviews? *Language Testing, 28*(2), 201–219. https://doi.org/10.1177/0265532210393704

Chalhoub-Deville, M., & Wigglesworth, G. (2005). Rater judgement and English language speaking proficiency. *World Englishes, 24*(3), 383–391. https://doi.org/10.1111/j.0083-2919.2005.00419.x

Charney, D. (1984). The validity of using holistic scoring to evaluate writing: A critical overview. *Research in the Teaching of English, 18*, 65–81.

Chun, C. W. (2008). Comments on "evaluation of the usefulness of the Versant for English test: A response": The author responds. *Language Assessment Quarterly, 5*(2), 168–172. https://doi.org/10.1080/15434300801934751

Council of Europe. (2001). *Common European framework of reference for languages: Learning, teaching, assessment.* Cambridge University Press.

Cumming, A. (1990). Expertise in evaluating second language compositions. *Language Testing, 7*, 31–51. https://doi.org/10.1177/026553229000700104

Davies, A., Brown, A., Elder, C., Hill, K., Lumley, T., & McNamara, T. (1999). *Dictionary of language testing.* Cambridge University Press.

Deygers, B., & Van Gorp, K. (2015). Determining the score validity of a co-constructed CEFR-based rating scale. *Language Testing, 32*(4), 521–541. https://doi.org/10.1177/0265532215575626

Ducasse, A., & Brown, A. (2009). Assessing paired orals: Raters' orientation to interaction. *Language Testing, 26*(3), 423–443. https://doi.org/10.1177/0265532209104669

Elder, C., Barkhuizen, G., Knoch, U., & von Randow, J. (2007). Evaluating rater responses to an online rater training program. *Language Testing, 24*(1), 37–64. https://doi.org/10.1177/0265532207071511

Elder, C., Knoch, U., Barkhuizen, G., & von Randow, J. (2005). Individual feedback to enhance rater training: Does it work? *Language Assessment Quarterly, 2*(3), 175–196. https://doi.org/10.1207/s15434311laq0203_1

Elder, C., McNamara, T., Woodward-Kron, R., Manias, E., McColl, G., Webb, G., & Pill, J. (2013). *Towards improved healthcare communication: Development and validation of language proficiency standards for non-native English speaking health professionals*. Final report for the OET Centre. https://minerva-access.unimelb.edu.au/handle/11343/55166

Erlam, R., Von Randow, J., & Read, J. (2013). Investigating an online rater training program: Product and process. *Papers in Language Testing and Assessment, 2*(1), 1–29.

Fulcher, G. (1987). Tests of oral performance: The need for data-based criteria. *ELT Journal, 41*(4), 287–291. https://doi.org/10.1093/elt/41.4.287

Fulcher, G. (1996). Does thick description lead to smart tests? A data-based approach to rating scale construction. *Language Testing, 13*(2), 208–238.

Fulcher, G. (2003). *Testing second language speaking*. Pearson.

Fulcher, G., Davidson, F., & Kemp, J. (2011). Effective rating scale development for speaking tests: Performance decision trees. *Language Testing, 28*(1), 5–29. https://doi.org/10.1177/0265532209359514

Harsch, C., & Martin, G. (2012). Adapting CEF-descriptors for rating purposes: Validation by a combined rater training and scale revision approach. *Assessing Writing, 17*(2), 228–250. https://doi.org/10.1016/j.asw.2012.06.003

Isaacs, T., & Thomson, R. I. (2013). Rater experience, rating scale length, and judgements of L2 pronunciation: Revisiting research conventions. *Language Assessment Quarterly, 10*(2), 135–159. https://doi.org/10.1080/15434303.2013.769545

Johnson, R. L., Penny, J., & Gordon, B. (2000). The relation between score resolution methods and interrater reliability: An empirical study of an analytic scoring rubric. *Applied Measurement in Education, 13*(2), 121–138. https://doi.org/10.1207/S15324818AME1302_1

Johnson, R. L., Penny, J., Gordon, B., Shumate, S., & Fisher, S. (2005). Resolving score differences in the rating of writing samples: Does discussion improve the accuracy of scores? *Language Assessment Quarterly, 2*(2), 117–146. https://doi.org/10.1207/s15434311laq0202_2

Kim, Y. H. (2009). An investigation into native and non-native teachers' judgements of oral English performance: A mixed methods approach. *Language Testing, 26*(2), 187–217. https://doi.org/10.1177/0265532208101010

Knoch, U. (2011). Investigating the effectiveness of individualized feedback to rating behaviour: A longitudinal study. *Language Testing, 28*(2), 179–200. https://doi.org/10.1177/0265532210384252

Knoch, U., Fairbairn, J., & Huisman, A. (2015). *An evaluation of the effectiveness of training Aptis raters online*. London: British Council.

Knoch, U., Fairbairn, J., & Jin, Y. (2021). *Scoring second language spoken and written performances: Issues, options and directions*. Equinox.

Knoch, U., McNamara, T., Woodward-Kron, R., Elder, C., Manias, E., Flynn, E., & Zhang, B. (2015). Towards improved language assessment of written health professional communication: The case of the Occupational English Test. *Papers in Language Testing and Assessment, 4*(2), 60–66.

Knoch, U., Read, J., & von Randow, J. (2007). Re-training raters online: How does it compare with face-to-face training? *Assessing Writing, 12*, 26–43. https://doi.org/10.1016/j.asw.2007.04.001

Lee, Y.-W., & Sawaki, Y. (2009). Cognitive diagnosis approaches to language assessment: An overview. *Language Assessment Quarterly, 6*(3), 172–189. https://doi.org/10.1080/15434300902985108

Linacre, J. M. (1989). *Many-faceted Rasch measurement*. MESA Press.

Lynch, B., & McNamara, T. (1998). Using G-theory and Many-facet Rasch measurement in the development of performance assessments of the ESL speaking skills of immigrants. *Language Testing, 15*(2), 158–180. https://doi.org/10.1177/026553229801500202

May, L. (2011). *Interaction in a paired speaking test: The rater's perspective*. Peter Lang.

McNamara, T. (1996). *Measuring second language performance*. Longman.

Messick, S. (1989). Validity. In R. L. Linn (Ed.), *Educational measurement* (3rd ed., pp. 13–103). Macmillan.

Mickan, P. (2003). *"What's your score?" An investigation into language descriptors for rating written performance*. https://www.ielts.org/-/media/research-reports/ielts_rr_volume05_report3.ashx

Myford, C. M., & Wolfe, E. W. (2003). Detecting and measuring rater effects using many-facet Rasch measurement: Part I. *Journal of Applied Measurement, 4*(4), 386–422.

Myford, C. M., & Wolfe, E. W. (2004). Detecting and measuring rater effects using many-facet Rasch measurement: Part II. *Journal of Applied Measurement, 5*(2), 189–227.

Pearson. (2020, July 23). Versant tests. https://www.versanttest.com/products/english.jsp

Pearson Education. (2008). *Versant English Test: Test description & validation summary*. Retrieved from Palo Alto, CA: Pearson Education.

Penny, J., & Johnson, R. (2011). The accuracy of performance task scores after resolution of rater disagreement: A Monte Carlo study. *Assessing Writing, 16*(4), 221–236. https://doi.org/10.1016/j.asw.2011.06.001

Turner, C. E., & Upshur, J. A. (2002). Rating scales derived from student samples: Effects of the scale maker and the student sample on scale content and student scores. *TESOL Quarterly, 36*(1), 49–70. https://doi.org/10.2307/3588360

Upshur, J. A., & Turner, C. E. (1995). Constructing rating scales for second language tests. *ELT Journal, 49*(1), 3–12. https://doi.org/10.1093/elt/49.1.3

Upshur, J. A., & Turner, C. E. (1999). Systematic effects in the rating of second-language speaking ability: Test method and learner discourse. *Language Testing, 16*(1), 82–111. https://doi.org/10.1177/026553229901600105

Weigle, S. C. (1998). Using FACETS to model rater training effects. *Language Testing, 15*(2), 263–287. https://doi.org/10.1177/026553229801500205

Wigglesworth, G. (1993). Exploring bias analysis as a tool for improving rater consistency in assessing oral interaction. *Language Testing, 10*(3), 305–323. https://doi.org/10.1177/026553229301000306

Winke, P. (2013). Rating oral language. In C. Chapelle (Ed.), *The encyclopedia of applied linguistics*. Blackwell: https://onlinelibrary.wiley.com/doi/10.1002/9781405198431.wbeal0993

Winke, P., Gass, S., & Myford, C. (2013). Raters' L2 background as a potential source of bias in rating oral performance. *Language Testing, 30*(2), 231–252. https://doi.org/10.1177/0265532212456968

Xi, X. (2012). Validity and the automated scoring of performance tests. In G. Fulcher & F. Davidson (Eds.), *The Routledge handbook of language testing* (pp. 438–451). Routledge.

Xi, X., & Mollaun, P. (2006). *Investigating the utility of analytic scoring for the TOEFL academic speaking test (TAST)*. Princeton University Press.

Xi, X., & Mollaun, P. (2009). How do raters from India perform in scoring the TOEFL iBT speaking section and what kind of training helps? TOEFL iBT Research Report RR-09-31. https://doi.org/10.1002/j.2333-8504.2009.tb02188.x

Yan, X. (2014). An examination of rater performance on a local oral English proficiency test: A mixed-methods approach. *Language Testing, 31*(4), 501–527. https://doi.org/10.1177/0265532214536171

Zechner, K., Chen, L., Davies, L., Evanini, K., Lee, C. M., Leong, C. W., Wang, X., & Yoon, S.-Y. (2015). Automated scoring of speaking tasks in the Test of English-for-Teaching (TEFT). http://doi.org/10.1002/ets2.12080

Zhang, Y., & Elder, C. (2011). Judgments of oral proficiency by non-native and native English speaking teacher raters: Competing or complementary constructs? *Language Testing, 28*(1), 31–50. https://doi.org/10.1177/0265532209360671

9.2

Scoring Second Signed Language Assessment

Tobias Haug, Eveline Boers-Visker, Wolfgang Mann, Geoffrey Poor, and Beppie Van den Bogaerde

Few studies have been published on practical or theoretical issues in signed language testing for adult second language (L2) or foreign language learners—let alone on scoring (e.g., Caccamise & Samar, 2009; Haug, 2017). One possible reason is the early stage of this field of research and its application. Another reason might be that institutions of higher education where signed languages are taught, including signed language interpreter training programs, have their own assessments in place. These instruments usually take the form of assessments that operate under the specific criteria or outcomes of a particular course; information about them is rarely published. There are a few studies documenting the development of a particular signed language test (e.g., the American Sign Language Sentence Reproduction Test; Hauser et al., 2008; Supalla et al., 2014) which mention issues related to scoring, such as inter- and intrarater reliability and rater training, although very briefly. In short, there is almost no study available in signed language testing that specifically addresses scoring issues.

With these limitations in mind, we take a closer look at the few studies available that include information on scoring signed language performance in adult learners. One assessment on which data on scoring issues is available is the Sign Language Proficiency Interview (SLPI; e.g., Newell et al., 1983) developed at the National Technical Institute for the Deaf (NTID), Rochester Institute of Technology (RIT) in the United States. The SLPI is an adaptation of the Language/Oral Proficiency Interview (OPI) for spoken English (Liskin-Gasparro, 1982) to American Sign Language (ASL). It was subsequently adapted to Sign Language of the Netherlands (*Nederlandse Gebarentaal* [NGT]; Van den Broek-Laven et al., 2014) and Swiss German Sign Language (*Deutschschweizerische Gebärdensprache* [DSGS]; Haug et al., 2019). The adaptation to NGT is called the NFA (*NGT Functional Assessment*). Apart

Tobias Haug, Eveline Boers-Visker, Wolfgang Mann, Geoffrey Poor, and Beppie Van den Bogaerde, *Scoring Second Signed Language Assessment* In: *The Handbook of Language Assessment Across Modalities*. Edited by: Tobias Haug, Wolfgang Mann, and Ute Knoch, Oxford University Press. © Oxford University Press 2022. DOI: 10.1093/oso/9780190885052.003.0027 from the SLPI, two other proficiency interviews for ASL were examined for this chapter: the ASL Proficiency Interview (ASLPI) developed at Gallaudet University in Washington, DC, and the Assessment of Signed Communication: American Sign Language (ASC:ASL), provided by the Educational Testing Service (ETS, 2014). For these last two interviews/test, very little information could be found; therefore the main discussion will be about the SLPI.

To guide the reader who is unfamiliar with these assessments, they will be briefly introduced in the following subsections, followed by a discussion on those topics.

THE SIGN LANGUAGE PROFICIENCY INTERVIEW

The SLPI is a video-recorded interview between the test-taker and the interviewer targeting functional language use (Caccamise & Samar, 2009); that is, the test-taker's ability to expressively and receptively communicate in ASL in different settings, such as in a signing environment at a university (e.g., Caccamise & Newell, 1999). Following the interview, the video-recordings are analyzed by trained SLPI raters, using the SLPI Rating Scale[1] that defines 11 discrete ASL levels ranging from "No Functional Skills" to "Superior Plus." The raters document the interviewee's language, both function and form, on a Rater Worksheet.[2] The Rater Worksheet is complemented by two documents to help with analysis, one using functional descriptors and one using descriptors for linguistic factors/form.[3] Further and more detailed examples on linguistic forms are provided in a separate guideline.[4] These scales are used to rate or judge the performance of the interviewee/test-taker, and the results and decisions are transferred to the Rater Worksheet.

The Rater Worksheet used in the rating process consists of three parts. In the first part, analyzing only function (1. Functional Range in the worksheet), the raters complete a 3-point functional scale ("above intermediate," "at intermediate," "below intermediate") to evaluate the overall signing of the test-taker. In the second part of the worksheet (2. Functional Descriptors), the raters select from the 11 functional descriptors the one that best matches the ASL level of the test-taker. In the third part of the rating scale (sections A. Vocabulary Knowledge through E. Candidate's Comprehension), focusing on sign form only, ASL skills are evaluated based on the candidate's vocabulary knowledge and use, production and fluency, use of grammatical features, discourse strategies, and overall comprehension. Each of these categories is further subdivided into different subcategories that focus on specific features. For instance, one category, "use of grammatical features," evaluates use of ASL grammar (e.g., directionality, morphological inflection, sentence structures, etc.). Upon completion, the test-taker is assigned a summative rating level, such as "Survival," "Intermediate

Plus," etc., based on the original OPI for spoken English (Liskin-Gasparro, 1982).

The different sections (A–E) in Part 3 of the rating sheet do not have a specific weight within the rating scale, but if a candidate performs very well in one area and badly in another, the overall rating will go down. The rating for vocabulary knowledge, for example, uses specific wording to describe the candidate's level of vocabulary knowledge. This specific wording corresponds to one of the functional levels (e.g., "very broad" corresponds to the level "Superior"). The observed examples of language use (lexical, grammatical, and discourse)—that is, the raw data—are written on the rating sheet. The raters then choose descriptors (e.g., good use, very clear, many, etc.) to describe the quality and quantity of the language in the sample. Finally, they match the descriptors with the appropriate level on the Rating Scale.

RELIABILITY ISSUES

Raters Training and Score Resolution Techniques

The National SLPI:ASL Leadership Board (NSLB) provides 4-day training workshops on administering the SLPI and use of the different rating procedures (Caccamise & Newell, 2009). The workshop trains participants in interviewing, rating, and sharing of results. A major focus of the training is on how to use the rating scale and what is meant by the concepts of form and function. It also develops participants' skills through many practice ratings, with the level of supervision and guidance decreasing as skills improve. The same training has been provided to the members of the NFA interview and rating teams in three RIT/NTID led training sessions between 2011 and 2014. In 2017, a Dutch trainer was trained by RIT/NTID to train new NFA raters.

The SLPI uses a variety of configurations for the rating process (Boers-Visker et al., 2015): a three-rater team procedure (synchronous or asynchronous) and a two-rater team procedure (synchronous or asynchronous). All configurations require at least two evaluators, and they must agree in their final decision (Caccamise & Newell, 2012a, p. 26). Caccamise and Newell (2008) describe the rating procedure as follows:

1. The three raters, using the SLPI scoring sheet, independently rate the interviewee's ASL skills. A fourth person can function as a coordinator between the raters.
2. If the raters' evaluations are only one rating level apart, they meet and, working together, fill out a raters' discussion worksheet, which is composed of the same categories and scales as the independent rating sheets. This step is followed by a comparison of the independent rating sheets with the one they have

filled out together. When the raters reach agreement on the final rating, the discussion scoring sheet becomes the official rating of the test-taker's performance. In case of any unsolvable disagreements, the raters can suggest that the test-taker be scored by another rater team or that another interview be scheduled.

3. If the first independent rating results in more than one rating level difference between the raters, the scoring sheet is returned to them (the results of the others are not shared) and raters view a short segment of the interview a second time and have the option to change their independent ratings.
4. If the raters are unable to reach agreement on a final rating, they discuss whether or not the interview is ratable and make a recommendation to the coordinator.
5. The SLPI Coordinator (1) may assign interview video to a second rating team if she or he believes the interview is ratable or (2) may decide the interview video is not ratable and inform the candidate that her or his interview is not ratable and that she or he should or may schedule another SLPI interview.

Steps 6 through 8 are local decisions made by each SLPI program.

6. When the raters are unable to agree on an official rating or think the interview is not ratable, the SLPI coordinator either informs the test-taker that the interview is not ratable and offers to schedule a new interview, or, when the SLPI coordinator thinks the interview is ratable, he or she will pass it on to another rating team.
7. In case a test-taker does not agree with the results or thinks that he or she did not perform well during the interview, it is possible to request a second round of rating or schedule a new SLPI.
8. If a re-rating is requested, the interview will be rated by another rater team. When they agree with the first raters' results, this will become the official rating. If they are not in agreement, the recording will be given to a third rating team. If the third team is in agreement with the first or second team, this will become the official agreement. In case of disagreement, a new SLPI will be scheduled.

Figure 9.2.1 summarizes the rating process of the SLPI.

The NFA only uses one of the configurations mentioned for the SLPI rating process: the two-rater (asynchronous) procedure. The two raters rate the NGT skills of the candidate independently using the NFA rating sheet and exchange their results (without intervention of a supervisor). If the raters are in agreement, their decision is the final rating awarded

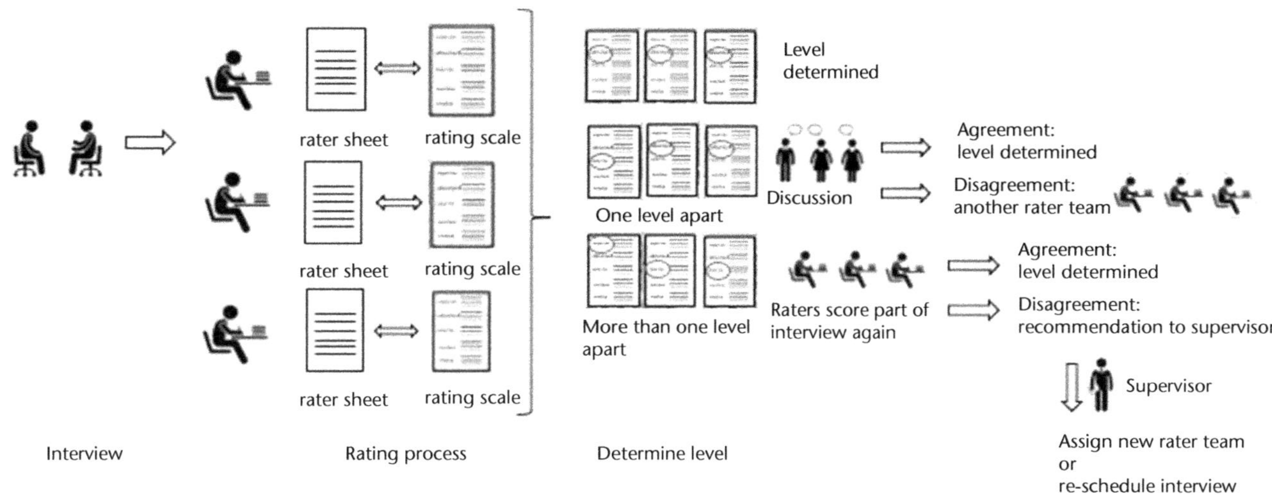

Figure 9.2.1 Rating process of the Sign Language Proficiency Interview.
From Boers-Visker (2014). First published in Van den Broek-Laven et al. (2014), *Papers in Language Testing and Assessment*.

to the candidate. If the raters are not in agreement, and the ratings do not differ by more than one level, the raters discuss their ratings and try to come to an agreement. If they reach agreement (i.e., one of the raters alters his or her rating and matches the other's rating), the agreed rating is awarded to the candidate. If the raters continue to disagree, a third rater scores the interview anew. If the rating of the third rater is the same as the rating of one of the two original raters, this rating will be the final rating. On very rare occasions, there are three different ratings (e.g., A2, B1, and B2). In this case the NFA trainer is consulted to detect the cause of the divergence. The NFA trainer is also consulted in cases where two raters differ by more than one level (e.g., rater 1 awards level A2 and rater 2 awards level B2). If the consultation of the NFA trainer does not result in a solution (i.e., the raters do not alter their original ratings), a new NFA will be scheduled. On rare occasions, the raters judge the interview to be unratable. If this happens, the candidate will be invited to be interviewed again. Candidates are always allowed to meet one of the assessors and receive feedback on their performance. The candidate is free to reject the invitation for a feedback session. Candidates were, by law, allowed to request a second opinion on their rating up until 2018, which rarely occurred (between August 2012 and January 2018, only three students requested a second opinion, out of 1,387 assessments).

In sum, the NFA differs from the SLPI in terms of the two-rater rating procedure, the levels of proficiency, and the adaption of the rating sheet itself to meet the features of NGT.

Identifying Rater Reliability

The SLPI was first developed in the early 1980s and has been used continuously since then at the NTID. So far, only one published peer-reviewed study has reported on the scoring reliability of the SLPI (Caccamise & Samar, 2009).

In the study on the scoring reliability of the SLPI (Caccamise & Samar, 2009), 160 SLPIs were included, which were rated by 34 trained SLPI raters of the NTID. Of these 160 SLPIs, 157 (98.1%) received an official agreed rating. For the remaining 3 interviews (1.9%), the rating teams could not come to an agreement, and no official rating was reported. A possible reason for no official rating is that the interview was not rateable because the interviewer did not do a good enough job. In those cases, the interview is rated by another team or a new interview is conducted. Only 8 (5%) of 160 test-takers requested a re-rating, which resulted in 6 resolved ratings of the 8 where an official rating could be reached. A common reason for re-rating was when the three raters were more than one level apart in their rating (see the previous section on "Rater Training and Score Resolution Techniques"). Interrater reliability was established such that 86.6% of the raters "provided first independent ratings that were either the same as or within one rating level [of 11 levels] of those of the other members of their rating team" (Caccamise & Samar, 2009, p. 39). Of the remaining 13.4% of the rated performances, a second independent rating by a new rating team resulted in 96.8% agreement; that is, raters judged candidates either the same or within one rating level difference and improved the rating by 10.2% (from the initial 86.6% to 96.8%). This was calculated by the percentage of agreement between the three raters for each SLPI.

The interrater reliability of the NFA has been monitored since this assessment was adapted from the SLPI in 2012. The NFA differs slightly from the SLPI with respect to the rating procedure. The video-recorded interview, which follows the same procedure as the SLPI, is analyzed by *two* trained raters. The raters use the NFA rating scale, which is an adapted version of the SLPI rating scale. This rating scale defines five discrete NGT levels, aligned to the levels described in the Common European Framework of Reference for Languages: Learning, Teaching, Assessment (CEFR; Council of Europe, 2001), ranging from "A1" to "C1/C2." There is no distinction between levels C1 and C2. There is not enough information on the exact differences between these two levels in NGT, and performing at level C1/C2 is extremely rare among students who take the test. (See Table 9.2.1 for a comparison of the 11 SLPI rating scale levels and the corresponding NGT FA CEFR-aligned levels.)

The rating procedure itself is similar to the SLPI rating procedure, except for the fact that the rating is performed by two raters instead of three and there is an adapted rating scale: the rater first indicates the functional skills of the candidate by selecting "above intermediate" (corresponding to above B1), "at intermediate" (corresponding to B1), or "below intermediate" (corresponding to below B1); he then selects the level that best matches the NGT level of the candidate based on functionality; and, finally, the rater focuses on form by evaluating the candidate's vocabulary knowledge and use; production and fluency; use of grammatical features; discourse strategies; and overall comprehension. The rating form to perform the latter is adapted for the features of NGT because this signed language differs from ASL with respect to some grammatical features. Based on the evaluation of function and form, the test-taker is assigned to an overall level of A1, A2, B1, B2, or C1/C2. Since 2012, interrater reliability studies have been carried out yearly to ensure the quality of the rater team. Figure 9.2.2 depicts, for each period the NFA has been administered, the instances of direct agreement, agreement after discussion, and requests for a third rater during 2014 and 2017 (calculated 5–6 times per year). Overall, the raters provided a final rating without request for a third rater in 80–100% of the ratings (mean: 94%). Percentages of direct agreement (i.e., the raters immediately agree and do not need a discussion to reach consent) are between 31% (2013–2014 T2) and 93% (2015–2016 T5), with a mean of

Table 9.2.1 Comparison of the 11 SLPI rating scale levels and the corresponding NGT FA CEFR-aligned levels

SLPI: Levels of the SLPI rating scale	NFA: Levels aligned with CEFR
Superior plus	C2
Superior	C1
Advanced plus	
Advanced	B2
Intermediate plus	
Intermediate	B1
Survival plus	
Survival	A2
Novice plus	
Novice	A1
No functional skills	No functional skills

From Boers-Visker et al., 2015.

68%, although it is worth mentioning that the number of NFAs is sometimes small (e.g., 2016–2017 T5 only consists of nine NFAs). During the period 2014–2017, new raters joined the team at two times. No decrease of agreement is noted (either direct or after discussion) on either occasions.

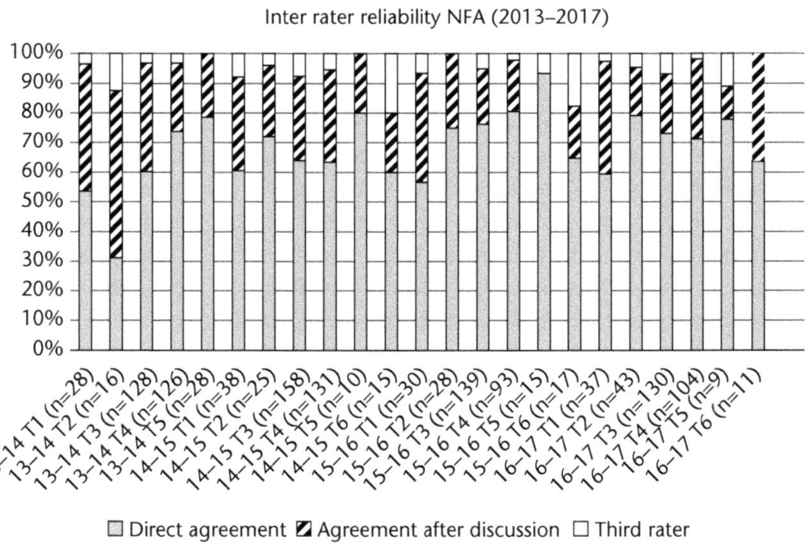

Figure 9.2.2 Overview of interrater reliability calculations during the period 2014–2017.

ASL PROFICIENCY INTERVIEW AND THE ASSESSMENT OF SIGNED COMMUNICATION: ASL

At Gallaudet University, the ASLPI is in use. For the ASLPI, no study in a peer-reviewed journal is available, but a short report on a reliability study is available at the university's website (Gallaudet University, 2020a). According to the website, inter- and intrarater reliability could be established based on 1,286 candidate interviews that were collected between 2008 and 2011. The ASLPI uses a holistic scale and dimension scores for (1) vocabulary, (2) grammar, (3) comprehension, (4) accent/production, and (5) fluency. Interrater reliability could be established across all possible evaluator pairs of the ASLPI, with .90 for the total score and holistic rating and between .80 and .86 for the dimension scores. Reliability was established by applying an *intraclass correlation* (ICC) (Gallaudet University, 2020a). Re-ratings of ASLPI support that a "new panel of evaluators and the original panel of evaluators resulted in reliable ratings" (Pearson r correlation between .89 and .92 and Spearman Rho of .88 to .90).

The fourth assessment is the ASC:ASL (ETS, 2014), provided by the ETS. The documentation does not provide any information on reliability or validity.

RATING SCALES

Rating Scale Development

Based on the available published literature, it is hard to make claims about rating scale development for signed language tests that evaluate adult L2 learners' proficiency. The SLPI seem to use holistic rating scales or a combination of a holistic and analytic scale, but no documentation is available about their development and construct representation. No claim can be made that the construct of "ASL proficiency" is represented in these rating scales.

Different types of scales are used for the proficiency interviews: whereas the ASLPI at Gallaudet University and the ETS version use holistic scales, the SLPI and the NFA use a combination of a holistic and an analytic scale, leaving more space for detailed information about the test-taker's performance.

As for the ASC:ASL (ETS, 2014), limited information is publicly available on this proficiency interview. According to the official ETS documentation, the interview is rated on a 5-point holistic rating scale, with 5 being the highest and 1 representing the lowest proficiency score. An example is "Level 5: The candidate consistently shows a very high level of proficiency in expressive and receptive communication in ASL" (ETS, 2014, p. 6), followed by a more elaborate description. No further information about that test could be obtained. The ASLPI uses a holistic rating scale from 0 to 5 (Gallaudet University, 2020b), but it also operates with dimension scores. No more information could be obtained from the ASLPI website. Similar to the SLPI, the ASLPI is based on the language proficiency evaluation that was "originally developed by the Foreign Service Institute (FSI) of the US Department of State" (Gallaudet University, 2020b). Whereas the ETS holistic scales use only a 5-point rating, the ASLPI uses levels in between (e.g., Level 4+), which does not, according to the ASLPI website, represent a midway level between Level 4 and 5, but rather means that the candidate does not fulfill all requirements of Level 5 (Gallaudet University, 2020c).

The construct on which the SLPI is based measures functional signed language skills at different proficiency levels. These levels are made explicit in the level descriptors, as for SLPI level "Superior" (Caccamise & Newell, 2012b), but the overall construct is not stated explicitly. The "Superior" level is defined as "*Able* to have a fully shared conversation, with in-depth elaboration for both social and work topics. Very broad signed language vocabulary, near native-like production and fluency, excellent use of signed language grammatical features, and excellent comprehension for normal signing rate."

Scale Validation

With regard to validation of the aforementioned rating scales, only the ASLPI provides some information on its website (Gallaudet University, 2020a). The construct of "ASL proficiency" is defined as consisting of the five dimensions of grammar, vocabulary, fluency, production/accent, and comprehension. The preliminary validity study concludes on the ASLPI website.

1. The five ASLPI dimensions appear representative of a single underlying construct, which is defined by five facets/dimensions
2. The dimensions relate to the underlying construct in a consistent manner
3. Rating for each ASLPI dimensions shows very little *systematic rater bias*
4. Each dimension contributed approximately equally to both the total score and the holistic rating
5. This provides construct validity evidence supporting the ASLPI definition of ASL proficiency

AUTOMATIC SCORING

To the best of our knowledge, the 3-year Swiss National Science Foundation–funded Scalable Multimodal Sign Language Technology for Sign Language Learning and Assessment (SMILE) project is the first of its kind to use signed language recognition technology for the purpose of automatic scoring in signed language assessment (Ebling et al., 2018). Due to the three-dimensional nature of signed languages, this requires a depth sensor and other cameras to recognize a produced sign and match it with a "base" form in order to provide feedback on whether the produced sign is correct or not. The SMILE project will also attempt to apply this technology to vocabulary assessment and a sentence repetition test.

FUTURE DIRECTIONS

From a research perspective, much more needs to be done to establish inter- and intrarater reliability in the use of rating scales and investigate construct representation in the rating scales as well as other aspects of scale validation. A deeper focus on rater training is also needed.

Interviewing techniques have quite an impact on candidates' performance, so studies on interviewer's language and back-channeling behavior is needed for reliability enhancement. Also, it is necessary to evaluate the function of the SLPI/NFA in educational programs with regards to other formative and summative assessment forms and their weight in the final language fluency evaluation of learners.

CONCLUSION

In this chapter, we addressed different issues of rating scales of signed language tests that assess adult L2 learners' proficiency. As a result of the limited information available on this topic, both on official websites as well as in publications, a "meta-discussion" of issues relevant to rating scales for signed language tests can only be tentative. This reflects the current state of research and application in the field of signed language assessment, which is emphasized at the beginning of this chapter and throughout this volume. Most of the issues addressed here are underresearched and require further attention.

NOTES

1. https://www.rit.edu/ntid/slpi/sites/rit.edu.ntid.slpi/files/page_file_attachments/RatingScale%20and%20Analyzing%20Function%202020a.pdf
2. https://www.rit.edu/ntid/slpi/sites/rit.edu.ntid.slpi/files/page_file_attachments/Rater_Worksheet_1RT.pdf
3. https://www.rit.edu/ntid/slpi/sites/rit.edu.ntid.slpi/files/page_file_attachments/Analyzing%20Form%202020.pdf
4. https://www.rit.edu/ntid/slpi/sites/rit.edu.ntid.slpi/files/page_file_attachments/Discussion%20and%20Grammar%20Guidelines.pdf

REFERENCES

Boers-Visker, E., Poor, G., & van den Bogaerde, B. (2015). The Sign Language Proficiency Interview (SLPI): Description and use with Sign Language of the Netherlands. Proceedings of the International Conference on Education of the Deaf. https://www.ecml.at/Portals/1/5MTP/Pro%20Sign%20II/documents/3.4.12_SLPI%20NFA%20Proceedings%20Paper%20Boers%20Poor%20vandenBogaerde%20paper.pdf

Caccamise, F., & Newell, W. (1999). *Section 13: An Overview of the Sign Communication Proficiency Interview (SCPI): History, Development, Methodology, & Use*. Manuscript, National Technical Institute for the Deaf, Rochester Institute of Technology.

Caccamise, F., & Newell, W. (2008). *PROGRAM Sign Language Proficiency Interview (SLPI) scheduling and interviewing procedures* (24th ed.). National Technical Institute for the Deaf, Rochester Institute of Technology.

Caccamise, F., & Newell, W. (2009). *Sign Language Proficiency Interview (SLPI) Notebook (NB). Section 1 (S1). Training workshop goals, principles, materials and procedures*. National Technical Institute for the Deaf, Rochester Institute of Technology.

Caccamise, F., & Newell, W. (2012a). *SLPI paper no. 1: SLPI notebook materials*. National Technical Institute for the Deaf, Rochester Institute of Technology.

Caccamise, F., & Newell, W. (2012b). *Section 3B: Sign Language Proficiency Interview: American Sign Language (SLPI: ASL). Individual rater and sharing of results procedure*. National Technical Institute for the Deaf, Rochester Institute of Technology.

Caccamise, F., & Samar, V. (2009). Sign Language Proficiency Interview (SLPI): Prenegotiation interrater reliability and rater validity. *Contemporary Issues in Communication Science and Disorders, 36*, 36–47.

Council of Europe. (2001). *Common European Framework of Reference for Languages: Learning, teaching, and assessment*. Cambridge University Press.

Ebling, S., Camgöz, N. C., Boyes Braem, P., Tissi, K., Sidler-Miserez, S., Stoll, S., Hatfield, S., Haug, T., Bowden, R., Tornay, S., Razavi, M., & Magimai-Doss, M. (2018). SMILE Swiss German Sign Language data set. *11th Language Resources and Evaluation Conference (LREC 2018)*, 4221–4229.

Educational Testing Service (ETS). (2014). *The Praxis Study Companion: Assessment of signed communication: American Sign Language*. ETS. https://www.ets.org/s/praxis/pdf/0632.pdf

Gallaudet University. (2020a, July 23). The American Sign Language Proficiency Interview: ASLPI research and statistics. https://www.gallaudet.edu/the-american-sign-language-proficiency-interview/aslpi/aslpi-research/validity-and-reliability-studies

Gallaudet University. (2020b, July 23). The American Sign Language Proficiency Interview. https://www.gallaudet.edu/the-american-sign-language-proficiency-interview/aslpi

Gallaudet University. (2020c, July 23). American Sign Language Proficiency Interview: ASLPI proficiency levels. https://www.gallaudet.edu/the-american-sign-language-proficiency-interview/aslpi/aslpi-proficiency-levels

Haug, T. (2017). Development and Evaluation of Two Vocabulary Tests for Swiss German Sign Language [Master thesis, Lancaster University]. https://doi.org/10.13140/RG.2.2.25397.17129
Haug, T., Nussbaumer, D., & Stocker Bachmann, H. (2019). Die Entwicklung von Instrumenten zur Überprüfung von kognitiven Fähigkeiten, gebärdensprachlicher Kompetenz und Dolmetschleistung von Gebärdensprachdolmetscherinnen. *Das Zeichen, 111*, 130–143.
Hauser, P., Supalla, T., & Bavelier, D. (2008). American Sign Language sentence reproduction test: Development and implications. In R. Müller de Quadros (Ed.), *Sign Languages: Spinning and unraveling the past, present and future. TISLR9, forty five papers and three posters from the 9th. Theoretical Issues in Sign Language Research Conference* (pp. 160–172). Editora Arara Azul. Petrópolis/RJ. Brazil.
Liskin-Gasparro, J. (1982). *Foreign language and proficiency assessment*. Educational Testing Service.
Newell, W., Caccamise, F., Boardman, K., & Ray Holcomb, B. (1983). Adaptation of the Language Proficiency Interview (LPI) for assessing sign communicative competence. *Sign Language Studies, 41*, 311–347.
Supalla, T., Hauser, P. C., & Bavelier, D. (2014). Reproducing American Sign Language sentences: Cognitive scaffolding in working memory. *Frontiers in Psychology, 5*. https://doi.org/10.3389/fpsyg.2014.00859
Van den Broek-Laven, A., Boers-Visker, E., & Van den Bogaerde, B. (2014). Determining aspects of text difficulty for the Sign Language of the Netherlands (NGT) Functional Assessment instrument. *Papers in Language Testing and Assessment—Special Issue, 1*, 53–75.

9.3

Discussion on Scoring Issues in Second Signed or Spoken Language Assessment

Tobias Haug, Ute Knoch, and Wolfgang Mann

In this chapter, we discuss some of the key issues related to scoring in spoken and in signed language assessment, with particular regard to any possible implications they might have on the other field.

SCORING NONVERBAL BEHAVIOR/ASPECTS OF LANGUAGE

One aspect of signed language assessment that has the potential to stimulate new research in spoken second language (L2) assessment is the scoring of nonverbal speaker behaviors. This aspect is rarely represented in the scoring criteria of spoken assessments and in many cases not even available to raters during the scoring process. The reason for this is that many assessments of spoken language are merely audio-recorded and rated later. Raters of signed language, on the other hand, have to also rely on nonmanual signals which are used for linguistic purposes (e.g., specific facial expressions to indicate a question) to successfully understand/interpret the message of the signer. This raises the question whether the "equivalents" of these nonmanual features in spoken languages (e.g., gestures) that serve different functions (e.g., to emphasize something) should feed into the scoring process of spoken language. We argue, therefore, for a broadening of the construct of spoken language assessment to also include elements of nonverbal communication in the scoring descriptors. This would be relevant to all cases of face-to-face spoken interaction, whereas the language assessments of call center personnel or pilots would make this less relevant. More research in this area is necessary, and we feel that signed language experts could contribute to this agenda.

Next, we are looking at aspects from spoken language assessment and their possible implications on signed language assessment. There are two topics of particular interest: (1) practical training of raters and (2) research on rating scale development and use.

Tobias Haug, Ute Knoch, and Wolfgang Mann, *Discussion on Scoring Issues in Second Signed or Spoken Language Assessment* In: *The Handbook of Language Assessment Across Modalities*. Edited by: Tobias Haug, Wolfgang Mann, and Ute Knoch, Oxford University Press. © Oxford University Press 2022. DOI: 10.1093/oso/9780190885052.003.0028

TRAINING OF RATERS FOR SIGNED LANGUAGE

With regard to practical training, signed language instructors who work in tertiary education will have experience in assessing adult learners, such as signed language interpreting students. However, we cannot automatically assume that language testing is part of each signed language teacher's curriculum. We are not aware of any more general training existing for raters of signed language tests; that is, training that is not for a specific assessment instrument, such as the Sign Language Proficiency Interview (SLPI) or the Sign Language of the Netherlands (*Nederlandse Gebarentaal* [NGT] FA; see Chapter 9.2), but training in a broader sense to help raters develop a common understanding (and use) of evaluation criteria. For instance, in a number of research projects related to assessing Swiss German Sign Language (*Deutschschweizerische Gebärdensprache* [DSGS]) in children and/or adults, training was offered for the use of specific rating scales but did not include general issues on language testing and assessment (e.g., what is the difference between a holistic and analytic scale?). To our knowledge, there is no research available that has investigated the effectiveness of rater training. This generates the need for research related to the development and use of rating scales. Furthermore, the fact that signed languages are nonstandardized languages (Adam, 2015) makes it more difficult to define, for example, a criterion of correctness. This can be quite challenging even on a very "simple" vocabulary translation test where, for example, a test-taker is asked to translate a German word into DSGS, and the raters decide if the sign produced is correct or incorrect (Haug et al., 2019). This becomes even more difficult given that we are still only now beginning to understand from recent research on DSGS what acceptable phonetic variants of signs are (Ebling et al., 2018).

APPLICATION OF STATISTICAL ANALYSIS IN SIGNED LANGUAGE TESTING

Recommendations from spoken language assessment in relation to key points made in the signed language assessment chapter are twofold: (1) the use of Rasch analysis and (2) the use of different rating scales. The first suggested area relates to the use of statistical analyses in estimating rater functioning and resolving rater discrepancies. Spoken language assessment has drawn on a number of statistics to estimate rater quality, many of which have been adopted from the broader field of educational assessment. In particular many-faceted Rasch analysis (Linacre, 1989) and generalizability theory (Brennan, 2001) have been used to discover systematic patterns in rating behavior and gain an understanding of the number of raters needed to arrive at reliable ratings.

In the case of the SLPI assessment, it may be possible to reduce the number of raters used and arrive at efficiencies in the rating procedures.

RESEARCH ON THE DEVELOPMENT OF RATING SCALES FOR SIGNED LANGUAGE ASSESSMENT

The second suggested area is related to rating scales. Signed language assessment researchers may want to examine whether it is possible to expand the construct currently represented in the rating scales for a particular test. This construct seems to be closely related to the one embodied by the Foreign Service Institute (FSI) rating scales used in spoken assessment. It would be worthwhile to explore whether there are particular linguistic aspects of signed languages that are not sufficiently captured in the kind of criteria currently used. For example, the notion of "interactional competence," or how well speakers are able to achieve a communicative outcome together, may be worth representing in the scale criteria. Once included in the rating scales, this may result in positive washback in terms of teaching and learning signed language.

Researchers in signed language assessment may also find it useful to experiment with a wider range of rating scales. Most scales currently used in signed language assessments seem to be holistic scales. These are useful if the test purpose is to place learners at a particular ability level without providing much feedback. In spoken assessment, analytic rating scales have been shown to result in higher reliability indices (e.g., Barkaoui, 2011) because raters are required to assess different linguistic aspects of the performance separately. In some circumstances, such as in classroom-based assessment contexts, diagnostic rating scales (e.g., checklists) may be useful to provide feedback to learners and provide information about learners to teachers (e.g., Jang & Wagner, 2014; Wagner, 2014).

Additional issues related to scoring that could build on the research carried out in spoken language include

1. Investigating raters characteristics' and how they influence the scoring results, as discussed by Knoch in Chapter 9.1.
2. Investigating if equivalents exist in signed language (assessment) to criteria such as "fluency" and "accent" in spoken language.
3. Investigating interviewer effect in signed language assessment formats like the SLPI.
4. Investigating how disagreements between signed language raters are solved.

Automatic scoring of signed production, based on automatic signed language recognition technology, is only starting to be used on the single-sign level (Ebling et al., 2018) and only as part of research projects rather than being implemented as scoring mechanism of an operational test. This technology is still in its infancy. Even though these technological advances, so far, are promising, there is still a long way before this technology can be used in high-stakes testing and to assess longer stretches of discourse (e.g., sentence repetition test, narrative tasks, interviews).

REFERENCES

Adam, R. (2015). Standardization of sign languages. *Sign Language Studies, 15*(4), 432–445. https://doi.org/10.1353/sls.2015.0015

Barkaoui, K. (2011). Effects of marking method and rater experience on ESL essay scores and rater performance. *Assessment in Education: Principles, Policy & Practice, 18*(3), 279–293. https://doi.org/10.1080/0969594X.2010.526585

Brennan, R. L. (2001). *Generalizability theory*. Springer.

Ebling, S., Camgöz, N. C., Boyes Braem, P., Tissi, K., Sidler-Miserez, S., Stoll, S., Hatfield, S., Haug, T., Bowden, R., Tornay, S., Razavi, M., & Magimai-Doss. (2018). *SMILE Swiss German Sign Language data set*. 11th Language Resources and Evaluation Conference (LREC 2018).

Haug, T., Ebling, S., Boyes Braem, P., Tissi, K., & Sidler-Miserez, S. (2019). Sign language learning and assessment in German Switzerland: Exploring the potential of vocabulary size tests for Swiss German Sign Language. *Language Education & Assessment*, 2(1), 20–40. https://doi.org/10.29140/lea.v2n1.85

Jang, E. E., & Wagner, M. (2014). Diagnostic feedback in the classroom. In A. Kunnan (Ed.), *The companion to language assessment* (pp. 693–711). John Wiley & Sons.

Linacre, J. M. (1989). *Many-faceted Rasch measurement*. MESA Press.

Wagner, M. (2014). Use of a diagnostic rubric for assessing writing: Students' perceptions of cognitive diagnostic feedback. Language Testing Research Colloquium, Amsterdam.

Topic 10

Discourse Analysis and Language Assessment

10.1

Discourse Analysis in Second Language Speaking Assessment

Kellie Frost

Discourse analysis has primarily been used in the field of language testing for the purposes of examining the appropriateness of task design and the generalizability of performances across different tasks, as well as for developing or refining rating scale criteria (see Lazaraton, 2013; McNamara et al., 2002, for overviews). Argument-based test validation frameworks (see Chapter 8.1) (Chapelle et al. 2010; Kane, 2006, 2012, 2013; Xi, 2008) emphasize the need for gathering empirical evidence in support of the chain of inferences made from test scores, including assumptions about the suitability of test constructs for generating conclusions about individuals' language capabilities in real-world interactions. While test validation procedures have traditionally relied heavily on statistical analyses of score data, it is increasingly recognized that discourse analytic methods are needed to properly interrogate the often complex relationships among task performances, scores, and real-world communication practices that are central to validity.

For language testers, discourse analysis provides a potential means of both characterizing actual language use in the real-world domains that test constructs are intended to represent and evaluating task design and the appropriateness of scoring criteria for tapping into such constructs. Discourse-based studies, for example, have identified important features of oral (and written) communication in higher education (Biber, 2006; Biber et al., 2002) and in some employment domains, such as healthcare professions (e.g., Sarangi & Roberts, 1999), where high-stakes language tests play key gatekeeping roles. Such studies provide a robust starting point from which to address various important validity questions, most notably the question of task authenticity, which involves interrogating the extent to which tasks elicit linguistic behaviors important to communicative success in real-world domains.

Two recent studies have addressed the question of the authenticity of high-stakes specific purpose tests in this way, one in relation to the Test of English as Foreign Language (TOEFL)-iBT speaking section (Brooks & Swain, 2014), a test of academic English proficiency used to

Kellie Frost, *Discourse Analysis in Second Language Speaking Assessment* In: *The Handbook of Language Assessment Across Modalities*. Edited by: Tobias Haug, Wolfgang Mann, and Ute Knoch, Oxford University Press. © Oxford University Press 2022. DOI: 10.1093/oso/9780190885052.003.0029 regulate access to English-medium universities, and the other in relation to the Occupational English Test (OET), which is used to assess if health professionals from non–English speaking backgrounds possess adequate English proficiency to function in the workplace (Woodward-Kron & Elder, 2016).

Brooks and Swain (2014) compared grammatical, lexical, and discourse-level features (cohesion and register) of oral performances produced by individuals on the TOEFL speaking section with their language use in the classroom and in interactions with other students outside the classroom. As Brooks and Swain note, the fact that speaking tasks in high-stakes tests such as TOEFL iBT are semidirect and monologic, which is a product of the constraints of its computer-based test delivery, creates an additional impetus for discourse-based evidence of the validity of extrapolations from test performances to performances in real-world academic contexts. Brooks and Swain's findings showed that performances differed in terms of grammatical complexity (the number of clauses contained in each unit of speech) and grammatical accuracy (the number of errors per clause) across all three contexts, with the highest levels of complexity and lowest levels of accuracy in the test context and the lowest complexity and highest accuracy in the out-of-class context. By contrast, on most of the discourse-level measures and some lexical measures, performances were comparable across the test and in-class contexts but not the out-of-class context, where the use of informal language, not surprisingly, was significantly higher than in the other two contexts, and the amount of coordination and subordination was significantly lower than in the other two contexts. These areas of "overlap and non-overlap of performances" suggest, according to the researchers, "a potential weak link in the interpretive argument chain" (p. 371).

In a similar vein, Woodward-Kron and Elder (2016) examine the extent to which test-taker performances on the speaking section of the OET elicited discourse features relevant to doctor–patient interactions in the medical profession. In this study, performances across two role-play simulations of a consultation between a doctor and a patient were compared, one from the OET test and the other from the Australian Medical Council clinical examination. Woodward-Kron and Elder argue that, given the difficulties associated with accessing actual doctor–patient consultations, the clinical examination offered a suitable means of capturing the real-world context as it provides "a strong representation of the values and requirements of the medical profession with respect to clinical interaction" (p. 254). The researchers analyzed the schematic structures of performance discourse and found that candidates produced moves involving domain-relevant communicative functions—"fostering the relationship, gathering information, providing information, making decisions and responding to emotions"

(p. 267) in similar stages across both the OET and clinical examination contexts. Although they also found interactional and lexicogrammatical differences across the two contexts, these were attributed, in some part, to differences in the language and approach used by the simulated patient in each task. The researchers concluded that the study supported the validity of the OET as a measure of the communication skills valued in the medical profession while acknowledging that findings offered little evidence to support claims that the language test elicited domain-relevant interactional skills.

Despite their value in evidencing the authenticity of test constructs, especially important in specific-purpose testing, studies examining the actual discourse produced in real-world communication contexts are scarce and usually, as in the two cases just described, retrospective. It is rarely the case that construct definitions and task design in speaking assessments are derived from evidence of actual discourse features and behaviors in real-world settings. Typically, at least in reputable, high-stakes academic and other specific-purpose testing, decisions about which discourse features to target for testing purposes are made on the basis of surveys of domain expert perspectives while decisions about how such features should be operationalized for measurement (i.e., how they are defined within rating scale criteria for scoring) are made by language testers, often on the basis of intuition.

By contrast, studies involving discourse analysis of test performances are numerous, and these have been crucial in shaping theoretical understandings of oral proficiency as well as test construct definitions and task design. Early discourse-based studies focused on the oral proficiency interview (OPI) (e.g., Lazaraton, 1992; van Lier, 1989; see McNamara et al., 2002, for a survey), a widely used test aimed at assessing test-takers' conversational abilities. These studies foregrounded the importance of empirically examining the discourse features elicited by test tasks as part of defining test constructs and evaluating their appropriateness. The OPI had been assumed to be a valid measure of interactional ability in conversations because of its face-to-face nature, which was thought to resemble natural conversation. As McNamara et al. (2002) point out, by using conversation analysis, van Lier (1989) and Lazaraton (1992) were able to show that features of performance elicited by the OPI did not correspond well to typical features of natural conversations. Findings from these studies indicated that the interactional event that emerged in response to the OPI task would be better characterized as a distinct type of formal interview and that scores therefore did not support interpretations about test-takers abilities to effectively engage in conversational interactions.

Following on from these early studies, discourse analysis in language testing research has shed important light on features of interaction relevant to task design (see Young & He, 1998), as well as the features of interaction-based talk between test-takers and between test-takers and interlocutors in face-to-face speaking tests, leading to a problematizing of the co-constructed nature of any oral performance and raising questions about the implications of this for the interpretability of test scores as measures of individual ability (see, e.g., Brown, 2000, 2003; Ducasse, 2009; Galaczi, 2008; Lazaraton, 1996; Lazaraton & Davis, 2008; May, 2009; McNamara, 1997; Taylor & Wigglesworth, 2009). Lazaraton and Davis (2008), for example, explore interactions between test-takers in paired oral assessments (using Cambridge English First [FCE] and Cambridge English Preliminary [PET]) to examine how test-taker identities—specifically, how test-takers position themselves as proficient or competent speakers—shape the nature of interactions and impact rater judgments. The researchers adopted a conversation analysis approach, transcribing features including turn-taking, overlapping speech, breathing, laughter, intonation, and rate of speech, with a view to examining how "macrosocial features of identity" (p. 317), such as legitimate, competent speaker versus novice or learner, were constructed through micro-level features of discourse in interaction. The authors suggest that test-takers not only bring ideas about their own proficiency identities into a task, but they also construct these in relation to their interlocuter within the interaction in ways that not only impact the nature of the interaction but also influence test scores.

Recognition of the co-constructed nature of speaking test performances involving paired test-takers or interviewers and test-takers has led to an increasing emphasis on identifying the features of interactional competence that distinguish test-takers at different speaking proficiency levels (see, e.g., Galaczi, 2014; Gan, 2010). Gan (2010) compared the interactional features of low- and high-scoring performances on a group oral assessment task used in a classroom setting. He found that high group discussions were characterized by a range of discourse moves, including suggestions, explanations, and challenges, as speakers engaged in contingent and constructive topic development. By contrast, low group interactions were structured according to the task prompt and were heavily constituted by negotiation of meaning moves, rather than topic development. Also focused on identifying interactional features at different proficiency levels, Galaczi (2014) used conversation analysis to examine the discourse produced in paired speaking test performances across four Common European Framework of Reference (CEFR) proficiency levels (B1 to C2). Her findings also highlighted differences in the nature of topic development, with mutuality and reciprocity between speakers increasing with proficiency. Lower proficiency pairs, for example, engaged in limited topic development and made abrupt topic shifts, whereas among higher proficiency pairs, Galaczi found that speakers displayed listener support through back-channeling and comprehension confirmations and cooperated to produce multiturn topics. More recently, Pallotti (2017), based on a study of native speaker interactions across six different oral tasks, argued that features of interaction, including the number of turn exchanges, the number of initiating moves required, and visual access (i.e., the possibility of making eye contact), influence task difficulty and are likely to be handled differently by second language (L2) learners at different levels of proficiency. She suggests a need to incorporate these aspects of interaction into speaking proficiency constructs and test task design.

Another area of research in which discourse analysis has been widely used, one similarly aimed at interrogating the nature of task difficulty, focuses on the impact of different task conditions on the accuracy, complexity, and fluency of oral discourse produced by learners across proficiency levels, with important implications for test construct definitions. One such condition which has received significant attention is pre-task planning time. The effects of planning time on performances has been widely researched in relation to language learning (see Skehan, 2014, for an overview) and has also been studied in language testing contexts (Elder & Iwashita, 2005; Wigglesworth, 1997, 2001; Wigglesworth & Elder, 2010). In L2 learning research, the effect of planning time is considered in terms of cognitive perspectives that emphasize the importance of limited working memory capacity in the process of L2 speaking (Robinson, 2001, 2007; Skehan, 1998, 2001, 2009). L2 users with lower levels of proficiency, it is assumed, are less able to rely on implicit, automatized knowledge than are higher proficiency language users and so face additional and competing cognitive demands during oral production. Research in L2 acquisition has shown that cognitive demands vary with task demands, influencing the accuracy, fluency, and complexity of learners' oral language (Robinson, 2001; Skehan & Foster, 1997, 1999, 2008). Based on such studies, planning time is generally thought to enable learners to better distribute limited attentional resources across different processing demands, leading to more fluent oral performances but having mixed effects on accuracy and complexity.

For language testers, the effect of planning time has implications for construct definitions and also for test fairness because task conditions should enable test-takers to produce their best performances but, at the same time, should not shroud distinctions between test-takers of different levels of proficiency. As in studies in the field of L2 acquisition, studies of the effect of planning time on language test outcomes have produced mixed results. While it is generally agreed that planning time leads to improvements in fluency, whether or not this task condition systematically impacts other discourse features or influences test score outcomes remains uncertain (Wigglesworth & Elder, 2010). Moreover, research suggests that rater judgments of performances under different task conditions are not necessarily consistent with discourse-based evidence of oral performance quality. For example, in an investigation of the effect of pre-task planning time versus no planning time on paired oral test performances, Nitta and Nakatsuhara (2014) found that while performances under the planning time condition were judged by raters to be more accurate, fluent, and complex, there were no differences between discourse-analytic measures of accuracy and complexity across the two conditions and a small reduction, rather than increase, in fluency with planning time. They also found that test-takers produced longer, monologue-like turns under the planning time condition, rather than interacting collaboratively to address test topics, which was the behavior the task was designed to elicit. The researchers speculated that efforts to produce longer utterances may have negatively impacted fluency and warned that planning time may undermine task validity, functioning instead to limit opportunities for test-takers to demonstrate their interaction skills.

In addition to investigating the impact of task conditions, discourse analysis methods have also been used as part of test validation efforts to examine how performances vary across different task types as well as whether different versions of the same task (i.e., parallel tasks) elicit comparable performances. Parallel tasks differ in terms of topic content only and are otherwise intended to be equivalent. In relation to different task types, an early study by Kormos (1999) analyzed the oral performance discourse elicited by role-plays compared to interviews, finding that role-play tasks tapped into more features of natural conversation. In relation to the TOEFL, Brown, Iwashita, and McNamara (2005) compared the discourse produced by test-takers in response to the various independent and integrated speaking tasks that comprise the speaking section of the test. Independent tasks only require test-takers to speak in response to a prompt, whereas integrated tasks require test-takers to first listen to and/or read stimulus texts and then incorporate content from these texts into their speaking performances. The latter was added to the TOEFL as a means of enhancing authenticity and better aligning the linguistic and cognitive demands made on test-takers with those relevant to the university context. Examining discourse measures of grammar, vocabulary, fluency, pronunciation, and rhetorical structure, Brown et al. found that independent tasks across different topics elicited comparable performances in terms of the discourse features examined and that the integrated tasks elicited different language use compared to the independent tasks, which, the researchers concluded, broadened the construct to better reflect the skills needed in university contexts. However, they also found that features of oral performance discourse in response to integrated tasks were specific to particular task versions. Thus, while their findings provided support for the inclusion of both task types as a means of capturing more aspects of academic oral proficiency, they also raised questions about the extent to which performances on this type of task can support inferences about performances on other, parallel tasks and, more importantly, in diverse higher education contexts.

Two more recent studies investigating the impact of stimulus text content on the discourse produced by test-takers in response to the integrated speaking tasks of the TOEFL-iBT also raise questions about the generalizability of test performances quality across different task versions (Crossley et al., 2014; Frost et al., 2020). Crossley, Clevinger, and Kim (2014) examined relationships between word-level properties of listening stimulus materials and test-takers recall and integration of source text words into their oral performances, as well as whether the latter influenced score outcomes. The researchers found that both the frequency of word occurrence and the location of words in particular clauses predicted their recall and integration by test-takers and that the use of words from the stimulus texts led to better scores, thereby providing important insights to address questions raised in earlier studies (as just discussed) about relationships among source text content, performance content, and test outcomes.

Frost et al.'s (2020) later study, which focused on the TOEFL reading-listening-speaking tasks, extended Crossley et al.'s focus on word-level properties of listening materials to examine if the way in which information was introduced, developed, and exemplified across both reading and listening texts impacted the content produced by test-takers at different levels of proficiency. The researchers compared test-taker performances across two supposedly parallel versions of the integrated speaking task in terms of the main ideas produced, the structure of responses in relation to the structure of input texts in terms of rhetorical "moves," and the accuracy with which idea units from source texts were reproduced. They found that while these content measures distinguished participants according to their level of speaking proficiency on one task version, on the other there were no real proficiency-related differences. The authors attributed the different findings across task versions to differences in the structure and idea development of the two sets of stimulus materials, which they argued placed different summarizing- and synthesizing-related demands on test-takers.

Discourse analysis of test-taker performances has also been used in the field of language testing to investigate the extent to which rating scale criteria and descriptors across different score bands correspond to the actual discourse produced by test-takers at different levels of proficiency (Brown et al. 2005; Douglas, 1994; Douglas & Selinker, 1992, 1993; Iwashita et al., 2008). These investigations relate to both the validity of construct definitions and the reliability of scoring procedures. For language testing purposes, discourse analysis can shed important light on threats to test validity that would otherwise remain hidden since rating scales are typically developed through intuition and expert opinion, with no guarantee that descriptors accurately represent the construct in question (Fulcher, 1996).

Early investigations in this area foregrounded the importance of incorporating discourse analysis methods into test validation procedures (Douglas, 1994; Douglas & Selinker, 1992, 1993). Douglas and Selinker (1992, 1993), for example, through a comparison of score data and qualitative analysis of discourse produced in speaking test performances, showed that raters can often arrive at similar scores for different reasons. Similarly, Douglas (1994) compared the grammar, vocabulary, fluency, content, and rhetorical organization of the oral discourse produced by speakers who received similar scores on a semi-direct speaking test and found little sign of a relationship between discourse quality and test scores. However, these studies did not examine rater perceptions, nor did the measures used mirror all scale criteria. It is thus possible that the discourse measures used failed to properly capture raters' interpretations of rating scale criteria and thereby may have failed to capture aspects of performance relevant to rater decision-making about scores.

Iwashita, Brown, McNamara, and O'Hagan (2008), in a subsequent study related to that conducted by Brown et al. (2005), used a discourse-analysis based methodology to investigate the relationship between test scores and actual performance discourse from 200 samples across independent and integrated tasks developed as part of the revised TOEFL. Findings showed that, for the most part, scores were supported by the discourse produced by test-takers and thereby provided support for the validity of the suite of tasks as a measure of speaking proficiency. However, as noted earlier in relation to Brown et al.'s (2005) study, Iwashita et al. (2008) noted that integrated task performances were contingent on stimulus context and raised questions about score generalizability.

FUTURE DIRECTIONS

While discourse-analytic methods have yielded significant insights, informing test validation processes as well as understandings of relationships between oral proficiency and task-related contextual factors, there remains, as already noted, a lack of discourse-based research into real-world oral communication practices, especially those engaged by speakers involved in culturally and linguistically diverse academic, employment, and social settings. Cultural and linguistic diversity is increasingly the norm in universities and workplaces, and communicative practices emerging in these contexts potentially conflict with conceptualizations of language proficiency, especially those related to oral communication, that underlie the constructs of the standardized international tests of English that function as gatekeeping devices in these contexts. Recent work by Canagarajah (2018), for example, based on a study of the communicative behaviors of scientists in multilingual laboratory settings, highlights the dynamic and fluid ways in which individuals draw on a range of semiotic resources, including objects, images, and fragments of various languages to produce meaning in complex and multidirectional ways. Canagarajah argues that workplace communication in culturally and linguistically diverse settings involves engaging professional knowledge and a diverse range of linguistic and other semiotic resources in ways that cannot be categorized in relation to dominant language norms or traditional notions of speaking, writing, reading, or listening proficiency.

Such research, much needed to better inform theoretical constructs and ensure that tests are well-aligned with real-world communication values and practices, also calls into question the usefulness of existing discourse-analytic tools, which either ignore nonlinguistic semiotic signs or consider them as secondary to the primary linguistic event of communication. There is a need for the development of novel "discourse" measures, encompassing the multimodal features of repertoires and practices most relevant to communication in increasingly diverse settings, that will better inform the adaptation of assessment designs to more effectively meet the decision-making purposes for which language tests are intended.

REFERENCES

Biber, D. (2006). *University language: A corpus-based study of spoken and written registers*. John Benjamins.

Biber, D., Conrad, S., Reppen, R., Byrd, P., & Helt, M. (2002). Speaking and writing at the university: A multidimensional comparison. *TESOL Quarterly*, *36*(1), 9–48. https://doi.org/10.2307/3588359

Brooks, L., & Swain, M. (2014). Contextualizing performances: Comparing performances during TOEFL iBT™ and real-life academic speaking activities. *Language Assessment Quarterly*, *11*(4), 353–373. https://doi.org/10.1080/15434303.2014.947532

Brown, A. (2000). An investigation of the rating process in the IELTS oral interview. In Tulloh, R (Ed.)., *IELTS Research Reports* (vol. 3, pp. 49–84). IELTS Australia.

Brown, A. (2003). Interviewer variation and the co-construction of speaking proficiency. *Language Testing*, *20*(1), 1–25. https://doi.org/10.1191/0265532203lt242oa

Brown, A., Iwashita, N., & McNamara, T. (2005). *An examination of rater orientations and test-taker performance on English-for-Academic-Purposes speaking tasks* (TOEFL Monograph Series MS-29). Educational Testing Service.

Canagarajah, S. (2018). Translingual practice as spatial repertoires: Expanding the paradigms beyond structuralist orientations. *Applied Linguistics*, *39*(1), 31–54. https://doi.org/10.1093/applin/amx041

Chapelle, C., Enright, M., & Jamieson, J. (2010). Does an argument-based approach to validity make a difference? *Educational Measurement: Issues and Practice*, *29*(1), 3–13. https://doi.org/10.1111/j.1745-3992.2009.00165.x

Crossley, S., Clevinger, A., & Kim., Y. (2014). The role of lexical properties and cohesive devices in text integration and their effect on human ratings of speaking proficiency. *Language Assessment Quarterly*, *11*(3), 250–270. https://doi.org/10.1080/15434303.2014.926905

Douglas, D. (1994). Quality and quality in speaking test performance. *Language Testing*, *11*(2), 125–144. https://doi.org/10.1177/026553229401100203

Douglas, D., & Selinker, L. (1992). Analyzing oral proficiency test performance in general and specific-purpose contexts. *System*, *20*(3), 317–328. https://doi.org/10.1016/0346-251X(92)90043-3

Douglas, D., & Selinker, L. (1993). Performance on a general versus a field-specific test of speaking proficiency by international teaching assistants. In D. Douglas & C. Chapelle (Eds.), *A new decade of language testing research* (pp. 235–256). TESOL Publications.

Ducasse, A. M. (2009). "Raters as scale makers for an L2 Spanish speaking test: Using paired test discourse to develop a rating scale for communicative interaction. In A. Brown & K. Hill (Eds.), *Tasks and criteria in performance assessment: Proceedings of the 28th Annual Language Testing Research Colloquium* (pp. 1–22). Peter Lang.

Elder, C., & Iwashita, N. (2005). Planning for test performance: Does it make a difference? In R. Ellis (Ed.), *Planning and task performance in a second language* (pp. 219–238). John Benjamins.

Frost, K., Clothier, J, Huisman, A, & Wigglesworth, G. (2020). Investigating the validity of an integrated listening-speaking task: A discourse-based analysis of test-takers' oral performances. *Language Testing*, 37 (1), 133–155. https://doi.org/10.1177/0265532219860750

Fulcher G. (1996). Does thick description lead to smart tests? A data-based approach to rating scale construction. *Language Testing*, *13*(2), 208–238. https://doi.org/10.1177/026553229601300205

Galaczi, E. D. (2008). Peer–peer interaction in a speaking test: The case of the First Certificate in English examination. *Language Assessment Quarterly*, *5*(2), 89–119. https://doi.org/10.1080/15434300801934702

Galaczi, E. D. (2014). Interactional competence across proficiency levels: How do learners manage interaction in paired speaking tests? *Applied Linguistics*, 35(5), 553–574. https://doi.org/10.1093/applin/amt017

Gan, Z. (2010). Interaction in group oral assessment: A case study of higher- and lower-scoring students. *Language Testing*, *27*(4), 585–602. https://doi.org/10.1177/0265532210364049

Iwashita, N., Brown, A., McNamara, T., & O'Hagan, S. (2008). Assessed levels of second language proficiency: How distinct? *Applied Linguistics*, *29*(1), 24–49. https://doi.org/10.1093/applin/amm017

Kane, M. (2006). Validation. In R. L. Linn (Ed.), *Educational measurement* (4th ed., pp. 17–64). MacMillan.

Kane, M. (2012). Validating score interpretations and uses. *Language Testing*, *29*(1), 3–17. https://doi.org/10.1177/0265532211417210

Kane, M. (2013). Validating the interpretations and uses of test scores. *Journal of Educational Measurement*, *50*(1),1–73. https://doi.org/10.1111/jedm.12000

Kormos, J. (1999). Simulating conversations in oral-proficiency assessment: A conversation analysis of role plays and non-scripted interviews in language exams. *Language Testing, 16*(2), 163–188. https://doi.org/10.1177/026553229901600203

Lazaraton, A. (1992). *A conversation analysis of structure and interaction in the language interview*. Unpublished doctoral dissertation, University of California, Los Angeles.

Lazaraton, A. (1996). Interlocutor support in oral proficiency interviews: The case of CASE. *Language Testing, 13*(2), 151–72. https://doi.org/10.1177/026553229601300202

Lazaraton, A. (2013). Discourse analysis in language assessment. In C. Chapelle (Ed.), *The encyclopedia of applied linguistics*. Blackwell.

Lazaraton, A., & Davis, L. (2008). A microanalytic perspective on discourse, proficiency, and identity in paired oral assessment. *Language Assessment Quarterly, 5*(4), 313–35. https://doi.org/10.1080/15434300802457513

McNamara, T. F. (1997). "Interaction" in second language performance assessment: Whose performance? *Applied Linguistics, 18*(4), 446–485. https://doi.org/10.1093/applin/18.4.446

McNamara, T. F., Hill, K., & May, L. (2002). Discourse and assessment. *Annual Review of Applied Linguistics, 22*, 221–242. https://doi.org/10.1017/S0267190502000120

May, L. (2009). "Co-constructed interaction in a paired speaking test: The rater's perspective," *Language Testing* 26, 397–421. https://doi.org/10.1177/0265532209104668

Nitta, R., & Nakatsuhara, F. (2014). A multifaceted approach to investigating pre-task planning effects on paired oral test performance. *Language Testing, 31*(1), 147–175. https://doi.org/10.1177/0265532213514401

Pallotti, G. (2017). Assessing tasks: The case of interactional difficulty. *Applied Linguistics*, 40(1), 176–197. https://doi.org/10.1093/applin/amx020

Robinson, P. (2001). Task complexity, cognitive resources, and syllabus design: A triadic framework for examining task influences on SLA. In P. Robinson (Ed.), *Cognition and second language instruction* (pp. 287–318). Cambridge University Press.

Robinson, P. (2007). Task complexity, theory of mind, and intentional reasoning: Effects on L2 speech production, interaction, uptake and perceptions of task difficulty. *International Review of Applied Linguistics, 45*(3), 237–257. https://doi.org/10.1515/iral.2007.009

Sarangi, S., & Roberts, C. (Eds.). (1999). *Talk, work and institutional order: Discourse in medical, mediation, and management settings*. De Gruyter Mouton.

Skehan, P. (1998). *A cognitive approach to language learning*. Oxford University Press.

Skehan, P. (2001). Tasks and language performance. In M. Bygate, P. Skehan, & M. Swain (Eds.), *Research pedagogic tasks: Second language learning, teaching, and testing* (pp. 167–185). Longman.

Skehan, P. (2009). Modelling second language performance: Integrating complexity, accuracy, fluency and lexis. *Applied Linguistics, 30*(4), 510–532. https://doi.org/10.1093/applin/amp047

Skehan, P. (2014). *Processing perspectives on task performance*. John Benjamins.

Skehan, P., & Foster, P. (1997). The influence of planning and post-task activities on accuracy and complexity in task based learning. *Language Teaching Research, 1*(3), 185–211. https://doi.org/10.1177/136216889700100302

Skehan, P., & Foster, P. (1999). The influence of task structure and processing conditions on narrative retellings. *Language Learning, 49*(1), 93–120. https://doi.org/10.1111/1467-9922.00071

Skehan, P., & Foster, P. (2008). Complexity, accuracy, fluency and lexis in task-based performance: A meta-analysis of the Ealing research. In S. Van Daele, A. Housen, F. Kuiken, M. Pierrard, & I. Vedder (Eds.), *Complexity, accuracy, and fluency in second language use, learning, and teaching* (pp. 207–226). Contactforum.

Taylor, L., & Wigglesworth, G. (2009). Are two heads better than one? Pair work in L2 assessment contexts. *Language Testing, 26*(3), 325–339. https://doi.org/10.1177/0265532209104665

Van Lier, L. (1989). Reeling, writhing, drawling, stretching and fainting in coils: Oral proficiency interviews as conversations. *TESOL Quarterly, 23*(3), 480–508. https://doi.org/10.2307/3586922

Wigglesworth, G. (1997). An investigation of planning time and proficiency level on oral test discourse. *Language Testing, 14*(1), 85–106. https://doi.org/10.1177/026553229701400105

Wigglesworth, G. (2001). Influences on performance in task-based oral assessments. In M. Bygate, P. Skehan, & M. Swain (Eds.), *Researching pedagogic tasks, second language learning, teaching and testing* (pp. 186–209). Longman.

Wigglesworth, G., & Elder, C. (2010). An investigation of the effectiveness and validity of planning time in speaking test tasks. *Language Assessment Quarterly, 7*(1), 1–24. https://doi.org/10.1080/15434300903031779

Woodward-Kron, R., & Elder, C. (2016). A comparative discourse study of simulated clinical roleplays in two assessment contexts: Validating a specific-purpose language test. *Language Testing, 33*(2), 251–270. https://doi.org/10.1177/0265532215607399

Xi, X. (2008). Methods of test validation. In E. Shohamy & N. H. Hornberger (Eds.), *Encyclopedia of language and education* (pp. 177–196). Springer Science+ Business Media LLC.

Young, R., & He, A. W. (Eds.). (1998). *Talking and testing: Discourse approaches to the assessment of oral proficiency*. John Benjamins.

10.2

Discourse Analysis in Second Language Signing Assessment: Sign Language Proficiency Interviews

Rachel McKee, Sara Pivac Alexander, and Wenda Walton

Increasing recognition of signed languages internationally has led to certain educational and employment contexts formalizing required standards of competence in signed language, prompting a demand for the measurement of signed language proficiency. The design and outcomes of several signed language proficiency assessment instruments and frameworks that can inform assessments have been documented, such as the Language Proficiency Interview for American Sign Language (ASL) (Newell et al., 1983a); the Common European Framework of Languages, adapted for signed languages[1] (Napier & Leeson, 2016, p. 105; see also Council of Europe, 2020); and the Sign Language Skills Classroom Observation (Reeves et al., 2000) but there has been relatively little analysis of their application. The Sign Language Proficiency Interview (SLPI) was first adapted from the Oral Proficiency Interview (OPI) for the purpose of benchmarking the ASL skill levels required of teaching faculty at the National Technical Institute for the Deaf (NTID), Rochester (Newell et al., 1983a), and has subsequently been widely used in North American deaf education as a screening tool for personnel and in other training and employment contexts requiring ASL competence (Caccamise et al., 1983; Caccamise & Samar, 2009). In the past decade, the SLPI has been adapted for other signed languages, including in the Netherlands (Van den Broek-Laven et al., 2014), South Africa, Kenya,[2] German Switzerland (Haug et al., 2019), and New Zealand. The structure of the SLPI (see Chapter 9.2) has not changed substantially since its development in the 1980s, and relatively minor modifications have been made in subsequent international adaptations. As yet, there is no published analysis of the ways in which interlocutors co-construct communication in the SLPI context. This chapter thus breaks new ground by examining a micro-level

Rachel McKee, Sara Pivac Alexander, and Wenda Walton, *Discourse Analysis in Second Language Signing Assessment: Sign Language Proficiency Interviews* In: *The Handbook of Language Assessment Across Modalities*. Edited by: Tobias Haug, Wolfgang Mann, and Ute Knoch, Oxford University Press. © Oxford University Press 2022.
DOI: 10.1093/oso/9780190885052.003.0030

aspect of discourse between fluent deaf interviewers and non-native (second language [L2]) SLPI candidates.

ACCOMMODATIVE FEATURES OF OPI DISCOURSE

The extent to which the discourse in proficiency interviews resembles situated discourse in the real world has been less studied than reliability of ratings, although this is fundamental to construct validity (Lazaraton, 1996). Van Lier (1989) was one of the first to scrutinize conversational naturalness in the OPI, showing that the interview process de-naturalizes discourse features of turn-taking and topic control, which are dominated by the interviewer. As reviewed by Knoch (Chapter 9.1), human variables in OPI ratings include the effects of rater and test-taker identity characteristics, the influence of interviewers on the discourse, and the relative contributions of each interlocutor in paired speaking tests. Contrary to prescribed LPI interview protocol, research evidence shows that OPI interviewers do accommodate their language to lower proficiency candidates in ways similar to natural native speaker (NS) and non-native speaker (NNS) interaction, posing a "threat" to the validity of the interview process and the subsequent rating (Ross & Berwick, 1992). Based on this finding, Ross (1992) undertook a microanalysis of linguistic accommodations by OPI interviewers, focusing on seven types of accommodative questions that occurred in 16 interviews at various levels, containing 598 interviewer questions (Ross, 1992, p. 177). The types were:

1. *Display question*. No genuine information gap—answer already known to interviewer
2. *"Or" question*. Suggests alternate response options
3. *Fronting*: One or more utterances set up a topic before the question
4. *Grammatical simplification*: Modifies syntax or semantic structure to simplify phrasing
5. *Slow-down*: Reduces speed of utterance
6. *Overarticulation*: Exaggerates stress or production of words or phrases
7. *Lexical simplification*: Chooses words that the interviewer believes are simpler

Ross analyzed antecedent triggers for accommodation (e.g., pause, unexpected response, poorly articulated response) to determine which factors had the most influence on eliciting accommodative question features. They were, in order (1) interviewee's response to the previous question, (2) structure of their response to previous question, (3) perceived proficiency level of the interviewee, and (4) whether or not the previous question was accommodated (Ross, 1992, p. 179). Ross suggests that these findings have implications for appreciating that performance results should be gauged in light of the co-constructed (i.e., interviewer-supported) nature of discourse and for training, stating, "analysis of instances of necessary versus superfluous uses of accommodation can make an interviewer-in-training more cognizant of discourse features that resemble genuine information-bearing conversational interaction" (p. 183). A subsequent study of OPI discourse similarly identified interlocutor support by interviewers in ways such as topic priming ("fronting"), supplying vocabulary, offering response options, collaborative completions, echoing and correcting, giving evaluative feedback, slowing down and overarticulating, and rephrasing questions (Lazaraton, 1996). As Lazaraton observes, while these features represent naturalness in the discourse, at the same time "interviewer speech modifications, unless systematic and consistent, add an element of uncontrolled variability to the assessment picture. Clearly, we want testing outcomes to be the result of candidate abilities and not a product of context" (Lazaraton, 1996, p. 154). Accordingly, guidelines for OPI and SLPI interviewers discourage accommodation behavior: interviewers are advised to maintain naturally paced language, to clarify by restating in full rather than modifying an utterance, and to avoid supplying vocabulary or response options in order to test the limits of the candidate's comprehension and expressive capacity (Buck, 1989, in Lazaraton, 1996, p. 155). This ideal is in tension with empirical findings on the occurrence of interviewer accommodations and, we would predict, with the style-shifting behavior of deaf individuals in negotiating communication encounters with lower proficiency, nondeaf signers.

LANGUAGE CONTACT AND "FOREIGNER TALK" ACCOMMODATION IN SIGNED LANGUAGES

Communities of deaf signed language users are invariably surrounded by a majority spoken/written language in which they are usually bilingual to varying degrees. Ongoing interaction between a spoken and signed language results in "bimodal" contact features in signed languages that manifest at the levels of syntax, morphology, lexicon, and bimodal production, in discourse between deaf individuals and between deaf and hearing interlocutors (Lucas & Valli, 1992; Quinto-Pozos & Adam, 2013). In particular, deaf signers often accommodate hearing (signing) interlocutors by adopting more contact features, such as English word order, reduced nonmanual and spatial inflectional morphology, fingerspelling more words, voiceless mouthing of sign "glosses," and more use of conventional gestures. Cokely (1983) identified that variation along an "ASL-English continuum" in deaf–hearing discourse (i.e., the use of more contact features) is an interplay of foreigner talk, judgments of proficiency, and learners' competence in the target language. If such accommodations are present in the context of SLPI discourse, this raises the question of how contact language features affect candidate responses and how such features should be treated by raters in relation to target language descriptors. In fact, the construct validity of an early iteration of the SLPI, called the Sign Communication Proficiency Interview (SCPI) (Caccamise et al., 1983; Newell et al., 1983a), was critiqued at the time on grounds of ambiguity of target language criteria that spanned a spectrum of signing styles from native ASL, to English-influenced "contact" styles of signing. Cokely (1983, p. 337) questioned "whether the SCPI as proposed by Newell et al. is possible or reasonable within a 'language in contact' situation," arguing that "native speaker" norms for intermediate varieties are elusive, unstable reference points for accuracy of form. In response, the SCPI originators acknowledged that communicative norms in a bilingual community are indeed more elastic and less predictable than in monolingual contexts (Newell et al., 1983b). This issue remains relevant to implementation of the SLPI. Sources of linguistic variability in interviewer discourse and how these affect proficiency ratings have not been studied in relation to the SLPI. In this chapter, we therefore take a first step toward this by reporting an empirical analysis of accommodative behavior by deaf interviewers working with candidates at differing levels of New Zealand Sign Language (NZSL) proficiency.

INVESTIGATING LINGUISTIC ACCOMMODATION IN THE CONTEXT OF THE NZSL-PROFICIENCY INTERVIEW

Adaptation of the SLPI for use in New Zealand began in 2015, to address the absence of NZSL standards for personnel in deaf education (Human Rights Commission, 2013). The NZSLPI project was supported by the Ministry of Education and implemented by universities with NZSL programs, in collaboration with Rochester Institute of Technology (RIT) as the owner of the SLPI tool. The original ASL rating rubrics were modified to reflect usage norms of NZSL, while descriptors for proficiency levels were retained from the original (as per Newell et al., 1983a) to maintain international parity. Procedural guides and rating forms were modified to improve usability for local assessors, including video links to NZSL grammar examples. Training in interviewing and rating techniques was conducted in three workshops by an SLPI expert from RIT. Key components of training included familiarization with the aims and construct of the SLPI, understanding formal and functional language criteria in the rating rubric and how to identify examples in data, interviewing techniques, and rating interviews independently and subsequently in groups to calibrate proficiency judgments across the 10 assessors. Since 2015, the NZSLPI has been piloted with approximately 100 candidates, interviewed and rated by 10 assessors. Data for this study are from that corpus of recorded interviews.

Interrater reliability was assessed after 60 candidates had been rated by pairs of independent raters, with consultation between them only as needed to resolve level differences. Krippendorff's alpha was applied to assess the mean difference between individual ratings of the same candidates. Krippendorff's alpha was calculated to be 0.914, indicating that the 10 raters overall had a high degree of agreement. This improved slightly by removing any one of four raters who generated more variance than the others, according to a set of Krippendorff's alpha values in a leave-one-out style, with each rater being removed in turn. Intrarater reliability was not analyzed. These results indicate that the NZSLPI assessment team to date produces reliable outcomes.

Data and Analysis

Nine recorded SLPI interviews were selected for this analysis, in three proficiency bands of low (novice/plus), mid (survival/intermediate), and high (advanced/superior). We selected a sample of three interviewers working with three candidates each in order to reduce the effects of individual variation between multiple interviewer styles and to ascertain whether interviewers' accommodative strategies differed by candidate proficiency level. Interviewers were three trained assessors who were NZSL-fluent deaf women, over 40 years of age. Eight of nine candidates were female. Eight work in the deaf education sector, and six undertook the SLPI as an employment requirement. Two of the high-proficiency candidates were qualified NZSL interpreters.

The prescribed SLPI interview time is 20 minutes, but these interviews ranged from 16:37 to 31 minutes. We analyzed only the first 20 minutes per interview, giving a total of 174 minutes across nine interviews. The three interviewers respectively contributed 56, 58, and 60 minutes of data.

Our focus was accommodative interviewer questions, and a total of 510 questions were identified. Using ELAN software,[3] all questions were transcribed using English glosses for signs, as well as mouthing that occurred without signs, where it contributed to eliciting or clarifying candidate responses. We coded the presence/absence of accommodation in each question and type of accommodation, and antecedent triggers for accommodated questions were also noted but not strictly categorized. Additional observations about the discourse were also noted. Nine initial accommodation question (AQ) types were based on Ross's (1992) taxonomy, modified for signed language; these are described in Table 10.2.1. We soon decided to omit "Display" questions because it was apparent that interviewers were often familiar with candidates' backgrounds due to close networks in the deaf sector and thus knew the answers to biographical and occupational questions, leading to many questions that were motivated purely by the interview "frame" (Ross, 1998) rather than genuine inquiry; as such, these

Table 10.2.1 Types and frequency of accommodated questions

Accommodated question (AQ) type	Definition and example (*translated from NZSL*)	Frequency of type (as a percentage of total AQs)
Display question	Interviewer asks for information which is already known to the interviewer, or which the interviewer believes the interviewee ought to know. E.g., *"What's your name?" "What are your job responsibilities?"*	*Not counted (see above)*
"Or" question	Interviewer asks a question and provides one or more options from which the interviewee may choose an answer. E.g., *"(you lived) over here (indicating on imaginary map) in the East, or down here in the South?"; "Is your walk on the flat or uphill?"*	23% (78)
Grammatical simplification	Interviewer modifies the syntactic or semantic structure of an utterance to make it easier to understand. E.g., *English word order, shorter sentence, make phrasing more distinct, use lexical signs instead of nonmanual features (NMF)* (e.g., *if for conditional, nothing*[a] *for neg rather than NMF); use (redundant) person pronouns with an inflected agreement verb.*	17% (56)
Overarticulation, signs	Exaggeration in production of signs—size or distinction of movement. Immediate repetition of the same phrase (adding redundancy). Exaggerated spatial (referential) contrast.	16 % (55)
Slow	Interviewer reduces speed of an utterance.	15% (52)
Lexical simplification	Interviewer chooses what is assumed to be a simpler or more familiar word or phrase. E.g., *way rather than system; know-neg rather than ignorant (colloq.); good rather than skilled; interest rather than hobby.*	14% (48)
Fronting	Interviewer foregrounds and/or establishes a topic before asking a question. E.g., *"You like reading. What kind of books do you like?"*	10% (34)
Over-articulation, mouthing	Interviewer attempts to clarify meaning by using more pronounced mouthing than normal, with or without a sign.	1.8% (6)
Fingerspelling	Interviewer attempts to clarify meaning of an unfamiliar sign or referent by fingerspelling it. E.g., PRO2 SAY TEACH fs-S-O-C-I-A-L SOCIAL . . ." ("You said you teach s-o-c-i-a-l, social . . .")	1.5% (5)
(Undetermined)	Ambiguous—could not agree on type	1.7% (3)
Total		100% (337)

Capitalized words represent glosses that represent actual signs used, as is conventional in sign linguistics literature. Glosses convey an approximate, typical English meaning for a particular sign form.

display questions were an accommodation to the context, rather than to candidates' language ability.

Of a total 510 questions identified, 66% (337) had accommodative features. Occurrences of AQ types are shown in descending order of frequency in Table 10.2.1 and described later.

"Or" questions, which suggest alternate responses, were the most common type at 23%. In these data, "or" questions generally appeared to have an intentionally accommodative function, modeling "this or that" response options, and many were articulated at a somewhat slower rate for clarity. "Or" accommodations were less frequent at higher levels, decreasing from 32 instances in the novice/novice plus range to 21 instances in the advanced/superior range. We note that alternate questions also occur between equal NS interlocutors and are not necessarily an accommodation strategy, but perhaps a product of the interviewer's need to prompt a response; this could be confirmed by looking at their frequency in natural NS conversations. At times we observed that "or" questions were introduced as a clarification ("Do you mean x or y?") and at times clearly complicated the language (or response options) that a candidate was presented with, rather than simplifying.

Simplification of grammar was the second most frequent accommodation at 17%. Examples included simplifying phrasing, elaborating a sequence of events, adding redundancy by repetition (e.g., "sandwich" questions with an initial and final interrogative), making subject or location references overt where they might typically be deleted, supplying lexical cues rather than relying on nonmanual grammar, or amplifying referential (spatial) contrasts. In one example, the interviewer asked the candidate when their sign language class started. To clarify that she was asking about a recent past timeframe, the interviewer simplified by elaboration: THIS YEAR. WHEN PAST, WHEN PAST? This was followed immediately by another AQ that offered "or" options framed by two "query" gestures of open, upturned hands: "palms-up JANUARY, FEBRUARY palms-up." The frequency of this grammatical accommodation type differs most between proficiency levels: at the highest level 3, different interviewers produced only one instance each of simplified grammar; at mid and low levels of proficiency, there are 24 and 31 instances, respectively.

Exaggerated articulation of signs (16%) and slow production rate (15%) were similarly frequent and often co-occurred. This overlap reflects the fact that expanding the size of signs to make them more distinct entails slower, more deliberate movement. "Exaggerated" and "slow" was determined impressionistically in relation to each interviewer's usual manner of signing with advanced-level candidates. We noticed that referential pointing, in particular, was often articulated more deliberately and held longer than in natural discourse, perhaps indicating interviewers' awareness that fleeting subject reference in connected SL can be difficult for NNS to perceive. The frequency of "slow signing" reduced with higher level candidates: 31 instances at novice level, 15 at survival/intermediate, compared to only 5 at advanced/superior. The frequency of overarticulated signs or repetition of utterances was similar at mid and high levels: 10 instances at advanced/superior levels, 12 at survival/intermediate, but much higher at novice level with 31 occurrences.

Lexical simplification was identified in 14% of questions. Simplification is a contextualized judgment because there are often vocabulary choices available to a signer, but we coded the use of high-frequency (more basic) signs as simplification in contexts where another, less frequent sign would be equally or more semantically precise. An example of lexical simplification via synonyms and elaboration occurred in this hypothetical question, "What would you like to see changed?," in which the interviewer seemed dubious that the candidate knew the signs PRETEND or IMAGINE by offering the simpler substitute WISH: "PRO2 PRETEND, PRO2+ IMAGINE WISH CHANGE IMPROVE WHAT PRO2, PRO2?" ("Pretend, imagine, **wish** you (can) change or improve (that). What (would you do?)"). Some questions coded as "or" type also suggest lexical simplification by unpacking the meaning of a less familiar sign, such as "when" in this example: "PRO2 GO-TO MORNING, NIGHT, WHEN?" ("Do you go there in the morning, at night, when?"). In another example, the interviewer spontaneously paraphrased with a more iconic sign (FLY) for a more opaque one (MOVE), asking: "WHEN PRO2 MOVE-TO, FLY-TO NZ?" ("When did you move here, fly to NZ?"). Lexical simplification reduced with increasing proficiency, with 26 instances at low level, 16 at mid-level, and 6 at high level.

Fronting of a topic (or "topic priming"; Lazaraton, 1996) occurred in 10% of AQs. Fronting gives supporting context by stating the topic of an upcoming question, for instance: "PRO2 fs-E LEARN. EXPLAIN-me g:palms-up" ("You do E-learning. Tell me what that is?"), or, "PRO2 fs-RTD. PRO2 HOW-MANY CHILDREN PRO2 TEACH?" ("You're a Resource Teacher of the Deaf. How many children do you teach?"). Fronting occurred more in the survival/intermediate range than in either the low or high levels of proficiency. The difference may not be significant, however, at 17 occurrences in the mid level compared with 12 at low level and 5 at high level.

Overarticulated mouthing occurred in 1.8% of questions, with no pattern of association with candidate levels. One interviewer produced four examples at two different levels, while two other interviewers only produced one each, at differing levels. Mouthing words with signs, especially nouns and adjectives, is usual in NZSL (McKee, 2016). Given this local norm, we coded only noticeably pronounced mouthing that appeared to be doing extra accommodation work, for example, in a phrase, TWO HOUR(s) (a) WEEK, where the interviewer apparently felt that the candidate was not quite familiar with the NZSL form of the time phrase and amplified their mouthing. More interestingly we observed interviewers' use of mouthing alone to confirm understanding of something a candidate had signed (e.g., mirroring back a fingerspelled name by mouthing it) or as back-channel ("right," "oh," "wow," "no"). Although the use of "solo" mouthing also occurs in natural NZSL discourse, its frequency in the SLPI data was noticeable and possibly reflected interviewers' effort to show understanding of candidates' signing. Fingerspelling as a form of AQ was seldom used; four instances occurred at the lowest level, one at mid-level, and none at the highest level. This distribution is interesting given that the low-proficiency candidates are generally least skilled at reading fingerspelling; fingerspelling as an accommodation is obviously prompted by their smaller NZSL vocabulary knowledge.

Overall, two-thirds of all questions (66%) had accommodative features, and the frequency of AQs corresponds with candidate level. Analysis shows that 51% (173/337) of questions at novice level are accommodated, 35% (117/337) at survival/intermediate level, and 15% (51/337) at advanced/superior level. AQs of every type are most prevalent with lower level signers and decrease with advancing proficiency, reflecting naturalistic NS behavior in communication with less, or more, proficient NNS, as also found by Ross (1992).

Triggers for AQs were not systematically quantified; however, our observation is that they paralleled those described for Ross's (1992) OPI data, including poorly articulated or unexpected candidate responses, pause (or blank face), and previous accommodations that reflect an interviewer's perception of the candidate's proficiency level.

Other Discourse Variables

Some accommodative features did not fit the original categories. Repetitions of an utterance—for example, "Where do you work? Where do you work?," were coded as overarticulation of signs, given that reiteration is an overproduction of the question, extending the candidate's opportunity to perceive it. Another accommodation was exhibited by one interviewer: when a candidate did not know a sign (used by the interviewer or to express a response), the interviewer would "teach" or supply the sign. Interviewers would sometimes substitute a better sign for the intended meaning. For example, a novice candidate (teacher) was asked how many children they taught, and replied FIVE CHILDREN; the interviewer responded with FIVE CHILDREN STUDENT, FIVE STUDENT. This type of interlocutor support exceeds the strict parameters of SLPI technique, yet is consistent with NS-NNS interaction in the real world, perhaps particularly so when the interviewer has another identity as a

SL teacher, which motivates their response to scaffold a learner. Such "language enrichment" responses suggest the potential of interlocutor identities or other roles to affect their approach to negotiating meaning in the interview; however, supplementing vocabulary can complicate assessment of the candidate's vocabulary knowledge (Lazaraton, 1996, p. 159).

Overlapping types of accommodation (e.g., slow + "or" question) occurred frequently, especially with lower proficiency signers. We did not consistently count co-occurrences as separate tokens of accommodation (coding only the more dominant feature in each case) because it seems unnatural to attempt to separate their production for analytic purposes. However, unpacking these clusters of features may be useful for interviewers to see which of their repertoire of accommodating strategies they are unconsciously producing.

Hyperpositive affect expressed through facial expression and body language was noted as an accommodation displayed mainly toward less proficient signers. Wide smiling ("over polite" from a NS perspective), encouraging head nods, and forward leaning occurred as back-channel in interviews with candidates at novice to intermediate levels. The affirming tone of these nonmanual behaviors contrasted with the behavior of the same interviewers with high level, and especially deaf, candidates, in which these signals were much reduced or absent. And, as described in OPI discourse (Lazaraton, 1996), we observed numerous instances of evaluative responses to a candidate's turn (GOOD, WOW, YAY, NICE) and interviewers affirming responses by echoing or correcting vocabulary used imperfectly by the candidate—strategies characteristic of NS–learner interaction, but not of equal interlocutors.

DISCUSSION AND IMPLICATIONS

Qualitative analysis of AQs reveals that trained SLPI interviewers use interlocutor support strategies that occur naturally in NS–NNS interaction, especially at lower proficiency levels. This highlights that SLPIs occur within a wider context of regular interaction between users of signed language and spoken language, leading interlocutors to draw on their communicative repertoires for interlanguage communication in the real world. For interviewers, these include a range of linguistic accommodations such as expanding the context, overarticulating signs and mouthing, selecting easier vocabulary, simplifying grammar, prompting response options, providing supportive back-channel, and responding to communicative "trouble" in facilitative ways. In this respect, interviewer behavior in SPLIs closely parallels features reported for spoken OPIs, and we can echo Lazaraton's observation that, "prescriptions and prohibitions about speech behaviour in language assessment situations ignore the fact that oral assessments do occur in an interactional context where participants have assigned 'roles' and behaviours that go along with them. These identities may conflict with other roles (e.g., 'the native speaker' 'tries to help' 'the non-native speaker') that are brought to, and may be difficult to shed in, the interview context." (Lazaraton, 1996, pp. 155–156). Findings in this study that these strategies do contribute to jointly constructed discourse is in tension with the SLPI guidelines to minimize interviewer collaboration in the interview. This evidence is potentially useful for the refinement of interview techniques in training by demonstrating accommodative tendencies to avoid.

The process of coding linguistic accommodation types highlighted for us the issue raised by Cokely (1983) in the early days of the SLPI, that the definition of evidence-based usage norms in relation to SL proficiency is a challenge, particularly in a language (such as NZSL) that exhibits variation at all levels of linguistic structure and that includes the use of contact styles that accommodate toward speakers of English. One small example in this study was determining gradient features such as mouthing: When was it an accommodation versus a "typical" contact language feature of NZSL? Lacking baseline data, we had to subjectively identify accommodation as instances where the interviewer mouthed a word more deliberately than adjacent mouthings or with more markedly English phrasing. Grammatical simplification was also difficult to judge in relation to a spectrum of acceptable usage. Ultimately, analytic decisions on many features were subjective and negotiated and took into account the overall demeanor of the interviewer: Did the style ("tone") look "accommodating" in contrast to other utterances? Similar challenges might arise with the assessment of candidates' language, which was beyond the scope of this study.

Our overall observation of interviews with candidates at different levels resonates with Cokely's (1983) point that functional competence might be less impeded by linguistic accuracy than a proficiency rating scale assumes. Hearing individuals who are not sophisticated signers but who interact regularly with deaf people can develop interlanguage strategies that are complemented by shared interactional context to achieve functionally effective communication; in several interviews we observed that communicative functionality was well ahead of accuracy of form. While the SLPI assessment criteria require both form and function to be taken into account, it seems that the uniquely bimodal affordances of code-blending (e.g., mouthing, speaking, or gesturing to supplement SL) contribute to interlanguage functionality in ways that distinguish SLPI discourse from other OPI contexts. We are not questioning the structural distinctiveness of native signed and spoken languages but acknowledge that the construct of assessing communicative competence for SL users is certainly complicated by the bimodal-bilingual conditions in which meaning is usually negotiated between signers and speakers.

FUTURE RESEARCH DIRECTIONS

Critically examining discourse characteristics of SLPIs highlights that many features of conversational discourse between NS signers are underdescribed as a baseline for evaluating the naturalness of interview discourse; for instance, how common is the use of collaborative strategies such as "or" questions, reformulation of questions, or unaccompanied mouthing as back-channel—all of which were frequent in NZSLPI data? Comparison of screen-mediated (e.g., Zoom) versus in-person interviews calls for investigation because SLPIs are increasingly likely to be technology-mediated for reasons of cost efficiency and service accessibility, especially in countries with smaller and dispersed populations.

In New Zealand, the SLPI was implemented primarily to measure the communicative competence of teachers to work with deaf children. With this application in mind, the manner in which interview discourse is collaboratively negotiated between an NS interviewer and NNS candidate is of real import: while a sophisticated adult (bilingual) SL user has the tools to negotiate meaning with a non-native hearing user of SL (e.g., by simplifying, supplying response options, lipreading, mouthing, etc.), a deaf child who is only developing proficiency in SL and English cannot deploy these strategies to the same extent, thus significantly reducing the (teacher) candidate's actual communicative effectiveness in a real-world context of working with a deaf child. Identifying and controlling the extent of linguistic accommodation by SLPI interviewers is thus consequential for maintaining the construct validity of its purpose and the benchmarks established by this type of assessment.

More fine-grained analysis of SLPI interview discourse is needed to investigate other ways in which interlocutors contribute to the co-construction of discourse and which of these support the validity and reliability of proficiency assessment. Although interviewers' linguistic accommodation facilitates the progress of an interview (as per natural conversation), it can also potentially affect raters' perception of language competence; for instance, Lazaraton (1996, p. 164) found that questions offering "or" response options in OPIs can restrict or confuse a candidate's opportunity to formulate a response and that interviewer initiated corrections, echoing, and repetitions may lower raters' perception of candidate comprehension. Given that accommodative behaviors increase with lower levels of candidate proficiency, Ross and Berwick (1992, p. 170) suggest that occurrences of accommodation could potentially be incorporated as a measure in rating proficiency, commenting that, "the concept of accommodation has not been a part of the framework of OPI thinking and has thus been ignored as a potential source of interview criteria." In the SLPI rating rubric, broad descriptors of the interviewers' rate of signing and frequency of repetitions are in fact included, which at least draws rater attention to these influences in the discourse. Future research should consider how specific collaborative behaviors of SLPI interviewers influence interview discourse: to what extent interviewers and to raters are conscious of accommodations, how they affect candidate language performance, and to what extent accommodation behaviors themselves might be considered a reliable indicator that contribute to judgments of candidate proficiency.

Finally, we reiterate the observations of previous researchers on spoken LPI discourse, that discourse analysis is an important resource not only in potential refinement of the assessment tool, but also in the training of interviewers to raise their awareness and control of the relative complexity of their language and their inclination to use accommodative strategies. Research evidence can also highlight contextual variables that affect interview outcomes, such as the identities and roles of interlocutors in the real world and the effect of habitual teacher–learner responses.

ACKNOWLEDGMENTS

The New Zealand Ministry of Education and Ministry of Social Development (Office for Disability Issues) funded the NZSLPI project from 2015 to 2019, from which this chapter arises. We acknowledge Geoff Poor of Rochester Institute of Technology for leading the implementation of the SLPI in New Zealand, and we thank the interviewers and candidates who are anonymous participants in the study.

NOTES

1. https://www.ecml.at/ECML-Programme/Programme2012-2015/ProSign/PRO-Sign-referencelevels/tabid/1844/Default.aspx
2. https://www.rit.edu/ntid/slpi/faq
3. https://tla.mpi.nl/tools/tla-tools/elan/

REFERENCES

Buck, C. (Ed.) (1989). *The ACTFL OPI: Tester training manual*. ACTFL.

Caccamise, F., W. Newell, & M. Mitchell-Caccamise (1983). Use of the SLPI for assessing the sign communicative competence of Louisiana School for the Deaf dormitory counselor applicants. *Journal of the Academy of Rehabilitative Audiology, 16*, 283–304.

Caccamise, F., & Samar, V. (2009). Sign Language Proficiency Interview (SLPI): Prenegotiation interrater reliability and rater validity. *Contemporary Issues in Communication Science and Disorders, 36*, 36–47.

Cokely, D. (1983). Comment on the SCPI. *Sign Language Studies, 41*, 337–343.
Council of Europe. (2020). *Common European framework of reference for languages: Learning, teaching, assessment. Companion volume*. Council of Europe Publishing. https://rm.coe.int/common-european-framework-of-reference-for-languages-learning-teaching/16809ea0d4
Haug, T., Nussbaumer, D., & Stocker Bachmann, H. (2019). Die Entwicklung von Instrumenten zur Überprüfung von kognitiven Fähigkeiten, gebärdensprachlicher Kompetenz und Dolmetschleistung von Gebärdensprachdolmetscherinnen [The development of instruments to assess cognitive abilities, sign language proficiency, and interpreting performance in sign language interpreters]. *Das Zeichen, 111*, 130–143.
Human Rights Commission. (2013). *A new era in the right to sign. Report of the New Zealand Sign Language enquiry*. Human Rights Commission.
Lazaraton, A. (1996). Interlocutor support in oral proficiency interviews: The case of CASE. *Language Testing, 13*(2), 151–172. https://doi.org/10.1177/026553229601300202
Lucas C., & Valli C. (1992). *Language contact in the American Deaf community*. Academic Press.
McKee, R. (2016). *New Zealand Sign Language: A reference grammar*. Bridget Williams Books.
Napier, J., & Leeson, L. (2016). *Sign Language in Action*. Palgrave Macmillan.
Newell, W., Caccamise, F., Boardman, K., & Holcomb, B. R. (1983a). Adaptation of the Language Proficiency Interview (LPI) for assessing sign communicative competence. *Sign Language Studies, 41*, 311–331.
Newell, W., Caccamise, F., Boardman, K., & Holcomb, B. R. (1983b). Authors' response. *Sign Language Studies, 41*, 344–352.
Quinto-Pozos, D., & Adam, R. (2013). Sign language contact. In R. Bayley, R. Cameron, & C. Lucas (Eds.), *Oxford handbooks of sociolinguistics*. Oxford University Press. https://doi.org/10.1093/oxfordhb/9780199744084.013.0019
Reeves, J., Newell, W., Holcomb, B. R., & Stinson, M. (2000). The Sign Language Skills Classroom Observation: A process for describing sign language proficiency in classroom settings. *American Annals of the Deaf, 145*(4), 315–341.
Ross, S. (1992). Accommodative questions in oral proficiency interviews. *Language Testing, 9*(2), 173–185. https://doi.org/10.1177/026553229200900205
Ross, S. (1998). Divergent frame interpretation in language proficiency interview interaction. In A. He (Ed.), *Talking and testing: Discourse approaches to the assessment of oral proficiency* (pp. 333–353). John Benjamins.
Ross, S., & Berwick, R. (1992). The discourse of accommodation in Oral Proficiency Interviews. *Studies in Second Language Acquisition, 14*(2), 159–176. https://doi.org/10.1017/S0272263100010809
Van den Broek-Laven, A., Boers-Visker, E., & van den Bogaerde, B. (2014). Determining aspects of text difficulty for the Sign Language of the Netherlands (NGT) Functional Assessment instrument. *Papers in Language Testing and Assessment, 3*(2), 53–75
van Lier, L. (1989). Reeling, Writhing, Drawling, Stretching, and Fainting in Coils: Oral Proficiency Interviews as Conversation. *TESOL*.

10.3

Discussion of Issues Related to Discourse Analysis in Signed and Spoken Language Assessments

Rachel McKee and Kellie Frost

The analysis of discourse in language proficiency interviews reveals many similarities and some issues that are specific to the modality and social context of spoken and signed languages. In this chapter, we comment on points of intersection and difference in the preceding two chapters to highlight how the exchange of insights from signed and spoken language research in this area can stimulate further inquiry and advance theory across both fields. The chapter begins with discussion of the ways in which discourse analysis in signed language, as presented by McKee et al. (Chapter 10.2), offers a potential way forward in addressing current challenges in speaking assessment related to capturing the multimodal and multilingual practices that characterize contemporary communication. We then move on to consider the need to develop evidence-based construct models of "baseline" authentic language use to inform signed language assessment design, and we reflect on ways that the discourse analysis work in speaking assessment, presented by Frost (Chapter 10.1), might contribute to this. In the last parts of the chapter we consider current research directions in characterizing multimodality as well as in defining communicative competence for the purpose of gatekeeping assessments, and we conclude with reflections on future directions in discourse analysis across modalities.

POSITIONING MULTIMODALITY AND MULTILINGUALISM AS THE NORM FOR SPEAKING ASSESSMENT PURPOSES

In the context of the NZSLPI, McKee et al. examine in Chapter 10.2 accommodation behaviors engaged by deaf interviewers, highly proficient in signed language, in interactions with test-takers—learners of signed language with a spoken first language (L1). In the field of

Rachel McKee and Kellie Frost, *Discussion of Issues Related to Discourse Analysis in Signed and Spoken Language Assessments* In: *The Handbook of Language Assessment Across Modalities*. Edited by: Tobias Haug, Wolfgang Mann, and Ute Knoch, Oxford University Press. © Oxford University Press 2022.
DOI: 10.1093/oso/9780190885052.003.0031

speaking assessment, interviewer accommodation, where it impacts the discourse produced by test-takers, is assumed to represent a source of construct-irrelevant variance because scores, which are intended to reflect test-taker speaking ability, are influenced at least in part by interlocutor behavior. This has led to debates in the field about how to account for the co-constructed nature of meaning in interaction, which, arguably, conflicts with the broad intention behind speaking testing—to provide a measure of an individual's oral proficiency (e.g., Brown, 2003; Galaczi, 2008; Lazaraton, 1996; Lazaraton & Davis, 2008; McNamara, 1997; Taylor & Wigglesworth, 2009).

While McKee et al. do not directly challenge the assumption that interviewer behaviors represent a potential threat to test validity in the context of signed language assessment, they posit that accommodation behaviors likely mirror the bimodal and bilingual nature of real-world interactions involving signed language, enabled by the fact that many deaf people have hearing parents and are thus exposed from an early age to the range of semiotic features associated with spoken language, such as gesture, mouthing, and other facial and bodily movements involved in meaning-making. In so doing, they highlight the importance of understanding the role of shared resources in facilitating effective communication between individuals from different language backgrounds and of different levels of proficiency in a lingua franca—in this case, signed language. McKee et al. also suggest that, given the inherently bimodal and bilingual nature of signed language interactions, an emphasis on communicative functionality is perhaps more relevant as a construct for assessment purposes than proficiency in any particular language variety.

These insights are highly relevant to current challenges in the field of speaking assessment, particularly in light of increasing linguistic and cultural diversity in contexts where language tests are widely used to regulate access to opportunities: universities and workplaces. In these contexts, where a spoken language often functions as a lingua franca between native and non-native speakers from diverse L1 backgrounds, achieving communication goals also likely depends on how different semiotic resources, particularly those that are shared, are engaged and utilized in interactions. This is consistent with recent arguments made by Canagarajah (2018), in light of evidence that effective communication in "English-speaking" workplaces depends on technical expertise at least as much, if not more, as proficiency in English, with images, objects, and fragments from different language repertoires all playing an important role. Nonetheless, in the field of speaking assessment, it is typically assumed that nonverbal features and the broader context of communication (i.e., the objects, spatial features, and the affordances they provide) are potentially supportive but not central to meaning-making, which has meant they are excluded from measurement constructs and are rarely, if ever, included in discourse-analytic studies. In the field of signed language assessment, discourse analysis necessarily calls for the inclusion of nonverbal features of communication and a foregrounding of the meaning-making work done through gesture, facial expressions, and various other symbols. In challenging a hierarchical view of communicative resources and in providing a set of analytic tools needed to capture a broader, more inclusive notion of "discourse," work in signed language assessment thus offers a way forward in expanding theoretical constructs in speaking assessment to capture more real-world relevant conceptualizations of language and of communication.

THE NEED FOR BASELINE EVIDENCE ABOUT SIGNED LANGUAGE DISCOURSE

In spoken language testing, Frost (Chapter 10.1) argues that evidence from the analysis of target language discourse in natural contexts provides an essential baseline for test authenticity—that is, assessment tasks that reflect real-world discourse demands and scoring criteria that correspond with real-world usage practices. A fundamental challenge for improving signed language assessment tools is the scarcity of published research on discourse and usage features in signed languages. Even below discourse level, there is insufficient application of available descriptive evidence about lexico-grammatical features to the design of signed language curricula, learning materials, and assessment tools; these commonly rely on received wisdom and intuition about which language features are typical and salient for learners (Fenlon, 2019; Johnston, 2012).

In spoken language testing, particularly for specific purposes, Frost notes that construct definition, task design, and criteria for scoring target features tend to be informed by specialist domain (e.g., medical) experts and language tester intuition rather than empirical studies of discourse features and behaviors in situated contexts. This is not to say that these sources of expertise necessarily lack integrity, but recent quantitative investigations in large corpora of authentic signed language discourse are making findings that challenge certain long-held generalizations and beliefs about the characteristics of signed languages. Examples include the surprising *in*frequency of "headshake" as a grammatical negator in Australian Sign Language (Auslan) (Johnston, 2018), lower than expected rates of inflection in verbs that are canonically taught as "agreement" verbs in Auslan and British Sign Language (BSL) (Fenlon et al., 2018), the prevalence of mouthing of words as a form of bimodal code-blending in numerous signed languages (Bank et al., 2016; Johnston et al., 2016; Nadolske & Rosenstock, 2007), and the identification of gestural elements in signed language discourse in common with multimodal aspects of spoken communication (e.g., Ferrara & Halvorsen, 2018; Schembri et al., 2005). These are all features that are subject to normative judgments in signed language tests, indicating that more usage-based evidence can refine measures of "good" or "typical" signed language use.

Without baseline evidence about typical usage, there is scope for inauthentic test content or misleading scoring criteria. For example, the rating rubric of the SLPI instrument discussed in Chapter 10.2 includes an unweighted list of grammar features to be rated; however this (a) potentially skews interview discourse away from a plausible "conversation" by the imperative to introduce topics that will elicit evidence of certain language structures (e.g., to prompt structures for describing locations and objects: "What does your house/oven/dog look like?") and (b) does not weight the relative frequency (i.e., actual communicative value) of the particular feature in natural usage. Similarly, the absence of lexical distribution data that reliably identify high- and low-frequency signs allows variability in scoring decisions about whether a candidate's vocabulary use is "basic" or "more advanced."[1]

Authenticity in signed language testing matters because deaf people's inclusion in society—in the contexts of family, school, workplace, or local community—increases when more people have functional skills in signed language. Motivated by this circumstance and by the fact that signed language has no written mode, signed language pedagogy tends to focus on interactive communication skills guided by functional-notional curricula that reflect everyday discourse situations. It is thus important that measurements of second language (L2) proficiency in signed languages, as in spoken languages, do elicit "linguistic behaviors important to communicative success in real world domains" (Frost, Chapter 10.1).

High-Stakes Testing

Frost's chapter discusses the importance of authenticity especially in high-stakes specific-purpose tests, such as those related to an occupational role (e.g., medical). This prompts us to observe that "high stakes" in relation to signed languages can be defined from the perspective of the minority (target) language community for whom L2 (hearing) signers inherently hold a different power status and are afforded different opportunities by acquiring competence in signed language. A common purpose of proficiency assessments such as the SLPI is to authorize candidates to assume professional roles that influence the lives of deaf people. From the deaf community's perspective, one "high-stakes" outcome of signed language assessment is to qualify individuals to work with deaf children as teachers. Because most deaf children have hearing parents, the acquisition of signed language is highly dependent on exposure to signed language models in the education system, and, moreover, the quality of that language use has major implications for a deaf child's educational experience. Benchmarking the signed language proficiency of professionals who become language models for deaf children is therefore considered "high stakes" for individual children and for language vitality at a collective level. However, we need more empirical investigation of how effectively the SLPI captures the construct of interactional competence in classrooms: How does a teacher's performance in a controlled situation with a deaf interlocutor who has an adult language repertoire compare with their ability to communicate with young deaf students (of diverse language profiles) about curriculum topics and situations that arise at school? Another high-stakes outcome of signed language assessment is the qualification of interpreters who facilitate language access for deaf individuals across multiple domains of their lives. In sum, deaf people's participation in society is, to a unique degree, mediated by non-native signers, and this is why it is particularly important that signed language assessment authentically mirrors discourse skills demanded by those real-world contexts. More research and likely innovation are needed to advance this.

Assessing Different Forms of Interaction

Given that signed language teaching methods emphasize interactive communication skills and that participation in group interaction in a visual language modality has some unique skills to be learned (e.g., visual turn-taking and attending), there is scope for research on how learners interact in groups at different levels and how interactive language competencies in different activity types could be assessed, as per Gan's (2010) study, described by Frost. Another interactive condition that could be explored in relation to signed language assessment is the (now common) use of computer-mediated interaction through online video applications such as Skype, Zoom, and Whatsapp for everyday personal communication and at events such as meetings, instruction, and interviews.

COMMUNICATION IS MULTIMODAL

Frost (Chapter 10.1) points out that the constructs of language proficiency that underlie assessment tools generally exclude multimodal, embodied dimensions of discourse, whereas contemporary research highlights "the dynamic and fluid ways in which individuals draw on a range of semiotic resources, including objects, images, and fragments of various languages to produce meaning in complex and multidirectional ways" (Frost, Chapter 10.1, p. xx). Since few people in society use signed languages, deaf people are typically adept in multimodal communication practices drawing on various resources including the physical context, such as pointing, gesturing, enacting, showing, mouthing words, and writing (Kusters et al., 2017). In encounters between deaf people and non-deaf people or L2 signed languages users, accommodation on both sides is the norm. We suggest that experience with these practices affects how successfully L2 signers can interact with deaf L1 signers in both real-world and simulated assessment contexts, even with gaps in target language form. Although expressive signed language assessments capture all visual elements by video-recording, this does not guarantee that multimodal features are considered, and indeed, they can create ambiguity for assessors. In our analysis of SLPI discourse, we noticed that even within the constraints of a structured conversation it was sometimes difficult to decide whether the use of multimodal behaviors by a candidate and/or interviewer, such as pointing, enactment, or mouthing, should be interpreted as deficiency of L2 form or as functional strategies that are familiar to deaf people. Theoretical interest in the intersection between signs and gestural elements, identified at the levels of lexicon, grammar, and discourse (e.g., Dudis, 2008; Ferrara & Hodge, 2018), is prompting interesting research on how this overlap affects L2 learners acquiring language in a visual modality (e.g., Emmorey et al., 2008). Findings may have implications for signed language assessment, including which skills are more cognitively demanding (or transferable) than others. The contribution of visible multimodal elements in spoken discourse could also be explicitly considered in the assessment of interactive oral language skills, and research from signed language may highlight potentially relevant features.

DEFINING COMPETENT LANGUAGE USE

In relation to the need to identify the norms that characterize typical features of signed language interactions for the purpose of decision-making about readiness for teaching deaf children, practices in English for specific-purpose testing provide a potentially useful parallel. In this area of research, speaking assessment tasks and scoring criteria have been developed, refined, and/or validated by eliciting expert 'insider" judgments of learner performances as a starting point to guide further discourse analytic studies. Elder et al. (2013) and Pill (2013), for example, showed a range of test-taker role-play performances to domain experts as a means of identifying discourse features most highly valued in the profession and of categorizing performances as meeting or being below acceptable standards. Discourse analysis of the kind undertaken by Woodward-Kron and Elder (2016), for example, then offers a means of verifying the commensurability of expert opinion and discourse evidence and of further characterizing the micro-level features of acceptable performances for assessment purposes. Rather than characterizing features of interactions between deaf signers, it might be more representative to conduct a similar type of needs analysis, beginning by examining and analyzing the discourse features of classroom interactions between competent L2 signers and deaf children and between L1 and L2 signers since everyday interactions typically involve bimodal and bilingual users. Expert signers (both L1 and L2 users) and domain experts (i.e., teachers) could then be consulted to identify the most important features of interaction to provide a baseline level of competence that is operationalizable for testing purposes and that is consistent with professional expectations and norms. This would also help in developing interviewer guidelines to limit behaviors that obscure the construct of interest in assessment situations by enabling finer-grained distinctions between those behaviors typically used to accommodate for a lack of interlocutor proficiency and cooperative communication strategies that are commonly used in interactions, regardless of perceptions of proficiency.

FUTURE DIRECTIONS

McKee et al.'s chapter addressed interviewer accommodation behaviors in SLPI discourse, a topic that has been previously examined in spoken languages but not in signed languages. As Frost discusses in her chapter, face-to-face language assessment entails co-constructed discourse, which raises questions about interpreting test scores as measures of individual ability without regard to the effects of interlocutor inputs. The NZSL study shows that interviewer accommodation behavior is a feature of interactive signed language assessment, as it is in spoken language oral assessment, and calls for further analysis of SLPI data in other signed languages.

Frost raises multimodal discourse analysis as a lens for understanding language practices in increasingly linguistically diverse and hybrid contexts (Blommaert, 2010). This also has relevance to the diversifying profile of younger deaf signed language users, many of whom have cochlear implants and bimodal-bilingual (spoken and signed) linguistic repertoires. In fact, many of this generation are L2 signers. The effects of bimodal language inputs (and delayed acquisition of signed language) on their morphosyntax, lexicon, and discourse practices are barely studied. This raises questions around the "target language" profile(s) that proficiency tests are oriented toward. Should they adhere to the notional norms of "native signers" as the reference point, or should (could?) they reflect changing usage practices of the wider signing community? Such questions are also potentially pertinent to the assessment of spoken English in diverse linguistic contexts (Blommaert, 2010). These issues are ideologically vexed but suggest the need for engagement with both theory and description in discourse analysis as a basis for designing "face-to-face" language assessment tools.

The above-mentioned issues highlight the comparatively short history of signed language assessment and the need for transfer of knowledge between signed linguistics and practices in signed language pedagogy and assessment. Our chapters have identified some challenges in refining and implementing discourse-based assessments that are common across in spoken and signed languages and signaled areas in which one field can draw insight from the other.

NOTE

1. However, a recent study reports that subjective native speaker judgments of sign frequency are reasonably congruent with distrubtional analysis of a corpus (Fenlon et al., 2014b).

REFERENCES

Bank, R., Crasborn, O., & Van Hout, R. (2016). The prominence of spoken language elements in a sign language. *Linguistics, 54*(6), 1281–1305. https://doi.org/10.1515/ling-2016-0030

Blommaert, J. (2010). *The sociolinguistics of globalization*. Cambridge University Press.

Brown, A. (2003). Interviewer variation and the co-construction of speaking proficiency. *Language Testing, 20*(1), 1–25. https://doi.org/10.1191/0265532203lt242oa

Canagarajah, S. (2018). Translingual Practice as Spatial Repertoires: Expanding the Paradigm beyond Structuralist Orientations. *Applied Linguistics, 39*(1), 31–54. https://doi.org/10.1093/applin/amx041

Dudis, P. (2008). Types of depiction in ASL. In R. M. de Quadros (Ed.), *Sign language: Spinning and unraveling the past, present and future* (pp. 159–190). Editora Arara Azul.

Elder, C., McNamara, T., Woodward-Kron, R., Manias, E., McColl, G., Webb, G., Pill, J., & O'Hagan, S. (2013). Developing and validating language proficiency standards for nonnative English speaking health professionals. *Papers in Language Testing and Assessment: An International Journal of the Association for Language Testing and Assessment of Australia and New Zealand, 2*(1), 66–70.

Emmorey, K., Borinstein, H. B., Thompson, R., & Gollan, T. H. (2008). Bimodal bilingualism. *Bilingualism, 11*(1), 43–61. https://doi.org/10.1017/S1366728907003203

Fenlon, J. (2019). Sign language linguistics and sign language teaching: Re-aligning the two fields. *Unpublished keynote address. Theoretical Issues in Sign Language Research Conference 13*. University of Hamburg.

Fenlon, J., Schembri, A., & Cormier, K. (2018). Modification of indicating verbs in British Sign Language: A corpus-based study. *Language, 94*(1), 84–118. https://doi.org/10.1353/lan.2018.0002

Fenlon, J., Schembri, A., Rentelis, R., Vinson, D., & Cormier, K. (2014). Using conversational data to determine lexical frequency in British Sign Language: The influence of text type. *Lingua, 143*, 187–202. https://doi.org/10.1016/j.lingua.2014.02.003

Ferrara, L., & Halvorsen, R. P. (2018). Depicting and describing meanings with iconic signs in Norwegian Sign Language. *Gesture, 16*(3), 371–395. https://doi.org/10.1075/gest.00001.fer

Ferrara, L., & Hodge, G. (2018). Language as Description, Indication, and Depiction. *Frontiers in Psychology, 9*, 716. https://doi.org/10.3389/fpsyg.2018.00716

Galaczi, E. D. (2008). Peer–peer interaction in a speaking test: The case of the First Certificate in English examination. *Language Assessment Quarterly, 5*(2), 89–119. https://doi.org/10.1080/15434300801934702

Gan, Z. (2010). Interaction in group oral assessment: A case study of higher- and lower-scoring students. *Language Testing, 27*(4), 585–602. https://doi.org/10.1177/0265532210364049

Johnston, T. (2012). Lexical frequency in sign languages. *Journal of Deaf Studies and Education, 17*(2), 163–193. https://doi.org/10.1093/deafed/enr036

Johnston, T. (2018). A corpus-based study of the role of headshaking in negation in Auslan (Australian Sign Language): Implications for signed language typology. *Linguistic Typology, 22*(2), 185–231. https://doi.org/10.1515/lingty-2018-0008

Johnston, T., van Roekel, J., & Schembri, A. (2016). On the conventionalization of mouth actions in Australian Sign Language. *Language and Speech, 59*(1), 3–42. https://doi.org/10.1177/0023830915569334

Kusters, A., Spotti, M., Swanwick, R., & Tapio, E. (2017). Beyond languages, beyond modalities: Transforming the study of semiotic repertoires. *International Journal of Multilingualism, 14*(3), 219–232. https://doi.org/10.1080/14790718.2017.1321651

Lazaraton, A. (1996). Interlocutor support in oral proficiency interviews: The case of CASE. *Language Testing, 13*(2), 151–72. https://doi.org/10.1177/026553229601300202

Lazaraton, A., & Davis, L. (2008). A microanalytic perspective on discourse, proficiency, and identity in paired oral assessment. *Language Assessment Quarterly, 5*(4), 313–35. https://doi.org/10.1080/15434300802457513

McNamara, T. F. (1997). "Interaction" in second language performance assessment: Whose performance? *Applied Linguistics, 18*(4), 446–485. https://doi.org/10.1093/applin/18.4.446

Nadolske, M. A., & Rosenstock, R. (2007). Occurrence of mouthings in American Sign Language: A preliminary study. In P. Perniss, R. Pfau, & M. Steinbach (Eds.), *Visible variation: Comparative studies on sign language* (pp. 35–61). Mouton de Gruyter.

Pill, J. (2013). *What doctors value in consultations and the implications for specific-purpose language testing*. PhD thesis, University of Melbourne.

Schembri, A., Jones, C., & Burnham, D. (2005). Comparing action gestures and classifier verbs of motion: Evidence from Australian Sign Language, Taiwan Sign Language, and Nonsigners' gestures without speech. *Journal of Deaf Studies and Deaf Education, 10*(3), 272–290. https://doi.org/10.1093/deafed/eni029

Taylor, L., & Wigglesworth, G. (2009). Are two heads better than one? Pair work in L2 assessment contexts. *Language Testing*, *26*(3), 325–339. https://doi.org/10.1177/0265532209104665

Woodward-Kron, R., & Elder, C. (2016). A comparative discourse study of simulated clinical roleplays in two assessment contexts: Validating a specific-purpose language test. *Language Testing*, *33*(2), 251–270. https://doi.org/10.1177/0265532215607399

Topic 11

Language Assessment Literacy in Second Language Assessment Contexts

11.1

Language Assessment Literacy in Second Spoken Language Assessment Contexts

Luke Harding, Benjamin Kremmel, and Kathrin Eberharter

Language assessment literacy (LAL) may be broadly defined as "a repertoire of competences that enable an individual to understand, evaluate and, in some cases, create language [assessments] and analyze [assessment] data" (Pill & Harding, 2013, p. 382). LAL has emerged as an important topic in the field of language assessment, with several studies addressing LAL requirements among language teachers, language assessment specialists, test score users, and other stakeholders (see Harding & Kremmel, 2016; Taylor, 2013). Among the various suggestions for taxonomies of LAL skills and abilities, there has been little discussion thus far concerning the specific *construct*-related knowledge required to conceptualize, develop, administer, and score language assessments, even though this type of construct knowledge may be crucial in newer types of assessments such as diagnostic assessment (Alderson et al., 2015) and dynamic assessment (Poehner & Lantolf, 2005). Acknowledging the importance of construct knowledge within language assessment literacy raises an important issue: as language modalities change, so must the construct-related LAL required of stakeholders. In addressing this issue, this chapter discusses, first, the broad elements of language assessment literacy that might be considered of core importance across different language modalities. It then focuses on the specific type of LAL that would need to be developed with respect to the construct of spoken language. Finally, methods for developing and improving construct knowledge related to spoken language among language assessment specialists, language teachers, and other stakeholders are discussed.

Luke Harding, Benjamin Kremmel, and Kathrin Eberharter, *Language Assessment Literacy in Second Spoken Language Assessment Contexts* In: *The Handbook of Language Assessment Across Modalities*. Edited by: Tobias Haug, Wolfgang Mann, and Ute Knoch, Oxford University Press.
DOI: 10.1093/oso/9780190885052.003.0032

APPROACHES TO DEFINING LANGUAGE ASSESSMENT LITERACY

With the rise of multiple forms of "literacies" in other disciplines, LAL emerged from a growing interest in "assessment literacy" within general education (see Brindley, 2001). At the beginning of the 1990s, assessment literacy was already being introduced as a feature of the American Federation of Teachers' (1990) standards for teachers and in the work of Stiggins (1991). Brindley (2001), however, provided one of the earliest discussions of assessment literacy specifically applied to the field of language education. He defined LAL as comprising five components: (1) knowledge about the social, educational, and political context and ethics of assessment; (2) theoretical knowledge about language proficiency as well as key concepts such as validity and reliability; (3) knowledge about how to construct and evaluate language tests; (4) knowledge about the role of assessment in the language curriculum; and (5) knowledge about how to put assessment into practice (Brindley, 2001).

As awareness of the relevance of LAL for teachers and other related stakeholder groups grew, conceptualizations of the nature and scope of LAL evolved in response (for a full discussion of the historical trajectory of LAL, see Harding & Kremmel, 2016). Early contributions to the LAL discussion proposed relatively simple models of LAL. Davies (2008), for example, outlined three core LAL elements: skills, knowledge, and principles. "Skills" related to the activities required to construct and analyze language assessments, "knowledge" to the theoretical underpinnings which informed practice, and "principles" to awareness of issues around test use and impact. This approach was reflected by Inbar-Lourie (2008), who framed these three areas as key questions to guide LAL development, maintaining that to become language assessment literate one would have to know or understand the "how-to" (skills), the "what" (knowledge), and the "why" (principles) of assessment.

Yet as discussions around LAL interrogated the notion of who needs LAL and how LAL needs may differ across stakeholder groups (see Jeong, 2013; Malone, 2013; Taylor, 2009), models of LAL necessarily became more complex. Fulcher (2012), for example, proposed an empirically based model that suggested a sequential hierarchy of competences: practical skills and knowledge as the foundation for theoretical knowledge, followed by ethical principles. Pill and Harding (2013) provided a different sort of developmental perspective, drawing on concepts from mathematics and science literacy, proposing a LAL continuum with several stages from "illiteracy" (i.e., no knowledge of "language assessment concepts and methods") to "multidimensional

LAL" (i.e., "knowledge extending beyond ordinary concepts including philosophical, historical, and social dimensions of assessment") (Pill & Harding, 2013, p. 383). This approach allowed for a clearer account of how LAL might differ across various stakeholder groups in terms of the developmental stages required.

Efforts to conceptualize LAL reached an important juncture in Taylor's (2013) discussion of papers in a special issue of *Language Testing*. Taylor synthesized key dimensions of LAL which featured in more traditional componential views of LAL with Pill and Harding's developmental stages, leading to a set of hypothetical radar charts depicting developmental needs across various LAL dimensions for different stakeholder groups (see Taylor, 2013, p. 410).

The diagrams, which effectively illustrate the relative importance and depth of different LAL dimensions required for different groups, have since provided useful templates for LAL research in various contexts (e.g., Baker & Riches, 2018; Yan et al., 2018). However, because these profiles were speculative when proposed by Taylor, Kremmel and Harding (2020) recently attempted to extend and empirically corroborate both the distinctiveness of the dimensions and the profiles themselves through a large-scale online survey ($N = 1{,}086$) that involved the views and responses of representatives of all stakeholder groups (see Kremmel & Harding, 2020, for a full discussion). Through this method, Kremmel and Harding arrived at a comprehensive, collaborative, and data-driven model of LAL that differed in some respects from Taylor's hypotheses but supported them in other ways. The model comprises nine dimensions, as displayed in Table 11.1.1. A description of the individual components is outlined in the following section.

Table 11.1.1 Nine dimensions of language assessment literacy (LAL)

Factor 1	Developing and administering language assessments
Factor 2	Assessment in language pedagogy
Factor 3	Assessment policy and local practices
Factor 4	Personal beliefs and attitudes
Factor 5	Statistical and research methods
Factor 6	Assessment principles and interpretation
Factor 7	Language structure, use and development
Factor 8	Washback and preparation
Factor 9	Scoring and rating

From Kremmel & Harding, 2020.

LANGUAGE ASSESSMENT LITERACY IN SPOKEN LANGUAGE ASSESSMENT

While Kremmel and Harding's dimensions are intended to be broad in scope, it is clear that the assessment of different language skills will require unique applications of knowledge within each of the categories. In the following sections, we explore each of the nine dimensions through the specific lens of spoken language assessment, mapping out the aspects of knowledge that might be of greatest importance in each case.

Developing and Administering Language Assessments

Assessment of spoken language raises a number of logistical challenges around the development and administration of language assessments for those with responsibilities in these areas. Development involves creating specifications and designing or selecting tasks or prompts through which to elicit spoken language. Good practice will be aided by knowledge of the relationship between aspects such as task complexity or planning time and performance (e.g., de Jong et al., 2012; Nitta & Nakatsuhara, 2014) and of guidelines around task quality. Equally as important, the development or modification of rubrics and rating scales (see Chapter 9.1) through which to judge spoken performance requires careful consideration of the fitness of a scale for its purpose (e.g., Galaczi & Khabbazbashi, 2016). Typically, administration of spoken language assessments—unless scored by computer—will require the use of human raters. This necessitates an understanding of both the features of benchmark performances which illustrate given scale points and also the range of methods through which raters may be trained most effectively to judge performances consistently. Finally, a key emerging issue among assessors of spoken language is decision-making around test-taker accommodations. Test-takers with hearing difficulties may require extra time, for example, and those with visual difficulties may require prompts in Braille (see O'Sullivan & Green, 2011).

Assessment in Pedagogy

A number of key elements of knowledge need to be considered in the dimension of LAL which concerns more pedagogical contexts (e.g., classroom assessment). First, in such contexts, assessment of spoken language is likely to be strongly connected to syllabus or curriculum goals. In such cases, it is important for those designing or using assessments (e.g., teachers) to have a clear understanding of how learning objectives (e.g., "use of a range of functional language") might be translated into assessment tasks. Another important consideration is knowledge of peer- and self-assessment, with respect to both methods and limitations. While these types of assessment can be important elements of more learner-centered assessment approaches (see Alderson et al., 2015), they must be used with full awareness of the potential for cognitive biases which may reduce their validity for more high-stakes decisions (Bejar, 2012).

Assessment Policy and Local Practices

In Kremmel and Harding (2020), this dimension of LAL is formed of considerations such as knowledge of "how to determine if a language assessment aligns with a local educational system" and "the assessment traditions in your local context." In interpreting this dimension from the perspective of spoken language assessment, it becomes clear that speaking assessments will often need to be designed with local concerns in mind. One example is the question of models and norms in grammatical usage; consideration must be given to local norms of spoken grammar in the design of rating scales and in rater training. At the same time, pedagogical traditions in specific local contexts might mean that "standard" British or American varieties are conferred with more "prestige", and these deeply embedded language ideologies will need to be addressed critically. Knowledge of local practices and traditions of this kind is an integral element of LAL for those who are responsible for designing speaking assessments in specific contexts, as well as for those who seek to implement international speaking assessments in environments where local practices exist.

Personal Beliefs and Attitudes

Knowledge of one's own personal beliefs and attitudes is a key component of reflective LAL practice. In the context of spoken language assessment, this would include considering one's own stance toward the usefulness of speaking assessment, the fairness and ethics of assessment, and how these might intersect with assessment practice.

Statistical and Research Methods

As with other types of assessment, LAL in spoken language assessment requires some research training and statistical skills in order to evaluate the quality and utility of assessments based on data. This may entail, as a minimum, an understanding of methods for calculating reliability (inter- and intrarater) and how different elements of the construct may be accorded different weightings in a total score depending on the purpose of the assessment. Beyond these more basic statistics, methods for exploring rater fit and consistency through methods such as many-facet Rasch measurement (MFRM) and generalizability (G) theory will be necessary for more sophisticated analyses. However, researching speaking—particularly analyzing the characteristics of spoken language performance—requires a wide-ranging set of skills which are not necessarily considered part of a standard training in language assessment. These might involve, for example, the use of corpus tools to analyze existing corpora of spoken language to determine the nature of spoken communication in a given domain. Alternatively, tools of speech science such as Praat (Boersma & Weenink, 2020) may be necessary for investigating the acoustic-phonetic characteristics of spoken performance data or in measuring a range of temporal fluency measures such as speech rate, mean length of run, and number of pauses per minute. A qualitative approach to investigating speaking examinations is *conversation analysis,* which may provide in-depth understanding of the test construct and the actual language use in interactive assessment tasks.

Assessment Principles and Interpretation

To a large extent, the key principles of language assessment—validity, reliability, fairness, justice—cut across multiple skill domains and filter down into many of the other dimensions discussed in this chapter. Ethical considerations are particularly important with respect to the assessment of spoken language because elements of speaking such as pronunciation have deeper connections with questions of identity and language ideologies (see Harding, 2013). Score interpretation, too, may be somewhat skill-dependent in that a score user will need to have some understanding of construct matters—the criteria on which candidates are judged—to come to a determination about how to use a score. For example, in the case of university admission, measures of language proficiency may take on a significant role. However, case studies such as O'Loughlin's (2011) have found that the administrative staff involved in decision-making may benefit from a deeper understanding of how proficiency tests are produced and scored and what inferences can be drawn from an applicant's language proficiency on the basis of that score.

Language Structure, Use, and Development

Arguably, the most skill-dependent element of LAL is the dimension which focuses on language. Teachers, assessment developers, and others who construct or use language assessments require a deep knowledge of the spoken language construct, which includes elements such as spoken grammar, vocabulary, pronunciation, fluency, discourse management, functional competence, pragmatics, and interactional competence. The latter is currently a "hot topic" in speaking assessment (see Plough et al., 2018, or Nakatsuhara et al., 2016) as the field grapples with the legacy of communicative competence and its applicability (and limits) for the assessment of speaking. Knowledge of these subcomponents of an overall speaking ability entails an understanding of the components of each, how these subcomponents develop, and how they vary across speech communities and communicative settings. While many professionals involved in language assessment may hold an (applied) linguistics background that provides a firm grounding for understanding the nature of spoken language, this may not be taken for granted. Relatedly, *language* has been an overlooked feature in many previous models of LAL competence (see Kremmel et al., 2017). Knowledge about language—theories of acquisition, variation, and change—is a key area where our field must continue to foster and develop LAL.

Washback and Preparation

Good practice in language assessment—particularly among teaching professionals—also involves a clear understanding of the influence of speaking assessment on teaching and learning and good (ethical) preparation practices. Often, LAL in this dimension will require both an understanding of the macro systems which connect teaching and learning with assessment and also a deep knowledge of the test format and construct itself. As Wall and Horák (2011) documented over the course of several years, changes to a language assessment suite, like the introduction of a speaking section to the TOEFL, may have a substantial impact on the amount of classroom time dedicated to developing speaking skills as well as the methods employed by the teachers.

Scoring and Rating

The final dimension is also an integral aspect of LAL for those involved in the assessment of spoken language. For human-rated speaking assessments, judging speaking (see Chapter 9.1) involves a wide range of issues which must be addressed through rater training. However, prior to rater training, it is important to be aware of the nature of different influences on rating processes. In terms of the cognitive processes that take place, the assessment of language is shaped by the features of the learner performance that raters notice and the features of the assessment scale or rubrics that raters use for their decision-making (i.e., the mental representations of the performance and the scale (Bejar, 2012). Not surprisingly, rater cognition research has explored all kinds of ways in which the perception of performances and use of rating scales may vary between raters. For example, based on their own L2 backgrounds, experience, or native language, raters may vary considerably in how they perceive learner accents (Huang et al., 2016) or weigh certain features described in the scale (Zhang & Elder, 2011). The design of the rating scale has also been found to influence rater behavior. The scale type—holistic or analytic—plays a fundamental role in shaping the raters' understanding of the test construct (Li & He, 2015) and rater decision-making processes (Barkaoui, 2010), while the layout of the rating scale may lead human raters to ascribe certain criteria more importance than others (Winke & Lim, 2015). While rater training is certainly helpful in guiding raters, it is important to acknowledge that including human raters in the assessment process will always introduce an element of variability that—particularly in the context of high-stakes testing—needs to be met by appropriate strategies (e.g., procedures for double-rating or score adjustment) (McNamara, 1996).

An emerging issue is the need for greater assessment literacy around automated scoring of speech, which includes an understanding of how algorithms work, what features of speech performance they measure (and which they do not), and how the validity of such measures is established and evaluated. As machine-scoring systems become more common—with all the attendant advantages and limitations—it is vital that score users develop knowledge about the mechanisms by which a score is produced.

FUTURE DIRECTIONS

It is clear that different stakeholder groups will have different priorities across each dimension of LAL, and future research should investigate in more detail what the specific needs are in different geographical or professional contexts. Alongside this, research will need to monitor the actual impact of increased LAL with regard to bringing about more informed discussions about language assessment-related matters, fair and just use of language assessment rooted in best practice, and beneficial consequences for individuals and communities in general as they pertain to language learning, language use, and communication.

Two issues that also emerge from this volume will deserve particular ongoing attention. First, the role of technology (see Chapters 12.1–12.3) and what influence the advances and opportunities in this area will have on language use, language learning, and, in particular, language assessment practice, theory, and validation. The second is what role the specific language modalities play in determining language assessment literacy requirements. We have endeavored to address this question in the current chapter, but further research will be required to map out LAL needs across different skill areas.

REFERENCES

Alderson, J. C., Brunfaut, T., & Harding, L. (2015). Towards a theory of diagnosis in second and foreign language assessment: Insights from professional practice across diverse fields. *Applied Linguistics*, *36*(2), 236–260. https://doi.org/10.1093/applin/amt046

American Federation of Teachers, National Council on Measurement in Education, and National Education Association. (1990). Standards for teacher competence in educational assessment of students. *Educational Measurement*, *9*(4), 30–32. https://doi.org/10.1111/j.1745-3992.1990.tb00391.x

Baker, B. A., & Riches, C. (2018). The development of EFL examinations in Haiti: Collaboration and language assessment literacy development. *Language Testing*, *35*(4), 557–581. https://doi.org/10.1177/0265532217716732

Barkaoui, K. (2010). Variability in ESL essay rating processes: The role of the rating scale and rater experience. *Language Assessment Quarterly*, *7*(1), 54–74. https://doi.org/10.1080/15434300903464418

Bejar, I. I. (2012). Rater cognition: Implications for validity. *Educational Measurement Issues and Practice*, *31*(3), 2–9. https://doi.org/10.1111/j.1745-3992.2012.00238.x

Boersma, P., & Weenink, D. (2020). Praat: Doing phonetics by computer [Computer program]. Version 6.1.20beta. http://www.praat.org/

Brindley, G. (2001). Language assessment and professional development. In C. Elder, A. Brown, K. Hill, N. Iwashita, T. Lumley, T. McNamara, & K. O'Loughlin (Eds.), *Experimenting with uncertainty: Essays in honour of Alan Davies* (pp. 126–136). Cambridge University Press.

De Jong, N., Steinel, M., Florijn, A. F., Schoonen, R., & Hulstijn, J. H. (2012). The effect of task complexity on functional adequacy, fluency and lexical diversity in speaking performances of native and non-native speakers. In A. Housen, F. Kuiken, & I. Vedder (Eds.), *Dimensions of L2 performance and proficiency: Complexity, accuracy and fluency in SLA* (pp. 121–142). John Benjamins.

Davies, A. (2008). Textbook trends in teaching language testing. *Language Testing*, *25*(3), 327–347. https://doi.org/10.1177/0265532208090156

Fulcher, G. (2012). Assessment literacy for the language classroom. *Language Assessment Quarterly*, *9*(2), 113–132. https://doi.org/10.1080/15434303.2011.642041

Galaczi, E., & Khabbazbashi, N. (2016). Rating scale development: A multistage exploratory sequential design. In A. J. Moeller, J. Creswell, & N. Saville (Eds.), *Second language assessment and mixed methods research* (pp. 208–222). Cambridge University Press.

Harding, L. (2013). Pronunciation assessment. In C. A. Chapelle (Ed.), *The encyclopedia of applied linguistics*. Wiley-Blackwell. https://doi.org/10.1002/9781405198431.wbeal0966

Harding, L., & Kremmel, B. (2016). Teacher assessment literacy and professional development. In D. Tsagari & J. Banerjee (Eds.), *Handbook of second language assessment* (pp. 413–428). De Gruyter/Mouton.

Huang, B., Alegre, A., & Eisenberg, A. (2016). A cross-linguistic investigation of the effect of raters' accent familiarity on speaking assessment. *Language Assessment Quarterly*, *13*(1), 25–41. https://doi.org/10.1080/15434303.2015.1134540

Inbar-Lourie, O. (2008). Constructing a language assessment knowledge base: A focus on language assessment courses. *Language Testing*, *25*(3), 385–402. https://doi.org/10.1177/0265532208090158

Jeong, H. (2013). Defining assessment literacy: Is it different for language testers and non-language testers? *Language Testing*, *30*(3), 345–362. https://doi.org/10.1177/0265532213480334

Kremmel, B., Eberharter, K., & Harding, L. (2017). *Putting language into language assessment literacy*. Paper presented at LTRC 2017 Bogota.

Kremmel, B., & Harding, L. (2020). Towards a comprehensive, empirical model of language assessment literacy across stakeholder groups: Developing the language assessment literacy survey. *Language Assessment Quarterly*, *17*(1), 100–120. https://doi.org/10.1080/15434303.2019.1674855

Li, H., & He, L. (2015). A comparison of EFL raters' essay-rating processes across two types of rating scales. *Language Assessment Quarterly*, *12*(2), 178–212. https://doi.org/10.1080/15434303.2015.1011738

Malone, M. E. (2013). The essentials of assessment literacy: Contrasts between testers and users. *Language Testing*, *30*(3), 329–344. https://doi.org/10.1177/0265532213480129

McNamara, T. F. (1996). *Measuring second language performance*. Addison Wesley Longman.

Nakatsuhara, F., May, L., Lam, D., & Galaczi, E. (2016). *Learning oriented feedback in the development and assessment of interactional competence. Cambridge Research Notes*, Issue 70.

Nitta, R., & Nakatsuhara, F. (2014). A multifaceted approach to investigating pre-task planning effects on paired oral test performance. *Language Testing*, *31*(2), 147–175. https://doi.org/10.1177/0265532213514401

O'Loughlin, K. (2011). The interpretation and use of proficiency test scores in university selection: How valid and ethical are they? *Language Assessment Quarterly*, *8*(2), 146–160. https://doi.org/10.1080/15434303.2011.564698

O'Sullivan, B., & Green, A. (2011). Test taker characteristics. In L. Taylor (Ed.), *Examining speaking: Research and practice in assessing second language speaking* (pp. 36–64). Cambridge University Press.

Pill, J., & Harding, L. (2013). Defining the language assessment literacy gap: Evidence from a parliamentary inquiry. *Language Testing*, *30*(3), 381–402. https://doi.org/10.1177/0265532213480337

Plough, I., Banerjee, J., Iwashita, N. (2018). Special issue on interactional competence. *Language Testing*, *35*(3).

Poehner, M. E., & Lantolf, J. P. (2005). Dynamic assessment in the language classroom. *Language Teaching Research*, *9*(3), 233–265. https://doi.org/10.1191/1362168805lr166oa

Stiggins, R. J. (1991). Assessment literacy. *Phi Delta Kappa*, *72*(7), 534–539.

Taylor, L. (2009). Developing assessment literacy. *Annual Review of Applied Linguistics*, *29*, 21–36. https://doi.org/10.1017/S0267190509090035

Taylor, L. (2013). Communicating the theory, practice and principles of language testing to test stakeholders: Some reflections. *Language Testing*, *30*(3), 403–412. https://doi.org/10.1177/0265532213480338

Wall, D., & Horák, T. (2011). *The impact of changes in the TOEFL® exam on teaching in a sample of countries in Europe: Phase 3, The role of the coursebook; Phase 4, Describing change*. Research Report. TOEFL iBT.

Winke, P., & Lim, H. (2015). ESL essay raters' cognitive processes in applying the Jacobs et al. rubric: An eye-movement study. *Assessing Writing*, *25*, 38–54. https://doi.org/10.1016/j.asw.2015.05.002

Yan, X., Zhang, C., & Fan, J. J. (2018). "Assessment knowledge is important, but . . . ": How contextual and experiential factors mediate assessment practice and training needs of language teachers. *System*, *74*, 158–168. https://doi.org/10.1016/j.system.2018.03.003

Zhang, Y., & Elder, C. (2011). Judgments of oral proficiency by non-native and native English speaking teacher raters: Competing or complementary constructs? *Language Testing*, *28*(1), 31–50. https://doi.org/10.1177/0265532209360671

11.2

Language Assessment Literacy in Second Signed Language Assessment Contexts

Eveline Boers-Visker and Annemiek Hammer

When compared to spoken language teaching, the practice of teaching signed languages as a subject is a relatively young domain of expertise. As a result, teachers of signed languages either adopt practices that have been proved effective for spoken language, or they rely on their intuition and experience (Quinto-Pozos, 2011). This also holds true for signed language assessment. Signed language assessment literacy ((S)LAL; i.e., knowledge and skills pertaining to construction and evaluation of signed language assessment) is a new area in signed language teaching and assessment but already exists in several teaching contexts. For instance, the Sign Language Proficiency Interview (SLPI; see Chapter 9.2) is implemented in different curricula internationally, and Haug et al. (2016) have formulated guidelines for signed language test development, evaluation, and use. Nevertheless, a general discussion on (S)LAL requirements for sign language teachers has not occurred. This chapter is a first attempt to address the issue raised in Chapter 11.1: How does modality change construct-related LAL required of sign language teachers?

We propose an (S)LAL-framework for classroom teachers based on experiences of teachers and teacher educators currently working in the field. We label this framework the Sign Language ASSessment–Design Matrix, or SLASS-DM. We have taken the five quality criteria for language assessment of Bachman and Palmer (1996) and related these to the construction of signed language assessments procedures. SLASS-DM is an overview of considerations, related to the Bachman and Palmer criteria, that teachers and/or developers can take into account when they construct and develop assessments, and rate and interpret scores on these assessments. In the remainder of this chapter, we explain the criteria of Bachman and Palmer and present our SLASS-DM.

Eveline Boers-Visker and Annemiek Hammer, *Language Assessment Literacy in Second Signed Language Assessment Contexts* In: *The Handbook of Language Assessment Across Modalities.* Edited by: Tobias Haug, Wolfgang Mann, and Ute Knoch, Oxford University Press. © Oxford University Press 2022. DOI: 10.1093/oso/9780190885052.003.0033

SETTING OUT QUALITY CRITERIA FOR SIGNED LANGUAGE ASSESSMENT LITERACY

(S)LAL involves knowledge about fundamental basic concepts such as validity and reliability and an awareness about the cautions that arise when developing assessments and conducting and interpreting scores on (signed) language assessments. Bachman and Palmer (1996, 2010) provided a practical guide for developing and using language assessments. They proposed five complementary test qualities. Language teachers need to find an appropriate balance among these qualities to construct a test that is fit for its purpose. These qualities relate to Brindley's (2001) LAL components, as outlined in Chapter 11.1, since both publications work from a similar perspective. Both agree that language assessment aims at measuring the individual's language ability, but language ability is affected by assessment design (see Bachman, 2007). As such, professional development in assessment starts off with knowledge on how to construct an assessment.

Reliability refers to the consistency of scores on an assessment despite the varied occasions in which the assessment is administered. A student's assessment result should be almost equal to assessment results obtained in an assessment targeting similar characteristics (e.g., student outcomes on multiple versions of a lexical assessment at a particular level should be comparable). *Validity* refers to the appropriateness of the judgment on the student's progress based on assessment outcomes. This justification is warranted by the evidence-based benchmarks in language proficiency. The assessment has to be in accordance with the student's level, and the type of assessment has to fit the type of knowledge or skill that is to be assessed. *Authenticity* has to do with the degree of correspondence between the characteristics of a given assessment and features of a situation outside the assessment itself. Outcomes of assessments should be generalized to some degree to situations in real life. *Interactiveness* is defined as the extent and type of student characteristics involved in accomplishing the assessment (e.g., metacognitive strategies, strategic competence, or topical knowledge). *Impact* relates to the impact the assessment has on students, but also on society and education. An important aspect of impact is *washback*, which refers to the effect of testing on teaching and learning; this is also known as the "teaching to the test" effect in education. *Practicality* is the correlation between the resources needed to construct and use an assessment and the resources available to construct and use the assessment.

On all criteria, except for interactiveness, we believe that considerations arise that are specific to signed language assessment procedures. In our view, student characteristics do not play out differently in students involved in spoken or signed language assessment procedures. However, anecdotal evidence from second language (L2) learners at our institute indicate high levels of anxiety prior to assessment (see also Sheridan, 2018). It is shown that anxiety negatively influences language competence as assessed by observers (McIntyre et al., 1997). Further research is needed to address this.

There is one fundamental issue that affects all criteria (except for interactiveness). In Chapter 11.1, it is stressed that deep knowledge of the language to be assessed is fundamental to teachers' LAL competence. However, the body of research into signed languages is far less when compared to spoken language. What complicates matters even further is the paucity in literature regarding signed language acquisition in adult learners. If this literature would be available, it could be used to set out milestones in L2 development that are to be measured with language assessments. Subsequently, outcomes on assessments could inform the student and the language teacher to what extent the student is actually developing their language proficiency. However, because of the small knowledge base of signed language development in L2 learners, language learning outcomes are not based on empirical data, but on language teacher perceptions (see, e.g., the use of the Common European Framework of Reference for Languages [CEFR] in signed language assessment, Chapter 9.2) (Figueras, 2012; Hulstijn, 2007).

SLASS-DESIGN MATRIX

Our SLASS-DM model is presented in Table 11.2.1. Horizontally, the two columns refer to different linguistic competencies: production and understanding. Vertically, each row represents a quality criterion as provided by Bachman and Palmer (1996, 2010) followed by aspects that must be taken into account when assessing signed language production and understanding.

Reliability

In spoken language tests, one can use audio recordings, which enables the test-taker to be (to some extent) anonymous. A signer, however, must be filmed (or rated while taking the test). This could potentially lead to *examiner bias:* raters could be influenced by the physical appearance of the student. In addition, the judgment of examiners might be influenced by perceptions of students' production skills experienced in classroom settings, since the field is dealing with a very small group of practitioners and students. In most practices the rater is the student's teacher as well.

Due to the scant research regarding signed language acquisition, rubrics stating what students need to show at a particular point in time are lacking. Moreover, designing clear rubrics is difficult because the visual-manual modality allows multiple ways to express

Table 11.2.1 Sign Language ASSessment–Design Matrix (SLASS-DM). An overview of issues that affect the quality of signed language assessment

	Signed language production	Signed language understanding
Reliability	Risk of examiner bias Difficult to achieve good agreement between examiners/ lack of rubrics Multiple ways of expressing similar meanings in signed language	Language variation affects understanding considerably Student response in glosses requires clear guidelines on gloss conventions Difficult to have comparable texts for assessment
Validity	Lack of clear norms based on evidence from L1 and L2-learners of signed language Interference of gestural behavior: risk of overestimating skills Risk of giving away grammatical information when using symbols (e.g., arrows to denote movement of action) Multiple ways of expressing similar meanings	Lack of clear norms based on evidence from L1 and L2 learners of signed language Risk of overestimating skills if amount of iconic signs and grammatical features is relatively high Risk of overestimating skills if amount of mouthings is high Risk of overdependency on memory skills (impossibility to watch and write simultaneously) Signed language from screen (2D) is different as compared to live (3D)
Authenticity	Risk of overattention to signed stories (easy to elicit by using cartoon or picture story)	Lack of authentic materials in general Lack of authentic materials that cover teaching content Lack of authentic materials that suit low language levels
Impact	No educational standard defined on level of proficiency at graduate level (national and international) Stakeholders vary greatly in level of signed language they expect from professionals (relatively small group of native-signers) External validity difficult to reach Risk of “washback” or teaching to the test	
Practicality	Time-consuming: recording time equals rating time (as opposed to scanning written text) Time-consuming, thus expensive	Time-consuming: recordings must be edited Making small adjustments to existing material difficult (as opposed to written texts) Time-consuming, thus expensive

similar meanings. For instance, in signed language narratives, the same event can be expressed from different perspectives (e.g., a description of a scene from an observer perspective or from the perspective of characters; i.e., *constructed action*). As a consequence, linguistic variation occurs and student' narratives are difficult to compare. In a similar vein, existing signed texts that are used for receptive assessments are hardly comparable with respect to linguistic level and variation, and there is a lack of empirical data to inform test developers how to determine aspects of text difficulty. This might have serious consequences for understanding the text and thus reliability in test outcomes.

Last, the type of response required by the student needs to be clear and transparent. If a student is asked, for example, to use glosses (i.e., the translation of a sign using the written form of the local spoken language) in a receptive vocabulary test, it should be clear for both students and raters (a) what are the conventions (e.g., is it compulsory to use small capitals, is a misspelled gloss accepted as long as the meaning of the sign is covered, etc.?) and (b) what are acceptable alternatives (i.e., a clear scoring guide with different possible glosses in case of signed language homonyms).

Validity

The validity of signed language assessment is increasingly improving because knowledge on signed language development and evaluation is evolving. Yet the justification of a particular level of language production or understanding is sometimes weak because there is not always sufficient evidence of what a student needs to show or how well at a particular time in his development. To put it in other words, it is difficult to define assessment outcomes based on the scarce data on signed language acquisition in adult learners. This is closely related to the lack of rubrics already pointed out in the section on reliability.

Signed languages have a certain amount of iconic signs (e.g., DRINK) or ways of expressing relations using space (e.g., giving something to an imaginary third person) that overlap with gestures produced by sign-naïve individuals (Ortega et al., 2017). As such, the use of these gestures/signs might not represent the students' linguistic knowledge (lexical or grammatical) of signed language. Similarly, some sign-naïve gesturers produce constructions that resemble classifier constructions to denote the movement or position of referents (Janke & Marshall, 2017; Schembri et al., 2005). This is illustrated in Figure 11.2.1A and 11.2.1B: the sign-naïve girl in Figure 11.2.1A uses a co-speech gesture with a flat handshape to indicate the movement of a rollercoaster-cart. This handshape resembles the handshape used in some signed languages to express the movement of vehicles, including rollercoaster-carts. The novel signer in Figure 11.2.1B, filmed during the first day of her education, gestures "eating an apple" and "taking a selfie," both

A B

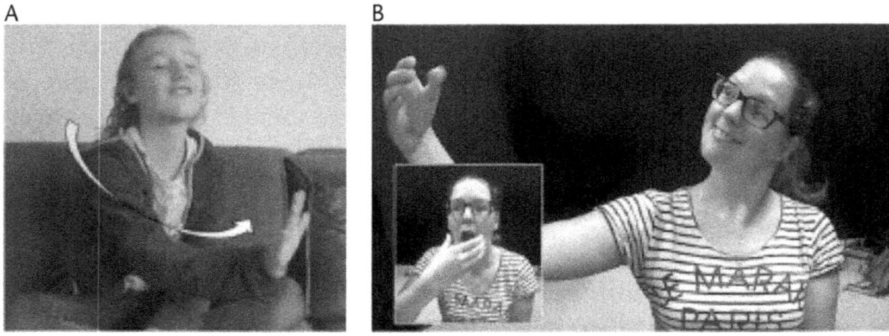

Figure 11.2.1 A,B: Examples of gestural behavior resembling signed language structures.
© Boers-Visker (2016, 2020).

resembling the signs used to express these actions. Thus, especially for lower-level leaners, one should be careful to not overrate student L2 development.

The way of presenting assessment stimuli might affect assessment outcomes (Hong et al., 2009). Research has shown that the way directional verbs are elicited affects the way students produce congruence between subject and objects (Boers-Visker & Pfau, 2020). Offering sentences in written form (i.e., as the first language [L1]) as a prompt elicited different responses as compared to video or pictures. Written sentences do not leave room for multiple interpretations, but the students' productions can be influenced by their L1. Video or pictures, on the other hand, are often prone to multiple interpretations, often leading to language productions that do not meet the desired target construction. In case of pictures aimed to elicit target signs that have gestural counterparts (e.g., THROW, GIVE), students' responses can be overestimated, as students can simply imitate the actions depicted. Figure 11.2.2 depicts a novel signer signing "give a present." It is difficult to determine whether the student signs the construction or simply is imitating the action depicted.

Moreover, some concepts are difficult to elicit using pictures (e.g., verbs like ASK, ANSWER, HELP).

As for assessment of receptive skills, the (amount of) overlap between signs and gestures could be used to guess the meanings of signs (see Ortega et al., 2017). Signs such as EAT, DRINK, CAR, BALL, or WRITE are highly iconic and have gestural counterparts that make it relatively easy to guess the meaning even if the learner did not acquire the sign yet. A similar situation holds for the mouthings that accompany signs in some signed languages, which enables the test-taker to guess the meaning of an unknown sign. This, and the fact that signed languages lack a written form, can affect validity. The latter forces assessment

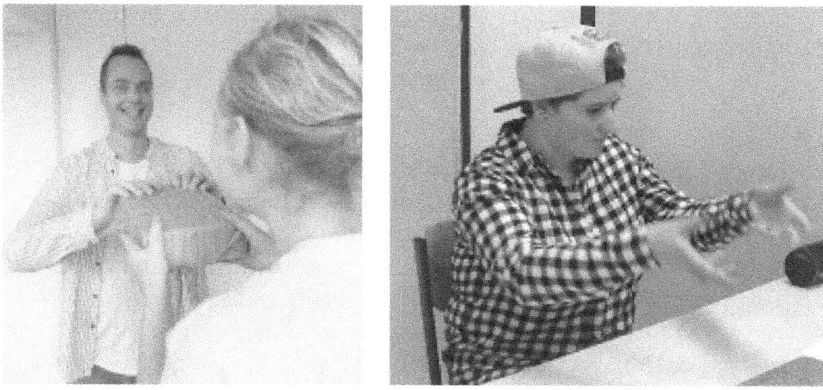

Figure 11.2.2 Example of signed/gestured construction (left: prompt; right: novel signer).
© Boers-Visker (2016, 2020).

developers to seek for solutions: one might use the local (written) spoken language (e.g., to write down answers after the presentation of a sign) or ask the student to sign their response (and risk missing information because the learner did *understand*, but was not able to *sign* the answer; i.e., the test measures receptive and productive skills). A third factor that can affect validity is overreliance on memory skills in case the video presentation is too long. Last, the two-dimensional nature of videos might cause problems for beginning learners (i.e., learners who are acquiring CEFR level A1 or A2).

Authenticity

The ultimate aim of assessing one's language ability is to determine whether the student can use the language in real communicative situations. As such, an assessment should be as authentic as possible. In reality, this is not always (or usually not) possible. Assessment developers should be aware of the limitations. It is tempting to use highly visual cartoons or picture stories to elicit signed language production. These are indeed very useful to elicit classifiers and constructed action, but might not elicit the student's ability to produce spontaneous language when encountering a deaf person (Boers-Visker, 2020). In addition, using cartoons or picture stories might result in a variety of (acceptable) responses, which might influence reliability. As for receptive skills, one can either use existing (thus authentic) materials or one can create materials. Authentic materials are not always available for signed languages, and, if they are, they are usually not created for the purpose of an assessment (e.g., signing rate is too high, grammatical/lexical level is too high). As a result, these materials do not always cover the teaching content and do not align with the level of beginning L2 learners due to high signing rate.

Impact

Although for some countries there are standards that provide level descriptions (e.g., CEFR levels; British Sign Language Qualification levels 1–6; K–12 American Sign Language Content Standards), a lot of countries lack such level descriptions. In addition, the expected language proficiency levels of (future) professionals greatly differs between stakeholders. For instance, while stakeholders involved in internships in our bachelor program for sign language teachers explicitly demand high proficiency levels (CEFR B2 level) of students upon application, the stakeholders involved in our bachelor program for signed language interpreter do not set level B2 at an internship threshold; interpreting skills and communication with the clients are much more at the foreground as compared to linguistic skills. The adjustment of the CEFR to include signed languages (Leeson et al., 2016) is a great contribution that enables curriculum and test developers to define levels. Yet much work has to be carried out to define the exact features that characterize the holistic descriptors, such as "shows a relatively high degree of grammatical control" (level B2; Council of Europe, 2001, p. 28). Caution is warranted not to focus on levels (e.g., A1 or B2) only, because language development is gradual rather than incremental. Although assessments focus on establishing a student's proficiency level, teaching should be more directed toward the small steps between levels. The washback effect that might occur is that teachers focus on how to get students from one level to the next as quickly as possible, taking steps that are not congruent with the actual learning process.

Practicality

The lack of a written form for signed languages brings some practical challenges (Boyes Braem, 2012). Signed languages cannot be written down, so assessing production always involves recording signed language production. Rating recorded signed language production takes at least as much time as the length of the actual recording. This contrasts with assessing written language, as teachers can quickly scan (and easily re-read) these texts. As for receptive tests, recording and editing is time-consuming, and making small adjustments is time-consuming as well (as often a new recording has to be made and edited). This makes signed language assessments relatively expensive to develop and score.

HOW TO USE THE SLASS-DESIGN MATRIX

The primary reason to set up the SLASS-DM is to offer a comprehensive overview of the issues that are specific to the quality of signed language assessments. The overview is helpful for young teachers to become more literate on testing, and it provides a state of the art on quality issues in signed language assessment. Hopefully, experienced teachers can relate their issues with respect to assessments to the issues mentioned in the SLASS-DM. In due time, we hope that good practices can be (internationally) shared that focus on the pitfalls outlined in the matrix and, as such, move signed language assessment literacy forward.

Sign language teachers can use the SLASS-DM to become aware of the specifics of signed language assessment. This awareness is a first step to address the topic of assessment literacy in teams of sign language teachers working in bachelor and master degree programs, but also in curricula for prospective sign language teachers. We believe that cooperation is key to reaching good quality in assessment: formulating learning objectives is a collective effort among teachers, researchers, and stakeholders; it takes too much time to develop assessment materials when done individually; and evaluation of assessment results can be too complex for individual teachers. The SLASS-DM can be used by teams of teachers to reflect on their assessments and pinpoint where they can improve.

FUTURE DIRECTIONS

Literacy in signed language assessment is in its earliest stages. At our institute, formal training on specific assessments (see Chapter 9.2) is offered to our teachers. This training is focused on increasing reliability when judging (productive) signed language levels of students. Moreover, teachers learn general principles of assessments in a training offered at our University of Applied Sciences. All in all, teachers have received more formal training on assessment over the past years.

Yet, in presenting the SLASS-DM, we want to take signed language assessment literacy to the next level. The difference in modality brings along issues in signed language assessment that every practitioner should be aware of. One issue that is placed in the foreground in this chapter is the risk of weak validity of signed language assessments (see Chapter 8.2) when teachers and developers define milestones that lack a solid evidence base. Students use assessment outcomes to monitor their development. If outcomes do not match with the actual language developmental path, then development might be hampered (i.e., negative impact of assessment). To reach good validity, research is needed to support learning objectives. This is beyond the process of choosing or developing an assessment, administering and scoring the assessment, and evaluating the outcomes (i.e., cycle of assessment). As such, to reach the next level, teachers are challenged to reflect on the issues raised in the SLASS-DM and researchers are challenged to assist in addressing these issues together with teachers. The SLASS-DM provides future avenues to increase our body of knowledge on signed language assessment literacy.

REFERENCES

Bachman, L. (2007). What is the construct? The dialectic of abilities and contexts in defining constructs in language assessment. Language Testing Reconsidered. https://books.openedition.org/uop/1563

Bachman, L., & Palmer, A. (1996). *Language testing in practice*. Oxford University Press.

Bachman, L., & Palmer, A. (2010). *Language assessment in practice*. Oxford Applied Linguistics.

Boers-Visker, E. (2020). Learning to use space: A study into the SL2 acquisition process of adult learners of Sign Language of the Netherlands (Doctoral Dissertation). University of Amsterdam.

Boers-Visker, E., & Pfau, R. (2020). Space oddities: The acquisition of agreement verbs by L2 learners of Sign Language of the Netherlands. *Modern Language Journal, 104*(4), 757–780. doi:10.1111/modl.12676

Boyes Braem, P. (2012). Evolving methods for written representations of signed languages of the deaf. In A. Ender, A. Leemann, & B. Waelchli (Eds.), *Methods in contemporary linguistics* (pp. 411–438). De Gruyter Mouton.

Brindley, G. (2001). Language assessment and professional development. In C. Elder, A. Brown, K. Hill, N. Iwashita, T. Lumley, T. McNamara, & K. O'Loughlin (Eds.), *Experimenting with uncertainty: Essays in honour of Alan Davies* (pp. 126–136). Cambridge University Press.

Council of Europe. (2001). The Common European Framework of Reference for Languages: Learning, Teaching, Assessment. https://www.coe.int/en/web/common-european-framework-reference-languages

Figueras, N. (2012). The impact of the CEFR. *ELT Journal, 66*(4), 477–485. https://doi.org/10.1093/elt/ccs037

Haug, T., Mann, W., Boers-Visker, E., Contreras, J., Enns, C., Herman, R., & Rowley, K. (2016, updated 2018). *Guidelines for sign language test development, evaluation, and use.* Unpublished document, retrieved from http://www.signlang-assessment.info

Hong, S., Hanke, T., König, S., Konrad, R., Langer, G., & Rathmann, C. (2009, July). *Elicitation materials and their use in sign language linguistics.* Poster presented at the Workshop "Sign Language Corpora: Linguistic Issues," London.

Hulstijn, J. H. (2007). The shaky ground beneath the CEFR: Quantitative and qualitative dimensions of language proficiency. *Modern Language Journal, 91*(4), 663–667. https://doi.org/10.1111/j.1540-4781.2007.00627_5.x

Janke, V., & Marshall, C. R. (2017). Using the hands to represent objects in space: Gesture as a substrate for signed language acquisition. *Frontiers in Psychology, 8*, 2007. https://doi.org/10.3389/fpsyg.2017.02007

Kemp, M. (1998a). Why is learning American Sign Language a challenge? *American Annals of the Deaf, 143*, 255–259.

Leeson, L., Bogaerde, B. van den, Rathmann, C., & Haug, T. (2016). *Sign languages and the Common European Framework of Reference for Languages: Common reference level descriptors*. European Centre of Modern Languages.

Miller, C., Hooper, S., Rose, S., & Montalto-Rook, M. (2001). Transforming e-assessment in American Sign Language: Pedagogical and technological enhancements in online language learning and performance assessment. *Learning, Media and Technology, 33* (3), 155–168.

Ortega, G., Schiefner, A., & Özyürek, A. (2017). Speakers' gestures predict the meaning and perception of iconicity in signs. In G. Gunzelmann, A. Howe, & T. Tenbrink (Eds.), *Proceedings of the 39th Annual Conference of the Cognitive Science Society (CogSci 2017)* (pp. 889–894). Cognitive Science Society.

Quinto-Pozos, D. (2011). Teaching American Sign Language to hearing adult learners. *Annual Review of Applied Linguistics, 31*, 137–158. https://doi.org/10.1017/S0267190511000195

Sheridan, S. (2018). *Composing the L2-M2 self: A grounded theory study on the concerns of adult Irish Sign Language learners*. PhD thesis, Trinity University, San Antonio, Texas. http://www.tara.tcd.ie/handle/2262/86194

Schembri, A., Jones, C., & Burnham, D. (2005). Comparing action gestures and classifier verbs of motion: Evidence from Australian Sign Language, Taiwan Sign Language, and nonsigners' gestures without speech. *Journal of Deaf Studies and Deaf Education, 10*(3), 272–290. https://doi.org/10.1093/deafed/eni029

11.3

Discussion of Issues Related to Language Assessment Literacy in Second Signed and Spoken Languages

Eveline Boers-Visker, Kathrin Eberharter, Annemiek Hammer, Luke Harding, and Benjamin Kremmel

FROM USER-GENERATED GUIDELINES FOR LANGUAGE ASSESSMENT TO LAL-NEEDS: SPOKEN LANGUAGE ASSESSMENT LEARNING FROM SIGNED LANGUAGE ASSESSMENT

It is clear in the chapter from signed language assessment that language assessment literacy (LAL) in this context—deemed (S)LAL by the authors—is still in a very nascent form. Although in the field of spoken language assessment there is a tendency to discuss LAL as being a "new" development and recent scholarship suggests that issues and constructs remain undertheorized, there has been much more written on LAL oriented toward spoken language (as surveyed in the Chapter 11.1), to the extent that LAL is now a core area of research and scholarship in the field. This does not yet seem to be the case for (S)LAL. However, Chapter 11.2 by Boers and Hammer presents an important step in this direction. LAL in spoken language assessment can learn a great deal from the signed language assessment chapter about the link between articulating guidelines for good practice and achieving good practice. Boers and Hammer describe the creation of the Sign Language Assessment Design Matrix (SLASS-DM), which is intended to raise awareness of "the specifics of signed language assessment." Drawing on Bachman and Palmer's (1996) qualities of test usefulness, they have outlined a range of common challenges for signed language assessment. Many of these overlap with issues that form core components of LAL, though some are unique to signed languages contexts (e.g.,

Eveline Boers-Visker, Kathrin Eberharter, Annemiek Hammer, Luke Harding, and Benjamin Kremmel, *Discussion of Issues Related to Language Assessment Literacy in Second Signed and Spoken Languages* In: *The Handbook of Language Assessment Across Modalities*. Edited by: Tobias Haug, Wolfgang Mann, and Ute Knoch, Oxford University Press. © Oxford University Press 2022. DOI: 10.1093/oso/9780190885052.003.0034 the need to be mindful of overestimating ability based on the use of iconic signs). More importantly, however, the act of thinking through known challenges is an important step in identifying training needs and in mapping out components that are relevant for a given context. In the SLASS-DM, we see an example of a user-generated resource that functions as a starting point for further discussion about LAL needs. This approach might be generalizable to other less-explored areas of LAL across both modalities.

Toward a Theoretically Motivated LAL in Signed Language Assessment

The chapter on signed language assessment literacy has an explorative character and, in that, demonstrates that assessment literacy has been barely touched on in the literature on signed language teaching and assessment. The SLASS-DM summarizes pitfalls in the construction of signed language assessments according to well-known literature on test quality. Essentially, the matrix brings together our years of experience on assessing students on their language proficiency. Chapter 11.1 by Harding, Kremmel, and Eberharter, however, shows that language assessment literacy in spoken assessment contexts has been theoretically much more evolved. It goes without saying that the field of signed language has to take note of these developments in order to move from experience-based LAL to theoretically motivated LAL.

In addition, Harding and colleagues raise the important question of who needs LAL and how LAL needs may differ across stakeholder groups. It is yet unclear who will be using the SLASS-DM. The matrix is of interest to teachers and students as well as test developers. The fact that stakeholders are not specifically defined might be due to the fact that, in the field of signed language teaching, the classroom teacher is the one who makes the assessment, tests the students, and scores the students' performance on the test. Signed languages, being minority languages, are taught in small-scale contexts involving only a small team of teachers who often take up multiple tasks in assessment. Yet, given the fact that teams are small, it is interesting to think through if all team members have to take up similar roles. The dimensions offered in Chapter 11.1 by Harding, Kremmel, and Eberharter provide a good starting point to discuss different roles and, as such, different areas of expertise in signed language assessment.

With respect to the nine dimensions presented in Chapter 11.1, because they are language-independent they can be applied to signed languages as well. However, there are additional considerations with respect to Factors 1, 6, 7, and 9 that are important to point out from the perspective of signed language assessment (see Table 11.3.1). The additional considerations stem from (a) the unique affordances offered by the visual-spatial modality to use the space around the body and to employ iconicity, (b) the fact that signed languages must be seen (i.e., the impossibility to be anonymous), and (c) a lack of research on signed language linguistic features and signed language acquisition. The latter can result in overreliance on the linguistic evidence found for other signed languages (e.g., American Sign Language) or scoring practices based on popular wisdom, as opposed to thoroughly researched descriptive grammars. All in all, the dimensions offer a good starting point for discussions on *who* needs *what* kind of expertise regarding language assessment and what are language-specific considerations.

A perennial challenge exists, however, in demonstrating how the identification of different LAL dimensions becomes of value for the practice of language assessment. Questions about which dimension is of priority to which stakeholder and what knowledge and/or skill pertains to which dimension are of interest. Answers on these questions will probably differ from one context to another. In addition to investigating the *needs* of different geographical and professional contexts, as mentioned by the authors, it is of interest to investigate how dimensions *can be used* to start up the discussion on language assessment literacy or to professionalize stakeholders within a specific context. To put it in other words, the dimensions can be used as a blueprint to LAL in a specific context, as demonstrated for signed language assessment in Table 11.3.1. To move the field of LAL forward it is not only beneficial to investigate the needs in different contexts, but also to know how to address these needs. This has the potential to bring together theory of LAL and everyday practice in language assessment.

FUTURE DIRECTIONS

The future directions for (S)LAL are well mapped-out in the signed language assessment chapter: to develop more assessment training and to facilitate more validation research. These are laudable aims; however, one lesson learned from spoken language assessment is that the path to achieving these aims is not always easy. Needs analyses of teachers (and other stakeholders) operating in situ would be an important first step in developing a more robust approach to (S)LAL. The SLASS-DM is a good departure point; it presents a series of potential pitfalls and challenges that should be avoided. What is not clear, at this point, is what teachers of signed languages already know about assessment and what they feel they need to know in order to perform their role effectively. Investigating needs may broaden the scope of inquiry from a more technical consideration of test quality (based on Bachman & Palmer, 1996) and may lead to wider considerations of local practices, existing beliefs about “good” and “bad” assessment, the sociopolitical nature of test use, and many other topics that may influence assessment practice. We therefore see the next step as moving from raising

Table 11.3.1 Language assessment literacy (LAL) dimensions and considerations for signed language assessment

LAL dimensions		Considerations for signed language assessments
1.	Developing and administering language assessments	*Design or selection of tasks/prompts* to elicit language must take into account the iconic features of signed languages and the employment of gestural behavior that resembles signing In *developing benchmark performances* to illustrate scale points, the (non)-anonymity of the test-takers must to be taken into account
6.	Assessment principles and interpretation	Modality-specific signed languages features might affect reliability and validity
7.	Language structure, use, and development	Paucity of research on (some) signed languages—few reference grammars are available Very limited knowledge on acquisition, in particular of L2/Ln signed language acquisition Lack of teacher preparation education in most countries
9.	Scoring and rating	Impossibility to be anonymous might influence scoring (e.g., test-takers physical performance or signs of insecurity cannot be hidden)

awareness of challenges to finding out what skills/knowledge teachers have and understanding how these develop in practice. Understanding (S)LAL needs and trajectories represents a very rich site for further research in the area.

From the two chapters (Chapters 11.1 and 11.2) and this subsequent discussion, it also seems obvious that a deeper level of collaboration between spoken and signed language assessment would be of great benefit to the language assessment literacy enterprise in general. For (S)LAL, cross-fertilization of ideas from LAL will help to rapidly shape an emerging area of inquiry. There is no need to reinvent the wheel because there is substantial overlap between many of the concerns that emerge for teachers (particularly) across both modalities. Rather, the wheel will only need to be modified to the extent that it would usually need to be modified when thinking about the LAL needs of teachers of particular languages. For example, it is clear that different spoken languages bring with them distinct challenges for assessment (e.g., the measurement of tone accuracy in assessing Mandarin, which may be less relevant in other languages). We would therefore suggest that (S)LAL should not be considered a completely distinct case; the chapter by Boers and Hammer illustrates this with their successful application of the Bachman and Palmer model to signed language assessment concerns. While there may be differences in the traditions that have informed assessment, the principles of good practice are very much shared. The concept of language assessment literacy includes all languages and all modes, and, while the respective language constructs are distinct, the central concerns related to assessment will be more or less the same. This is in keeping with the direction taken in LAL research more latterly, which seeks to identify core components of LAL while at the same time trying to understand the specific contextual needs of language educators and tailor LAL training accordingly. Naturally, a deep understanding of the construct is crucial to LAL, and, in both modalities, there is more work to be done on transferring research on language acquisition and use into LAL models.

REFERENCE

Bachman, L., & Palmer, A. (1996). *Language testing in practice*. Oxford University Press.

Topic 12

Use of New Technologies in Second Language Assessment

12.1

New Technologies in Second Language Spoken Assessment

Phuong Nguyen and Volker Hegelheimer

Face-to-face speaking tests are considered the oldest form of assessment for second language (L2) spoken ability (Weir et al., 2013). Although face-to-face (i.e., direct) speaking assessment has offered many benefits, such as the potential to elicit direct evidence of interactional competence and generate positive washback on learning, it also has many disadvantages. Specifically, it can be logistically complex and resource-intensive to administer and score face-to-face spoken performance. It is also inconvenient to administer face-to-face speaking tests to students in geographically remote areas. Additionally, it can be difficult to achieve consistent administration and scoring (Davis et al., 2017).

However, recent technological developments have allowed researchers and test developers to investigate more practical alternatives to face-to-face speaking assessment. In fact, the past decade has witnessed a growth of semi-direct speaking tests; that is, tests where test-taker speech is elicited with technology-delivered prompts and scored by human raters, and automated speaking tests, which are both delivered and scored by the computer. In classroom assessment, language instructors have utilized recent advancements in multimedia recording to assess their students' oral proficiency. Because of the increasing popularity of these emerging technologies, it is necessary to evaluate the potential merits and problems associated with technology-based L2 oral proficiency assessment.

This chapter provides an overview of the use of new technologies in L2 speaking assessment in task design, test delivery and administration, and scoring of spoken responses in high-stakes testing and classroom assessment. Specifically, this chapter includes a discussion of commonly used video-conferencing and communication applications, several app-based assessments included in popular learning tools, and virtual environments, along with state-of-the-art technologies currently used for scoring examinees' speech. We will also outline opportunities and inherent challenges presented by these technologies when they are used in different phases of the testing cycle. We conclude the chapter

Phuong Nguyen and Volker Hegelheimer, *New Technologies in Second Language Spoken Assessment* In: *The Handbook of Language Assessment Across Modalities*. Edited by: Tobias Haug, Wolfgang Mann, and Ute Knoch, Oxford University Press. DOI: 10.1093/oso/9780190885052.003.0035 with notes on future directions for the use of new technologies in L2 speaking assessment.

TECHNOLOGIES USED FOR TASK DESIGN, TEST DELIVERY, AND ADMINISTRATION

Today, many English language proficiency tests exploit new technologies to develop their specialized systems used to design and deliver spoken language tests. These tests mainly utilize their specialized testing platform to administer the speaking tasks via the internet to examinees who are required to speak into a microphone, record, and store their responses to be rated by human examiners. Examples of such test include the speaking component of the Business Language Testing Service (BULATS), developed and owned by Cambridge ESOL; the Canadian Academic English Language (CAEL); the Canadian English Language Proficiency Index Program (CELPIP) for immigration, refugee, and citizenship purposes, both developed by Paragon Testing Enterprises; and the Test of English as a Foreign Language (TOEFL) iBT Speaking test developed by the Educational Testing System (ETS). In addition to using technology as a platform to administer speaking tests and record test-takers' responses, language testing agencies can also develop automatic speech scoring systems to assess test-takers' spoken production. For example, Duolingo developed a computer-adapted test which is administered on the computer or mobile devices using the device's screen, camera, keyboard, speakers, and microphone. The test, which claims to assess general L2 speaking ability, requires test-takers to read aloud a written sentence presented on the screen. Because the test is computer-adaptive, the test-taker's speech sample is scored automatically and instantly by the computer using a proprietary algorithm. It should be noted, however, that because of the nature of the speaking task (i.e., sentence read-aloud), the Duolingo English test measures a very limited construct of English spoken proficiency.

Additionally, various technologies can be employed to design innovative task types and deliver the tests to assess students' L2 oral proficiency in low-stakes testing. These technologies can be classified into three groups: web-based applications, video-conference tools, and technologies for assessment in virtual environments.

Many web-based applications—programs accessed over a network connection using HTTP and often run in a web browser—can be used to deliver and administer L2 speaking tests. Web-based applications can be developed as assessment management systems which specialize in assessment solutions for educational purposes and allow for question authoring, item bank management, and assessment creation (e.g., Questionmark Perception and Learnosity) or educational, multimedia platforms which serve as learning tools for instructors and students to create or share files (e.g., VoiceThread). For instance, Questionmark Perception (https://www.questionmark.com), designed to deliver assessments to a variety of devices including smartphones, tablets, and touchscreen devices, allows test developers and instructors to author, deliver, and report on survey, quizzes, and tests. Although this application is not designed specifically for speaking assessment, it allows the test developer to present the speaking prompt to test-takers and ask them to upload their responses. In fact, this application was employed in a study by Kiddle and Kormos (2011) who compared students' spoken performance and perception in a direct face-to-face speaking test with those in the online version of the test. Questionmark Perception allows the test developer to include stimulus such as images, audio, or video. Test-takers can see the time allowed for each task, record their responses on a voice recording application, and upload the recordings for rating. Similar to Questionmark, Learnosity (https://www.learnosity.com/) offers many task types and functions. For example, the audio/video player and audio/video recorder functions enable instructors and students to ask and answer questions as they would in a real-life scenario, and therefore, these could be employed for assessing students' oral communication skills. Specifically, the test developer could embed audio or video files in the stimulus. Test-takers' spoken responses can be easily captured by the audio or video recorder supported by Learnosity. In addition to assessment management systems, VoiceThread (https://www.voicethread.com/), a web-based asynchronous voice tool, can also be used for L2 speaking assessment. Instructors can ask students to record and post their audio or video responses to speaking tasks which employ images, audio files, and videos as their stimuli. VoiceThread has been explored as a means for formative assessment and found to be beneficial to classroom assessment, especially formative assessment (Herlihy & Pottage, 2013). These applications, although designed as independent platforms, can be integrated into other learning management systems such as Moodle and Instructure Canvas.

Another group of applications useful to lower-stakes L2 speaking assessment is video-conferencing tools. Although these tools are less widely used for assessing L2 oral proficiency compared to their application in language learning, recent studies have shown that they can be employed to design tasks that elicit L2 learners' spoken proficiency (Kim & Craig, 2012; Nakatsuhara et al., 2017), especially interactional competence (Davis et al., 2017). For example, Adobe Connect web conferencing (https://www.adobe.com/products/adobeconnect.html) is a virtual meeting tool that enables the test developer to administer a speaking test to multiple examinees. It allows the examiner (i.e., the host) and the test-takers to share images, prerecorded videos, or live web camera videos from a computer or any mobile devices. The examiner can make recordings of the interaction, which show exactly what participants heard and saw, and archive them for rating. This application has been explored in Kim and Craig (2012) who compared examinees' scores and their attitudes across the two testing modes (face-to-face vs. computer-based) of a speaking interview. Another example is Zoom (https://zoom.us/). A free, basic Zoom account allows for an unlimited number of meetings, each of which can last up to 40 minutes. Similar to Adobe Connect, Zoom supports simultaneous screen sharing, voice-recording, and screen capture. The "waiting room" feature in Zoom, similar to a waiting room at a doctor's office, allows the examiner to control which test-taker to converse with first and which test-takers should remain in the waiting room. This function is very useful for group speaking tests in which test-takers are involved in both individual and group tasks. In their study, Nakatsuhara et al. (2017) investigated the application of Zoom for delivering and conducting the International English Language Testing System (IELTS) speaking test as well as the differences between the standard face-to-face and computer-mediated modes. The researchers found evidence supporting the use of Zoom for L2 speaking assessment, arguing that Zoom could be used as a parallel alternative to the standard face-to-face mode for the IELTS. Another useful video-conferencing application is Skype (https://www.skype.com), which can be accessed from a computer, mobile phone, or table. Skype-to-Skype service supports unlimited communication between groups of multiple users in the form of audio, video calls, or conference callings in addition to messaging. Skype Interviews allows examiners to schedule an interview and share multimedia files with one or more examinees, which is also useful for integrated group speaking tests. In fact, Skype has been investigated and incorporated in a system for oral proficiency assessment in a study by Davis et al. (2017) who evaluated the feasibility of using Skype for speaking tasks requiring interaction between a moderator and participants in different locations. They reported that most participants expressed positive attitudes to the tasks and technology. However, one disadvantage of Skype is that it does not support call recording, which requires the test developer to rely on a third-party application if they wish to make audio recordings or screen captures for later rating.

Other applications useful for L2 speaking assessment include Facebook's WhatsApp and Messenger, Viber, and Google Hangouts. These applications are free, although it is mandatory that participants must provide a standard cellular number to get service from WhatsApp and Viber, while users must have a Facebook or a Gmail account to access Facebook Messenger or Google Hangouts. Participants can access these applications either from a computer or other mobile devices and send text massages, make voice and video calls, and send multimedia files to one or multiple other participants. However, a third-party application is needed to record conversations between participants. Among these applications, only WhatsApp has been explored for L2 speaking assessment in the study conducted by Tarighat and Khodabakhsh (2016) who examined the feasibility of using WhatsApp on mobile phones to assess students' speaking proficiency and suggested that the application should be used as a complementary assessment form in the formative assessment of students' oral proficiency.

The final group of technologies, relatively new and limited in their use, can be potentially used for L2 speaking assessment in lower stakes testing. These are virtual environments. In these virtual worlds, test-takers are represented by an avatar and are able to interact in real time with examiners or other test-takers via internet-connected computers or devices. To date, Second Life, an off-the-shelf virtual environment, is the most commonly explored for L2 learning and, to some degree, L2 speaking assessment. An example of the use of such a system can be found in Park's (2018) study in which the researcher developed virtual interactive tasks to assess aviation English proficiency in air traffic controllers. The tasks in this study involved listening to simulated pilots' radiotelephony transmissions, watching animated helicopters landing and departing, reading flight plans and weather information, and orally responding to pilots in seven prototype aviation English tasks simulated in Second Life (Park, 2018). Figure 12.1.1 illustrates the virtual interactive aviation English test environment simulated in Second Life.

However, since commercially available virtual environments are rarely designed specifically for assessing L2 oral communication, it is common that test developers must build virtual environments for

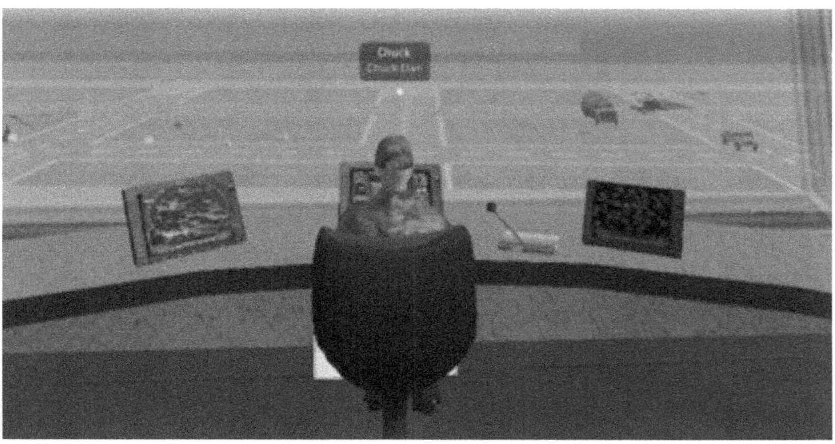

Figure 12.1.1 View from the air traffic control tower simulated in Second Life. Used with permission from the author.

the test purpose and assist with delivering L2 oral communication assessments. For instance, Ockey et al. (2017) built their virtual environment based on Metamersive Interactive Learning Space developed by Indusgeeks Solutions, an adaptation of Second Life and other virtual environments that allow conferences in the 3D environment. Other technologies used to develop the system included Unity3D, a cross-platform game engine; Autodesk 3D Studio Max, a 3D computer graphics program for creating 3D animations, models, and images; C+ programming language; Vivox plugin; and the Metamersive-based application from Indusgeeks for voice communication.

While the applications just discussed make it more convenient to administer an L2 spoken assessment, they might introduce additional challenges for human raters who are also in charge of administering the test. For example, when using conference applications for L2 speaking assessment, raters have to simultaneously navigate the interface to present the stimuli to test-takers or record their responses in addition to giving instructions to test-takers and attending to their performance if they are to provide a fair assessment of their speaking ability. This requires further training and practice to prevent raters from cognitive overload. In the case of live rating, raters must also be trained on how to resolve technical issues that might arise during test administration.

TECHNOLOGIES USED FOR SCORING SPOKEN RESPONSES

Recent advancements in natural language processing have enabled the development and utilization of automatic speech recognition (ASR) systems in scoring examinees' spoken language. An ASR system inputs a digitized acoustic signal and produces the best estimate of text corresponding to the input signal. To date, the most advanced ASR systems are SpeechRater, owned by ETS to score English speech, and the Versant testing system, owned by Pearson to score speech of various languages such as English, Arabic, Dutch, French, and Spanish. These systems are *speaker-independent* (i.e., systems trained with a corpus of model speakers' spoken language to recognize future user's speech) and *continuous* (i.e., intended to process longer phrases and utterances) (Wachowicz & Scott, 1999). However, SpeechRater and the Versant testing system adopt different approaches to automating the scoring of L2 spoken language.

SpeechRater was developed to score spontaneous speech produced by prospective test-takers of the TOEFL iBT Speaking (Xi et al., 2008; Zechner et al., 2009). The development of this system is based on free, extended speech elicited through communicative speaking tasks. Learners' spoken production for each speaking task is first decoded by a speech recognizer. After that, based on the output produced by the speech recognizer, 29 scoring features representative of four aspects of spoken performance, namely fluency, pronunciation, vocabulary diversity, and grammatical accuracy, are extracted. These features are then analyzed in the scoring model built on a multiple regression model to arrive at a score for the task. Xi et al. (2008) presented a very detailed description of this technology. This system is currently being used for scoring the TOEFL Practice Online (TPO), a low-stakes practice test product.

Adopting an approach that differs from SpeechRater, the Versant testing system was developed to assess highly constrained speech produced in response to tasks such as reading aloud, repeating sentences, building sentences, giving antonyms, and so on. An augmented ASR system, a speech recognizer built with Cambridge University Engineer Department's Hidden Markov Model Toolkit (HTK) (Bernstein & Cheng, 2007), is employed to analyze examinees' performance and handle variations in non-native speech. This system provides lexical units; spectral measures; and time-aligned, detailed transcriptions of examinees' responses. Linguistic measures (based on words used in the spoken responses and the pace, fluency, and pronunciation of those words in phrases and sentences) representative of the content and manner of examinees' speech are then extracted based on statistical models and combined into four subscores—sentence mastery, vocabulary, fluency, and pronunciation—using advanced statistical modeling techniques (Bernstein & Cheng, 2007; Bernstein et al., 2010).

More details about the ASR systems for scoring L2 spoken language are presented in Knoch's Chapter 9.1.

OPPORTUNITIES AND CHALLENGES OFFERED BY NEW TECHNOLOGIES FOR THE ASSESSMENT OF L2 SPOKEN LANGUAGE

The new technologies discussed in the previous sections have offered many opportunities as well as challenges for L2 spoken language assessment. Specifically, they provide language test developers with opportunities pertaining to logistics, test reliability, task authenticity, and the potential to assess new constructs of L2 spoken proficiency. Nevertheless, these emerging technologies also present challenges in terms of test security and the constructs measured by L2 speaking tests.

Opportunities

Undoubtedly, the application of new technologies has made it more convenient and less labor-intensive to administer L2 speaking assessments and score examinees' spoken performance. The use of video-conference tools or virtual environments, for example, helps overcome the issue of test-takers and examiners who are not conveniently available in the same location and also helps reduce the cost for testing venues. ASR systems for scoring spoken responses, although labor-intensive and costly to develop, make scoring more time-efficient and, in the long run, become more cost-effective because of potential cost reductions in hiring and training human raters. Furthermore, with new technologies, stimuli for the speaking tests such as presentations, audio files, and videos can be uploaded, stored, and integrated easily, and examinees' spoken responses can be recorded, stored, and shared with raters conveniently. All of these help reduce the cost of production and assembly of test forms and transmission and of the storage of stimuli and response files.

The second advantage of new technologies is that they can help enhance the reliability of the test scores, which therefore contributes to the validity of test score interpretation and use. In fact, the use of ASR systems for scoring spoken responses helps enhance rating consistency, which is hard to achieve with human raters because raters can be a source of test score variability (Barkaoui, 2010a, 2010b; Brown, 1995; Cumming, 1990; Orr, 2002; Shi, 2001). In fact, automatic scoring can help maintain score consistency or reliability across items and over time (Bernstein, 2013). In addition, delivering L2 speaking assessments on the computer using web-based applications or specifically developed platforms also allows for consistent administration of the tests, thus contributing to enhancing test fairness among test-takers.

Additionally, new technologies allow for the development of innovative task types that are more authentic. For instance, given that stimuli in the form of audio files or videos can be easily presented to test-takers through web-based or video-conferencing applications, test developers are able to include integrated speaking tasks that are more similar to communication tasks in the real world, where often one speaks in response to some input or one can get visual cues from facial expressions of the other person. This provides a more robust, authentic medium for L2 speaking assessment. Similarly, the interactive virtual tasks that were developed for the aviation English test (Park, 2018) replicated real-world scenarios that air traffic controllers would encounter in their daily job. Such tasks could be as useful for assessing English for specific purposes in other fields, such as business and tourism. As test-takers' language proficiency should be ideally assessed in an authentic task and situation (Alderson, 2010; Douglas, 2013), the fact that new technologies can facilitate the design of authentic tasks is undeniably a significant benefit for L2 speaking assessment.

More importantly, as emerging technologies have transformed the test delivery systems and supported the creation of innovative assessment tasks that assess new language constructs (Chapelle, 2008; Chapelle & Douglas, 2006), they are also expected to foster the design of innovative speaking tasks that can measure new constructs in L2 spoken language. For example, video-conferencing tools enable language testers to measure the spoken proficiency of many test-takers concurrently and create tasks requiring discussion and collaboration among them. Also, examiners and test-takers are able to access the vocal and facial cues of one another. All of these allow for a more reliable assessment of interactional competence (i.e., the ability to comprehend spoken input and produce language that appropriately responds to the input by negotiating meaning, taking turns, etc.), an important aspect of oral proficiency (Louma, 2004; Ockey, 2018; Nakatsuhara et al., 2018). Although interactional competence can be assessed during face-to-face speaking tasks, it can be assessed more conveniently with the help of video-conferencing technologies and virtual environments.

Challenges

Along with these advantages, however, new technologies also pose some challenges to the assessment of L2 spoken proficiency. In terms of test security, technology-mediated L2 speaking assessment might facilitate cheating or hacking of the testing systems, especially in high-stakes testing. Ironically, technological developments also make it easier for test-takers to cheat using digital recorders, smart watches, and screen capture applications, to name but a few, to record test item information. Therefore, it is critical that developers, especially of high-stakes tests, should have stringent protocols to maintain the security of their test materials, test delivery systems, and scoring systems (Crooks & Kane, 1996) as well as to ensure that assessments are administered in secure, standardized environments (Roever, 2001). The test administration process should be monitored carefully by collecting test-takers' identity information onsite using photos, facial recognition, biometric scanning, and so on. When technology-mediated L2 speaking assessments are administered to test-takers in locations other than the testing site, webcams could be used to ensure the identity of registered test-takers. However, when test-takers are required to upload their responses to speaking test tasks through web-based applications, it is impossible for the instructor/test developer to prevent students from cheating unless the test is administered with the instructor's surveillance. In such cases, the test scores should be used for low-stakes decisions or classroom assessment.

The second challenge is related to the construct that an L2 speaking test aims to measure. Many researchers have argued that the effects of the delivery medium on the nature of the construct being measured is the fundamental issue since the advent of computer-based language testing (Chapelle & Douglas, 2006; Douglas, 2013; Douglas & Hegelheimer, 2007). When new technologies are employed in test task design, test delivery, or administration, test developers need to consider the technology being used when defining the construct for their test (Douglas, 2013). In fact, discussing the concept of language ability,

Chapelle and Douglas (2006) proposed that language ability should be redefined to include "the ability to select and deploy appropriate language through the technologies that are appropriate for a situation" (p. 107). If the aim of a test is to make inferences about test-takers' ability to engage appropriately in discussions in academic contexts, then video-conferencing tools are more appropriate than web-based applications as the medium for test administration. In other words, test developers must take into account what technologies are most appropriate for the test purposes and include these technologies in the test construct definition. Additionally, the construct being measured is also affected by the scoring system used to score test-takers' responses. The limitations of current ASR systems narrow the construct being assessed and threaten the validity to the claims made based on the test results (Chapelle & Chung, 2010). Norris (2001) argued that it is challenging to capture the complexities of speaking performances using ASR systems. In fact, current ASR systems are not efficient in capturing aspects such as content, appropriateness of word choice or expression use, and development of ideas and are mainly developed to score monologic speech. In this case, the argument that test-takers can interact appropriately cannot be substantiated when such an ASR system is used as the sole rater for the test. Therefore, test developers must be cautious and consider the limitations of ASR systems when making inferences about test-takers' spoken ability.

In addition to the challenges pertaining to test security and construct, most available technologies can only allow for the use of restricted task types, which might lower the validity of the test score interpretation. For example, QuestionMark and VoiceThread are beneficial for assessing individual speech, although the video/audio functions are useful for integrated speaking tasks. These technologies might not be appropriate if the test aims to measure interactional competence. Instead, Skype or Zoom could be a more suitable solution. In contrast, although Skype and Zoom are flexible in allowing the examiner to present stimuli to test-takers through screen sharing, it is challenging to use audio or video recordings as stimuli and share them to a group of test-takers. In fact, there is no technology that can be appropriate for all types of speaking tasks. The test developer should decide on a certain application depending on the purpose of their test and the resources available.

FUTURE DIRECTIONS

Given that emerging technologies create many potentials as well as present challenges in L2 spoken language assessment, more research will be done in the future to explore their application for test design, delivery, administration, and scoring. With the development of new technologies, speaking tasks continue to be more authentic through the integration of multimedia stimuli, thus strengthening the relationship between stimuli employed in the speaking test tasks and those in real-world tasks (Douglas & Hegelheimer, 2007). Additionally, the use of video-conferencing applications is expected to be more common in L2 speaking assessment because of (1) their low-cost or sometimes no-cost service and (2) their ability to allow access to participants' facial cues and group discussion, thus enabling the assessment of interactional competence. As L2 oral proficiency is defined as the use of verbal language to communicate with others (Fulcher, 2003), implying that oral proficiency includes the ability to comprehend spoken input and appropriately respond to the input by negotiating meaning, taking turns, etc., speaking tests that can assess interactional competence are more likely to be valid indicators of oral proficiency than those that do not. Also, the future may witness more application of virtual reality systems in L2 spoken assessment since technological advancements will enable these systems to thrive and continue to be used by language test developers. It is also possible that more L2 speaking tests will be delivered on mobile and tablet devices, especially for low-stakes testing.

In addition, ASR systems will continue to be perfected and employed to score spoken responses in high-stakes testing. These systems will be more accurate when analyzing test-takers' acoustic input, especially that of non-native accents. They will also be able to extract linguistic features not captured by current systems, such as idea organization or lexical appropriateness.

CONCLUSION

This chapter has shown that a variety of new technologies have been employed in various stages of the testing cycle to assess L2 spoken language both in high- and low-stakes testing. These technologies have offered great potentials in test task design, test delivery and administration, and examinees' response scoring, making it convenient and less labor-intensive to assess the L2 speaking ability of test-takers living in different physical locations. Advancements in video-conferencing technologies and virtual environments also enable the design of speaking tasks that are more representative of those in the target language use domain as well as the possibility of assessing new constructs in L2 spoken proficiency. The use of automatic scoring has yielded more time-efficient, consistent evaluation of L2 spoken speech.

Despite of some challenges posed by new technologies, the integration of new technologies in L2 spoken assessment will remain an ongoing area of research. Limitations of current technologies for scoring or test security will be mitigated through future research. Language test developers and researchers will continue to explore technologies that can efficiently assess learners' L2 speaking ability so that they can make valid inferences about L2 spoken proficiency based on test scores.

REFERENCES

Alderson, J. C. (2010). A survey of aviation English tests. *Language Testing*, *27*(1), 51–72. https://doi.org/10.1177/0265532209347196

Barkaoui, K. (2010a). Explaining ESL essay holistic scores: A multilevel modeling approach. *Language Testing*, *27*(4), 515–535. https://doi.org/10.1177/0265532210368717

Barkaoui, K. (2010b). Variability in ESL essay rating processes: The role of the rating scale and rater experience. *Language Assessment Quarterly*, *7*(1), 54–74. https://doi.org/10.1080/15434300903464418

Bernstein, J. (2013). Computer scoring of spoken responses. In C. A. Chapelle (Ed.), *The encyclopedia of applied linguistics* (pp. 857–863). Wiley-Blackwell.

Bernstein, J., & Cheng, J. (2007). Logic, operation, and validation of a spoken English test. In V. M. Holland & F. P. Fisher (Eds.), *The path of speech technologies in computer assisted language learning* (pp. 174–194). Routledge.

Bernstein, J., Van Moere, A., & Cheng, J. (2010). Validating automated speaking tests. *Language Testing*, *27*(3), 355–377. https://doi.org/10.1177/0265532210364404

Brown, A. (1995). The effect of rater variables in the development of an occupation-specific language performance test. *Language Testing*, *12*(1), 1–s15. https://doi.org/10.1177/026553229501200101

Chapelle, C. A. (2008). Utilizing technology in language assessment. In E. Shohamy (Ed.), *Encyclopedia of language education*, vol. 7: *Language testing and assessment* (2nd ed., pp. 123–134). Springer.

Chapelle, C. A., & Chung, Y. R. (2010). The promise of NLP and speech processing technologies in language assessment. *Language Testing*, *27*(3), 301–315. https://doi.org/10.1177/0265532210364405

Chapelle, C. A., & Douglas, D. (2006). *Assessing language through computer technology*. Cambridge University Press.

Crooks, T., & Kane, M. T. (1996). Threats to the valid use of assessment. *Assessment in Education: Principles, Policy, and Practice*, *3*(3). 265–286. https://doi.org/10.1080/0969594960030302

Cumming, A. (1990). Expertise in evaluating second language compositions. *Language Testing*, *7*(1), 31–51. https://doi.org/10.1177/026553229000700104

Davis, L., Timpe-Laughlin, V., Gu, L., & Ockey, G. (2017). Face-to-face speaking assessment in the digital age: Interactive speaking tasks online. In J. M. Davis, J. M. Norris, M. E. Malone, T. H. McKay, & Y.-A. Son (Eds.), *Useful assessment and evaluation in language education* (pp. 115–130). Georgetown University Press.

Douglas, D. (2013). ESP and assessment. In B. Paltridge & S. Starfield (Eds.), *The handbook of English for specific purposes* (pp. 367–383). John Wiley & Sons.

Douglas, D., & Hegelheimer, V. (2007). Assessing language using computer technology. *Annual Review of Applied Linguistics*, *27*, 115–132. https://doi.org/10.1017/S0267190508070062

Fulcher, G. (2003). *Testing second language speaking*. Cambridge University Press.

Herlihy, D., & Pottage, Z. (2013). Formative assessment in a Web 2.0 environment: Impact on motivation and outcomes. *Cambridge English Language Assessment Research Notes, 53*, 9–18. https://www.cambridgeenglish.org/Images/142798-research-notes-53-document.pdf

Kiddle, T., & Kormos, J. (2011). The effect of mode of response on a semidirect test of oral proficiency. *Language Assessment Quarterly*, *8*(4), 342–360. https://doi.org/10.1080/15434303.2011.613503

Kim, J., & Craig, D. A. (2012). Validation of a video-conferenced speaking test. *Computer Assisted Language Learning*, *25*(3), 257–275. https://doi.org/10.1080/09588221.2011.649482

Louma, S. (2004). *Assessing speaking*. Cambridge University Press.

Nakatsuhara, F., Inoue, C., Berry, V., & Galaczi, E. (2017). Exploring the use of video-conferencing technology in the assessment of spoken language: A mixed-methods study. *Language Assessment Quarterly*, *14*(1), 1–18. https://doi.org/10.1080/15434303.2016.1263637

Nakatsuhara, F., May, L., Lam, D., & Galaczi, E. (2018). Learning-oriented feedback and interactional competence. *Cambridge Research Notes, 70,* 4–67. https://www.cambridgeenglish.org/Images/517543-research-notes-70.pdf

Norris, J. M. (2001). Concerns with computerized adaptive oral proficiency assessment. *Language Learning & Technology*, *5*(2), 99–105. http://llt.msu.edu/vol5num2/norris/default.html

Ockey, G. J. (2018). Oral language proficiency tests. In J. L. Liontas (Ed.), *The TESOL encyclopedia of English language teaching* (vol. 3). Wiley-Blackwell. https://doi.org/10.1002/9781118784235.eelt0234

Ockey, G. J., Gu, L., & Keehner, M. (2017). Web-based virtual environments for facilitating assessment of L2 oral communication ability. *Language Assessment Quarterly*, *14*(4), 346–359. https://doi.org/10.1080/15434303.2017.1400036

Orr, M. (2002). The FCE Speaking test: Using rater reports to help interpret test scores. *System*, *30*(2), 143–154. https://doi.org/10.1016/S0346-251X(02)00002-7

Park, M. (2018). Innovative assessment of aviation English in a virtual world: Windows into cognitive and metacognitive strategies. *ReCALL*, *30*(2), 196–213. https://doi.org/10.1017/S0958344017000362

Roever, C. (2001). Web-based language testing. *Language Learning & Technology*, *5*(2), 84–94. http://llt.msu.edu/vol5num2/roever/default.html

Shi, L. (2001). Native- and nonnative-speaking EFL teachers' evaluation of Chinese students' English writing. *Language Testing*, *18*(3), 303–325. https://doi.org/10.1177/026553220101800303

Tarighat, S., & Khodabakhsh, S. (2016). Mobile-Assisted Language Assessment: Assessing speaking. *Computers in Human Behavior, 64*, 409–413. https://doi.org/10.1016/j.chb.2016.07.014

Wachowicz, K. A., & Scott, B. L. (1999). Software that listens: It's not a question of whether, it's a question of how. *CALICO Journal, 16*, 253–276.

Weir, C. J., Vidakovic, I., & Galaczi, E. D. (2013). *Measured constructs: A history of Cambridge English Examinations, 1913–2012*. Cambridge: Cambridge University Press.

Xi, X., Higgins, D., Zechner, K., & Williamson, D. M. (2008). Automated scoring of spontaneous speech using Speechrater v1.0 (ETS Research Report No. RR-07-02). http://www.ets.org/research/researcher/RR-08-62.html

Zechner, K., Higgins, D., Xi, X., & Williamson, D. (2009). Automatic scoring of non-native spontaneous speech in tests of spoken English. *Speech Communication, 51*(10), 883–895. https://doi.org/10.1016/j.specom.2009.04.009

12.2

New Technologies in Second Language Signed Assessment

Sarah Ebling, Necati Cihan Camgöz, and Richard Bowden

In this chapter, two signed language technologies and their application to signed language assessment are introduced. The modality-specific challenges of these technologies are discussed, which originate in the complex, multichannel nature of signs and the lack of a standardized writing system.

While the quantity of language resources (corpora, lexicons, etc.) available for signed languages differs from country to country, it is generally significantly lower than that available in a country's spoken language. Automatic signed language processing, a subfield of natural language processing (NLP), provides a way to reduce this imbalance, comprising, among others, applications such as signed language recognition (SLR; the identification of the form and meaning of signs) and signed language animation (the creation of virtual signers). For each of these applications, important contributions have been made in the past decades, but the existing body of research is still considerably smaller than that of the field of automatic spoken language processing, not to mention the research contributions on applying these technologies in signed language assessment.

Many current automatic signed language processing systems pursue a statistical approach; for example, they derive probabilities from previously created pairings of signed language videos and corresponding transcriptions (in the case of SLR). Creating such data is time-consuming; in particular, providing a written, machine-readable record of signed language is highly labor-intensive. In the largest signed language corpus acquisition project to date, the German Sign Language (*Deutsche Gebärdensprache* [DGS]) Corpus Project,[1] the ratio between transcribed time and transcription time has been shown to be

Sarah Ebling, Necati Cihan Camgöz, and Richard Bowden, *New Technologies in Second Language Signed Assessment*
In: *The Handbook of Language Assessment Across Modalities.* Edited by: Tobias Haug, Wolfgang Mann, and Ute Knoch,
Oxford University Press. © Oxford University Press 2022. DOI: 10.1093/oso/9780190885052.003.0036

1:600 (i.e., 1 minute of signing takes 600 minutes to transcribe and annotate) (Thomas Hanke, personal communication, October 17, 2018). To account for the physical form of signs, the Hamburg Notation System for Sign Languages (HamNoSys) (Prillwitz et al., 1989) is often used. It consists of approximately 200 symbols describing the manual components, which include hand shape, hand position (with finger direction and palm orientation as subcomponents), location, and movement. The symbols together constitute a Unicode font. Figure 12.2.1 shows the HamNoSys notation of the sign VOLK ("PEOPLE") in Swiss German Sign Language (*Deutschschweizerische Gebärdensprache* [DSGS]) that contains one instance of each manual component.

Apart from these manual components, nonmanual components of signing (such as head and shoulder movements, eyebrow movements, direction of eye gaze, etc.) exist that are capable of assuming functions at all linguistic levels (Crasborn, 2006). No HamNoSys symbols exist for encoding nonmanual aspects of signing; instead, this information is specified in an XML extension of the notation system commonly using the Signing Gesture Markup Language (SiGML) (Elliott et al., 2000). SiGML provides an inventory of XML attribute values for expressing nonmanual information such as "(both) eyebrows raised" or "head nod" (Hanke, 2001).

As in other areas of NLP, data-driven approaches (i.e., those based on machine learning) typically assume that "more data is better data" (Mercer, 1993, p. 18). However, compared to spoken language systems which may be trained on millions of sequences, automatic signed language processing systems that are trained on datasets of the order of thousands of sequences can be expected to work well only if they operate on restricted domains, for example, that of weather reports or public transportation information.

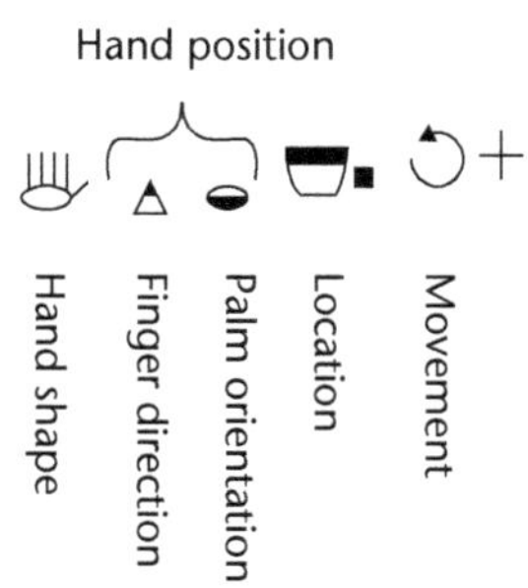

Figure 12.2.1 HamNoSys notation of the DSGS sign volk ("people").
From Ebling (2016).

SIGNED LANGUAGE TECHNOLOGIES

This section first looks at technology for SLR using computer vision to recognize the signs produced by a human signer, followed by the converse problem of signed production: using avatars to generate synthetic sign sequences. It then links these technologies to signed language assessment.

Signed Language Recognition

SLR, the ability of a computer to process and recognize an incoming stream of sign video, has been studied by computer vision researchers for the past two decades (Starner et al., 1998), and it has produced several real-life applications such as TESSA (Cox et al., 2002), a post office translation application; Dicta-Sign (Efthimiou et al., 2012), a signed language wiki system; and HospiSign (Camgöz et al., 2016b), a hospital information kiosk for the deaf, as well as searchable signed language dictionaries (Cooper et al., 2011a; Elliott et al., 2011). However, most of these prototypical systems to date focused on isolated signs (which has a potential application in vocabulary assessment of signed languages). To address the full remit of the technology, SLR approaches are required that can recognize continuous sign streams; for example, to recognize a signed utterance in a sentence repetition test.

There are various factors that contribute to previous work focusing on isolated signs. First and foremost is the fact that the collection and annotation of continuous SLR data is a laborious task. Although there are datasets available from linguistic sources (Hanke et al., 2010; Schembri et al., 2013) and signed language interpretation can be exploited from broadcast footage (Cooper & Bowden 2009; Buehler et al., 2009), such data tend to be only partially annotated (e.g., lacking timing information or detailed information on the pose of the signer). This has resulted in many researchers collecting their own isolated signed language datasets (Ong et al., 2012; Camgöz et al., 2016a; Yin et al., 2016) in controlled environments with limited vocabulary.

Another factor is that, until recently, a dataset that is shared among researchers to serve as a baseline for SLR has not been established. This has led researchers to work on their own small datasets specific to their applications (Ong et al., 2014; Camgöz et al., 2016a; Wang et al., 2016; Zafrulla, Brashear et al., 2011a), making most of the research incomparable and hence robbing the field of competitive progress.

With the recent developments in the field of artificial intelligence (AI) that have overcome the limitations in annotation (Buehler et al., 2009; Cooper et al., 2012; Pfister et al., 2013; Koller et al., 2013) and breakthroughs in estimating the pose of human bodies in images and video (Cao et al., 2017; Charles et al., 2014; Wei et al., 2016), working on linguistic data and signed language interpretations from broadcast footage has become a feasible option. These developments were followed by Forster et al.'s release of the RWTH-PHOENIX-Weather-2012 dataset (Forster et al., 2012) and its extended version RWTH-PHOENIX-Weather-2014 (Forster et al., 2014), which contained DGS interpretations of weather forecasts. The PHOENIX dataset has quickly become a baseline for continuous SLR.

Because signs are spatio-temporal constructs, generally all SLR methods consist of two steps: (1) extraction of spatial features from video frames and (2) temporal modeling of these representations. Legacy approaches (Cooper & Bowden 2010; Cooper, Pugeault, et al., 2011) relied heavily on hand-crafted features to represent manual and nonmanual aspects of the sign. These features are then modeled using graphical models or template-based approaches to capture temporal changes in the sign sequence (Cooper & Bowden, 2007; Ong et al., 2012; Ong et al., 2014).

With the recent development of efficient and successful *deep learning* methods, which can learn spatio-temporal representations from data with minimal human intervention, SLR researchers have swiftly adopted the latest AI tools, specifically, approaches based on convolutional neural networks (CNNs) and recurrent neural network (RNNs) (Koller, Ney et al., 2016; Koller, Zargaran et al., 2016; Koller et al., 2017; Camgöz et al., 2017; Cui et al., 2017). Automatic signed language assessment can profit from these new methods applied to SLR.

Although there has been major progress in the field of SLR, such as realizing continuous SLR and training using partially annotated data, there are still several challenges to overcome. One of these challenges is signer-independent recognition, which focuses on approaches that can be trained on one person and that generalize to others. Koller et al. (2017) compared their method's performance on both signer-independent and signer-dependent setups. Yin et al. (2016) proposed using hand-crafted features, which were designed to be signer-independent, and reported comparative signer-dependent and -independent results on isolated SLR. The current state of research suggests that to be able to scale to signer-independent continuous recognition, the SLR community needs to collaborate with signed language linguists to utilize the vast amounts of annotated high-quality data available (Camgöz et al., 2017).

Another research topic that has not been fully explored is the explicit modeling of signed language modalities (i.e., manual and nonmanual). Although there is a large body of work in the literature focused on hand shape estimation (Camgöz et al., 2017; Koller, Ney, et al., 2016), mouthing recognition (Koller, Ney, & Bowden, 2015), and facial expression analysis (Moore & Bowden, 2009), there is very little work (Aran, Burger et al., 2009) that explicitly combines them to model the sign as a whole, to realize SLR. This is of great importance for assessing signed language performance in learners at the sentence level and higher.

Signed Language Animation

Signed language animation, the process of creating a signing avatar, is a young field of research, looking back on only about 20 years of existence. Signed language animations are typically created through one of three approaches: animation by hand (traditional animation), motion capturing, or animation from linguistic description. Animation by hand consists of manually modeling and posing an avatar character in a software such as Maya, 3ds Max, or Blender. This procedure is highly labor-intensive but generally yields excellent results. A signing avatar may also be animated based on information obtained from motion capture, which involves recording a human's signing. While the quality tends to be high, major drawbacks of this approach are the long calibration time and the extensive post-processing required. Recordings of motion capture are also difficult to edit and combine to form the novel utterances needed in automatic translation systems (Gibet et al., 2011). An alternative is animation from linguistic description, where animated signs are created from a notational script, which means that, at execution time, there is access to the structure of signs at whatever level of detail the underlying notation system offers. While this approach is highly flexible, it typically results in the lowest quality (Ebling, 2013; Ebling & Glauert, 2016; Kipp et al., 2011). A fourth approach to signed language animation is sometimes distinguished from the other approaches, *procedural animation* (McDonald et al., 2017). This approach consists of modelling sign movements mathematically.

An animation system developed for American Sign Language (ASL), *Paula*, relies on a combination of hand animation and procedural animation (McDonald et al., 2017). Individual hand-animated signs are used as a motion base, with procedural transitions established between them to form sentences. Procedural techniques are also used for individual supporting movements or processes on the body (e.g., torso or ambient motion) coordinated to other body movements like the arm motions of a sign (McDonald et al., 2016).

SIGNED LANGUAGE TECHNOLOGIES IN L2 SIGNED LANGUAGE ASSESSMENT

The combination of signed language technology and L2 signed language assessment has not yet been explored to a great extent. Here, we present two ongoing projects related to SLR. The next section introduces work in combining signed language animation with mathematics assessment and L1 signed language assessment, respectively, that can be taken as indicators of where future work in applying signed language animation to L2 signed language assessment is likely to lead.

SLR in L2 Signed Language Learning and Assessment

At the moment, signed language education is conducted in a traditional manner, with students being taught by Deaf signers or hearing professional tutors who are licensed to teach signed language. However, classes tend to be on a weekly basis and are limited by the number of tutors available. An automated signed language assessment system could improve signed language education by allowing students to practice on their own and receive faster feedback. Furthermore, such a system would also give tutors the chance to go through more material during lectures by eliminating the need for repetitive assessment and feedback to each student.

As SLR methods are designed to be able to distinguish between signs and classify them, they are ideal tools to employ for automatic signed language assessment. There have been a few examples of SLR being adapted to use in signed language education. SignTutor (Aran, Ari et al., 2009) is one of the earlier applications, which utilized webcams and color gloves to provide feedback to ASL learners. Their system integrated hand shape, hand motion, and nonmanual head features to analyze and recognize signs from a small vocabulary of 19 signs. More recently, Zafrulla, Brashear, et al. (2011b) proposed CopyCat, a computer-assisted system with a user-friendly interface for Deaf children to encourage ASL practice. The system incorporated a video camera and color gloves with accelerometers attached to the wrists. Authors evaluated their system on 59 different phrases that are composed of a vocabulary of 19 signs (Zafrulla et al., 2010).

Another important component of automated signed language assessment systems is how the feedback is conveyed to the user. In their recent study, Huenerfauth et al. (2017) conducted a study to investigate how to best present video-based feedback to ASL learners. Their findings indicate that augmenting feedback into the learner's own sign video improved the user interaction. They also suggest that providing the correct ASL face and hand feature with the feedback resulted in better user learning experience.

As part of a 3-year project in Switzerland, Scalable Multimodal Sign Language Technology for Sign Language Learning and Assessment (SMILE),[2] developed a prototype of an automated signed language assessment system for L2 learners of Swiss German Sign Language (*Deutschschweizerische Gebärdensprache,* [DSGS]). The system assesses isolated signed language production in L2 learners of DSGS. The prototype focuses on a small set of isolated signs and has both practice and test modes. During practice, learners can perform a sign and are given direct feedback on how to improve by comparison against a reference sign. During test mode, a sequence of signs are recorded and

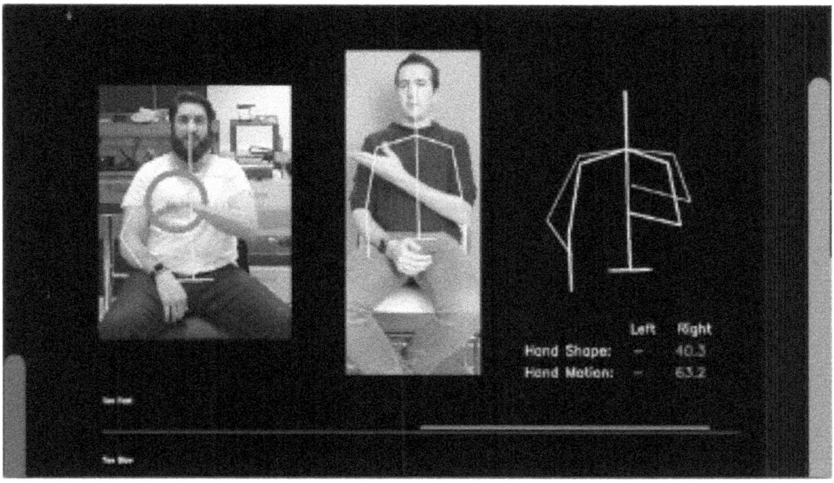

Figure 12.2.2 Screenshot of the SMILE assessment prototype.
From Project SMILE and University of Surrey (2019).

an overall score returned to the user. For each sign, the system additionally provides feedback on which aspects of the sign production need improvement. The system currently only focuses on the manual components of the sign (hand shape, location, motion, and speed of production). Figure 12.2.2 shows the interface of the application.

Signed Language Animation in Assessment

Ebling et al. (2017) created animations of DSGS signs by utilizing the Paula avatar as part of a receptive skills test (RST) for DSGS (Haug & Perrollaz, 2015). The DSGS RST is completed by Deaf children between ages 4 and 11 years. The test assesses morphological constructions of DSGS such as spatial verb morphology, negation, number, distribution, and verb agreement with 46 items. In its original form, an item consists of a video of a human signer performing a DSGS sequence, such as BÄR KLEIN ("BEAR SMALL"), APFEL VIELE ("APPLE MANY"), or BUB SCHAUEN-oben ("BOY LOOK-upward"). Test-takers are asked to pick the correct item among three or four images; that is, the image that best matches the content previously signed (single-selection multiple-choice items). Figure 12.2.3 shows the options given for the sequence APFEL VIELE, where B is the targeted response. The rationale behind including animations in a signed language test is that signed language avatars have the potential to increase motivation and interest in young learners of signed language, evoking the *persona effect* (Lester et al., 1997) that has been observed in pedagogical agents for children in spoken languages. While the acceptance of the individual animations has been assessed (Ebling et al., 2017), an evaluation of the comprehensibility of the animations in their designated context, the DSGS RST, among the target group remains to be carried out.

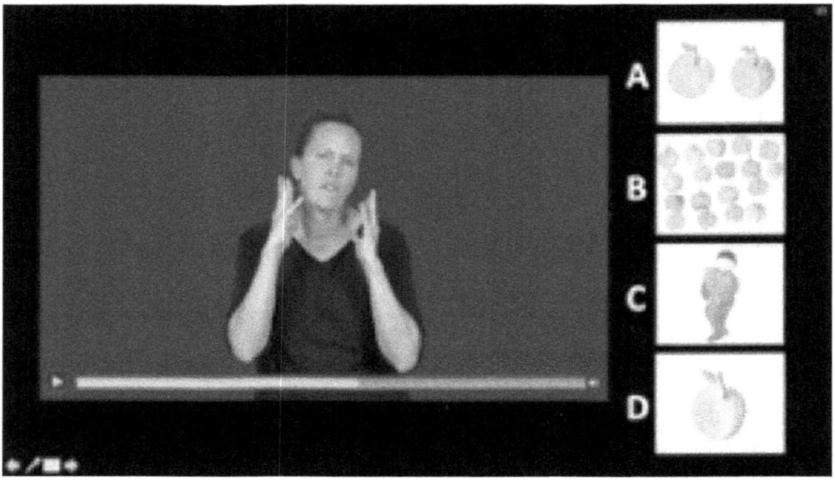

Figure 12.2.3 Item apfel viele ("apple many") in the DSGS Receptive Skills Test. From Haug & Perrollaz (2015).

Hansen et al. (2018) investigated both comprehension and acceptance of ASL animations in a mathematics test. The authors presented a total of 31 Deaf/hard-of-hearing US high-school and post-high school participants with 10 pre-college mathematics items. The items had the form of single-selection multiple-choice items with five answer options. Each item was shown to each participant in three conditions: with the English content (1) replaced by human-signed ASL, (2) replaced by avatar-signed ASL, and (3) unmodified (no signing involved). Not presenting the English original alongside the ASL content was motivated by the authors' intent to determine the comprehensibility and acceptance of the latter in isolation; in an authentic test scenario, the two modalities would likely co-occur.

The English-only condition (Condition 3) was always presented last; half of the participants saw Condition 1 first, the other half Condition 2. Participants were asked to solve the mathematics items as well as to provide an English translation of the signed content in Conditions 1 and 2. Translations were rated by human experts. As a proxy for comprehension, the authors investigated the results of both the actual mathematics task and the translation task. Notwithstanding order effects resulting from the repeated-measures design, the authors observed no significant difference in the mathematics scores in relation to signing mode (human signer vs. avatar). Similarly, no significant association between the scores of the translation task and the signing mode was found. Thus, with regard to comprehension (as operationalized by the mathematics and translation scores), no statistical difference as a function of signing mode was found. Regarding acceptance, the participants expressed a clear preference for human signing as opposed to avatar signing and judged the quality of the human signing to be superior to that of the avatar signing. Participants criticized the lack of facial expression and body movements in the avatar.

FUTURE DIRECTIONS

The field of automatic signed language assessment is still in its infancy. Similar to the historical progress of SLR, automatic signed language assessment has started by focusing on isolated signs and manual features. However, with the availability of datasets such as the SMILE Dataset (Ebling et al., 2018), the field will gain more attention from both computational linguists and computer vision researchers.

Following the footsteps of SLR, the next step for automatic signed language assessment is to move to the continuous domain, where nonmanual features are more prominent. To achieve continuous automatic signed language assessment, researchers will require more data. However, annotating continuous sequences with both manual and nonmanual feature is a laborious task and considerably more complex than working on isolated signs. One way to overcome this problem might be to exploit the recent development in the field of image synthesis using generative adversarial networks (A generative adversarial network is composed of two neural networks: a generative network and a discriminative network. These work together with one network trying to fool the other such that accuracy improves; see Goodfellow et al., 2014). Current state-of-the-art in the field is able to generate images of humans in unseen poses with promising performance (Ma et al., 2017; Siarohin et al., 2018), and preliminary work (Stoll et al., 2018) has already demonstrated its utility in the generation of sign. Using these methods, researchers could generate vast amounts of variant-acceptable sequences from prototypical signs. Another solution could lie in utilizing the currently available avatar-based signed language production systems and combining them with recent machine learning approaches (Shrivastava et al., 2017), which can transform simulated avatars into real-life appearing images.

Whether it is automatic SLR or signed language animation, one area that all research fields need is more explicit modeling of signed language linguistics. There is to date relatively little linguistic study at the scale required for machine learning on the fundamental building blocks and grammar of sign (e.g., the combined use of different articulators, sign syntax, and grammatical constructs such as the use of syntactic/topographic space and placement).

NOTES

1. https://www.sign-lang.uni-hamburg.de/dgs-korpus/index.php/dgs-korpus.html
2. https://www.idiap.ch/project/smile

REFERENCES

Aran, O., Ari, I., Akarun, L., Sankur, B., Benoit, A., Caplier, A., . . . Fanard, F. X. (2009). SignTutor: An interactive system for sign language tutoring. *IEEE Multimedia, 16*(1), 81–93. https://doi.org/10.1109/MMUL.2009.17

Aran, O., Burger, T., Caplier, A., & Akarun, L. (2009). A belief-based sequential fusion approach for fusing manual signs and non-manual signals. *Pattern Recognition, 42*(5), 812–822. https://doi.org/10.1016/j.patcog.2008.09.010

Buehler, P., Zisserman, A., & Everingham, M. (2009). Learning sign language by watching TV (using weakly aligned subtitles). In *IEEE Conference on Computer Vision and Pattern Recognition (CVPR)*, 2961–2968. https://doi.org/10.1109/CVPR.2009.5206523

Camgöz, N. C., Hadfield, S., Koller, O., & Bowden, R. (2017). SubUNets: End-to-end hand shape and continuous sign language recognition. In *IEEE International Conference on Computer Vision (ICCV)*, 3075–3084. https://doi.org/10.1109/ICCV.2017.332

Camgöz, N. C., Kındıroğlu, A. A., & Akarun, L. (2016b). Sign language recognition for assisting the deaf in hospitals. In M. Chetouani, J. Cohn, & A. A. Salah (Eds.), *Human Behavior Understanding* (vol. 9997, pp. 89–101). Springer International. https://doi.org/10.1007/978-3-319-46843-3_6

Camgöz, N. C., Kindiroglu, A. A., Karabuklu, S., Kelepir, M., Ozsoy, A. S., & Akarun, L. (2016a). BosphorusSign: A Turkish Sign Language recognition corpus in health and finance domains. In N. Calzolari, K. Choukri, T. Declerck, S. Goggi, M. Grobelnik, B. Maegaard, J. Mariani, H. Mazo, A. Moreno, J. Odijk, & S. Piperidis (Eds.), *International Conference on Language Resources and Evaluation (LREC)* (pp. 1383–1388). European Language Resources Association (ELRA).

Cao, Z., Simon, T., Wei, S.-E., & Sheikh, Y. (2017). Realtime multi-person 2D pose estimation using part affinity fields. 2017 IEEE Conference on Computer Vision and Pattern Recognition (CVPR), 1302–1310. https://doi.org/10.1109/CVPR.2017.143

Charles, J., Pfister, T., Everingham, M., & Zisserman, A. (2014). Automatic and efficient human pose estimation for sign language videos. *International Journal of Computer Vision, 110*(1), 70–90. https://doi.org/10.1007/s11263-013-0672-6

Cooper, H., & Bowden, R. (2009). Learning signs from subtitles: A weakly supervised approach to sign language recognition. *2009 IEEE Conference on Computer Vision and Pattern Recognition*, 2568–2574. https://doi.org/10.1109/CVPR.2009.5206647

Cooper, H., Holt, B., & Bowden, R. (2011). Sign language recognition. In T. B. Moeslund, A. Hilton, V. Krüger, & L. Sigal (Eds.), *Visual analysis of humans* (pp. 539–562). Springer London. https://doi.org/10.1007/978-0-85729-997-0_27

Cooper, H., Ong, E.-J., Pugeault, N., & Bowden, R. (2012). Sign language recognition using sub-units. *Journal of Machine Learning, 13*, 2205–2231.

Cooper, H. M., & Bowden, R. (2007). Sign language recognition using boosted volumetric features. *Proceedings MVA2007 IAPR Conference on Machine Vision Applications* (pp. 359–362). https://www.cvl.iis.u-tokyo.ac.jp/mva/proceedings/2007CD/papers/08-33.pdf

Cooper, H. M., & Bowden, R. (2010). Sign language using linguistically derived sub-units. *Proceedings of the 4th Workshop on Representation and Processing of Sign Languages: Corpora and Sign Language Technologies*, LREC 2010 (pp. 57–61). https://www.sign-lang.uni-hamburg.de/lrec2010/lrec_cslt_01.pdf

Cooper, H. M., Pugeault, N., & Bowden, R. (2011a) Reading the signs: A video based sign dictionary. *Proceedings IEEE International Conference on Computer Vision Workshops (ICCV)* (pp. 914–919). https://doi.org/10.1109/ICCVW.2011.6130349

Cox, S., Lincoln, M., Tryggvason, J., Nakisa, M., Wells, M., Tutt, M., & Abbott, S. (2002). Tessa, a system to aid communication with deaf people. *Proceedings of the Fifth International ACM Conference on Assistive Technologies—Assets '02*, 205. https://doi.org/10.1145/638249.638287

Crasborn, O. (2006). Nonmanual structures in sign language. In K. Brown (Ed.), *Encyclopedia of language & linguistics* (pp. 668–672). Elsevier.

Cui, R., Liu, H., & Zhang, C. (2017). Recurrent convolutional neural networks for continuous sign language recognition by staged optimization. *2017 IEEE Conference on Computer Vision and Pattern Recognition (CVPR),* 1610–1618. https://doi.org/10.1109/CVPR.2017.175

Ebling, S. (2013). Evaluating a Swiss German Sign Language avatar among the Deaf community. In *Proceedings of the 3rd International Symposium on Sign Language Translation and Avatar Technology (SLTAT).* Chicago, IL. www.zora.uzh.ch/85717/1/CAMERA_READY_sltat2013_submission_14.pdf

Ebling, S. (2016). *Automatic translation from German to synthesized Swiss German Sign Language* [Dissertation, Universität Zürich]. http://www.cl.uzh.ch/dam/jcr:8c0f6d30-05dc-4e31-9324-0ed7ef74214b/ebling_diss.pdf

Ebling, S., Camgöz, N. C., Braem, P. B., Tissi, K., Sidler-Miserez, S., Stoll, S., Hadfield, S., Haug, T., Bowden, R., Tornay, S., Razavi, M., & Magimai-Doss, M. (2018). SMILE Swiss German Sign Language Dataset. In *Proceedings of the 11th International Conference on Language Resources and Evaluation (LREC) 2018*. The European Language Resources Association (ELRA). https://aclanthology.org/L18-1666

Ebling, S., & Glauert, J. (2016). Building a Swiss German Sign Language avatar with JASigning and evaluating it among the Deaf community. *Universal Access in the Information Society, 15*(4), 577–587. https://doi.org/10.1007/s10209-015-0408-1

Ebling, S., Johnson, S., Wolfe, R., Moncrief, R., McDonald, J., Baowidan, S., Haug, T., Sidler-Miserez, S., & Tissi, K. (2017). Evaluation of animated Swiss German Sign Language fingerspelling sequences and signs. In M. Antona & C. Stephanidis (Eds.), *Universal access in human-computer interaction, LNCS* (pp. 1–13). Springer.

Efthimiou, E., Fotinea, S.-E., Hanke, T., Glauert, J., Bowden, R., Braffort, A., Collet, C., Maragos, P., & Lefebvre-Albaret, F. (2012). The Dicta-Sign Wiki: Enabling Web Communication for the Deaf. In K. Miesenberger, A. Karshmer, P. Penaz, & W. Zagler (Eds.), *Computers helping people with special needs* (pp. 205–212). Springer. https://doi.org/10.1007/978-3-642-31534-3_32

Elliott, R., Cooper, H., M., Ong, E., J., Glauert, J., Bowden, R., & Lefebvre-Albaret, F. (2011). Search-by-example in multilingual sign language databases. *Proceedings of the 2nd Sign Language Translation and Avatar Technology Workshop (SLTAT)*. http://vhg.cmp.uea.ac.uk/demo/SLTAT2011Dundee/

Elliott, R., Glauert, J. R. W., Kennaway, J. R., & Marshall, I. (2000). The development of language processing support for the ViSiCAST project. *Proceedings of the Fourth International ACM Conference on Assistive Technologies—Assets '00* (pp. 101–108). https://doi.org/10.1145/354324.354349

Forster, J., Schmidt, C., Hoyoux, T., Koller, O., Zelle, U., Piater, J. H., & Ney, H. (2012). RWTH-PHOENIX-Weather: A large vocabulary sign language recognition and translation corpus. In N. Calzolari, K. Choukri, T. Declerck, M. Doğan, B. Maegaard, J. Mariani, A. Moreno, J. Odijk, & S. Piperidis (Eds.), *Proceedings International Conference on Language Resources and Evaluation (LREC)* (pp. 3785–3789). European Language Resources Association (ELRA).

Forster, J., Schmidt, C., Koller, O., Bellgardt, M., & Ney, H. (2014). Extensions of the sign language recognition and translation corpus RWTH-PHOENIX-Weather. In N. Calzolari, K. Choukri, T. Declerck, H. Loftsson, B. Maegaard, J. Mariani, A. Moreno, J. Odijk, & S. Piperidis (Eds.), *Proceedings of the 9th International Conference on Language Resources and Evaluation (LREC)* (pp. 1911–1916). European Language Resources Association (ELRA).

Gibet, S., Courty, N., Duarte, K., & Naour, T. L. (2011). The SignCom system for data-driven animation of interactive virtual signers: Methodology and evaluation. *ACM Transactions on Interactive Intelligent Systems, 1*(1), 6.

Goodfellow, I., Pouget-Abadie, J., Mirza, M., Xu, B., Warde-Farley, D., Ozair, S., Courville, A., & Bengio, Y. (2014). Generative adversarial nets. In Z. Ghahramani, M. Welling, C. Cortes, N. D. Lawrence, & K. Q. Weinberger (Eds.), *Advances in neural information processing systems 27* (pp. 2672–2680). Curran Associates, Inc.

Hanke, T. (2001). ViSiCAST Deliverable D5-1: Interface definitions. Technical report, ViSiCAST project. http://www.visicast.cmp.uea.ac.uk/Papers/ViSiCAST_D5-1v017rev2.pdf

Hanke, T., König, L., Wagner, S., & Matthes, S. (2010). DGS corpus & Dicta-Sign: The Hamburg studio setup. *Proceedings of the 4th Workshop on the Representation and Processing of Sign Languages: Corpora and Sign Language Technologies,* 106–109. www.lrec-conf.org/proceedings/lrec2010/workshops/W13.pdf

Hansen, E. G., Loew, R. C., Laitusis, C. C., Kushalnagar, P., Pagliaro, C. M., & Kurz, C. (2018). Usability of American Sign Language videos for presenting mathematics assessment Content. *Journal of Deaf Studies and Deaf Education,* 23(3), 284–294. https://doi.org/10.1093/deafed/eny008

Huenerfauth, M., Gale, E., Penly, B., Pillutla, S., Willard, M., & Hariharan, D. (2017). Evaluation of Language Feedback Methods for Student Videos of American Sign Language. *ACM Transactions on Accessible Computing, 10*(1), 2:1–2:30. https://doi.org/10.1145/3046788

Haug, T., & Perrollaz, R. (2015). Verständnistest Deutschschweizer Gebärdensprache. Unpublished test, Interkantonale Hochschule für Heilpädagogik.

Kipp, M., Nguyen, Q., Heloir, A., & Matthes, S. (2011). Assessing the deaf user perspective on sign language avatars. *The Proceedings of the 13th International ACM SIGACCESS Conference on Computers and Accessibility,* 107–114. https://doi.org/10.1145/2049536.2049557

Koller, O., Ney, H., & Bowden, R. (2013). May the force be with you: Force-aligned signwriting for automatic subunit annotation of corpora. *2013 10th*

IEEE International Conference and Workshops on Automatic Face and Gesture Recognition (FG), 1–6. https://doi.org/10.1109/FG.2013.6553777

Koller, O., Ney, H., & Bowden, R. (2015). Deep learning of mouth shapes for sign language. *2015 IEEE International Conference on Computer Vision Workshop (ICCVW)*, 477–483. https://doi.org/10.1109/ICCVW.2015.69

Koller, O., Ney, H., & Bowden, R. (2016). Deep hand: How to train a CNN on 1 million hand images when your data is continuous and weakly labelled. *2016 IEEE Conference on Computer Vision and Pattern Recognition (CVPR)*, 3793–3802. https://doi.org/10.1109/CVPR.2016.412

Koller, O., Zargaran, S., & Ney, H. (2017). Re-Sign: Re-Aligned End-to-End Sequence Modelling with Deep Recurrent CNN-HMMs. *2017 IEEE Conference on Computer Vision and Pattern Recognition (CVPR)*, 3416–3424. https://doi.org/10.1109/CVPR.2017.364

Koller, O., Zargaran, S., Ney, H., & Bowden, R. (2016). Deep sign: Hybrid CNN-HMM for continuous sign language recognition. *Proceedings of the British Machine Vision Conference 2016*, 136.1–136.12. https://doi.org/10.5244/C.30.136

Lester, J. C., Converse, S. A., Kahler, S. E., Barlow, S. T., Stone, B. A., & Bhogal, R. S. (1997). The persona effect: Affective impact of animated pedagogical agents. *Proceedings of the SIGCHI Conference on Human Factors in Computing Systems—CHI '97*, 359–366. https://doi.org/10.1145/258549.258797

Ma, L., Jia, X., Sun, Q., Schiele, B., Tuytelaars, T., & Van Gool, L. (2017). Pose guided person image generation. In I. Guyon, U. V. Luxburg, S. Bengio, H. Wallach, R. Fergus, S. Vishwanathan, & R. Garnett (Eds.), *Advances in neural information processing systems 30* (pp. 406–416). Curran Associates, Inc.

McDonald, J., Wolfe, R., Johnson, S., Baowidan, S., Moncrief, R., & Guo, N. (2017, July 14). An Improved Framework for Layering Linguistic Processes in Sign Language Generation: Why there should never be a "brows" tier [Presentation]. HCI International 2017, Symposium on Sign Language Translation and Avatar Technology, Vancouver, BC, Canada.

McDonald, J., Wolfe, R., Moncrief, R., & Baowidan, S. (2016). A computational model of role shift to support the synthesis of signed language. 12th Theoretical Issues in Sign Language Research (TISLR), Melbourne, Australia, January 4-7 (2016).

Mercer, K. C. R. (1993). Introduction to the special issue on computational linguistics using large corpora. *Computational Linguistics*, *19*(1), 1–24.

Moore, S., & Bowden, R. (2009). The effects of pose on facial expression recognition. *Proceedings of the British Machine Vision Conference 2009*, 79.1–79.11. https://doi.org/10.5244/C.23.79

Ong, E.-J., Cooper, H., Pugeault, N., & Bowden, R. (2012). Sign language recognition using sequential pattern trees. *2012 IEEE Conference on Computer Vision and Pattern Recognition*, 2200–2207. https://doi.org/10.1109/CVPR.2012.6247928

Ong, E.-N., Koller, O., Pugeault, N., & Bowden, R. (2014). Sign spotting using hierarchical sequential patterns with temporal intervals. *2014 IEEE Conference on Computer Vision and Pattern Recognition*, 1931–1938. https://doi.org/10.1109/CVPR.2014.248

Pfister, T., Charles, J., & Zisserman, A. (2013). Large-scale learning of sign language by watching TV (using co-occurrences). In T. Burghardt, D. Damen,

W. Mayol-Cuevas, & M. Mirmehdi (Eds.), *British Machine Vision Conference (BMVC)*, 1–11. http://dx.doi.org/10.5244/C.27.20

Prillwitz, S., Leven, R., Zienert, H., Hanke, T., & Henning, J. (1989). *HamNoSys: Version 2.0: An introductory guide*. Signum.

Schembri, A., Fenlon, J., Rentelis, R., Reynolds, S., & Cormier, K. (2013). Building the British Sign Language corpus. *Language Documentation & Conservation, 7*, 136–154.

Shrivastava, A., Pfister, T., Tuzel, O., Susskind, J., Wang, W., & Webb, R. (2017). Learning from simulated and unsupervised images through adversarial training. *2017 IEEE Conference on Computer Vision and Pattern Recognition (CVPR)*, 2242–2251. https://doi.org/10.1109/CVPR.2017.241

Siarohin, A., Sangineto, E., Lathuiliere, S., & Sebe, N. (2018). Deformable GANs for pose-based human image generation. ArXiv:1801.00055 [Cs]. http://arxiv.org/abs/1801.00055

Starner, T., Weaver, J., & Pentland, A. (1998). Real-time American sign language recognition using desk and wearable computer based video. *IEEE Transactions on Pattern Analysis and Machine Intelligence, 20*(12), 1371–1375. https://doi.org/10.1109/34.735811

Stoll, S., Camgöz, N. C., Hadfield, S., & Bowden, R. (2018). Sign language production using neural machine translation and generative adversarial networks. *Proceedings of the 29th British Machine Vision Conference (BMVC 2018)*. 29th British Machine Vision Conference (BMVC 2018), Northumbria University, Newcastle Upon Tyne, UK.

Wang, H., Chai, X., Hong, X., Zhao, G., & Chen, X. (2016). Isolated sign language recognition with Grassmann Covariance Matrices. *ACM Transactions on Accessible Computing, 8*(4), 1–21. https://doi.org/10.1145/2897735

Wei, S.-E., Ramakrishna, V., Kanade, T., & Sheikh, Y. (2016). Convolutional pose machines. *2016 IEEE Conference on Computer Vision and Pattern Recognition (CVPR)*, 4724–4732. https://doi.org/10.1109/CVPR.2016.511

Yin, F., Chai, X., & Chen, X. (2016). Iterative reference driven metric learning for signer independent isolated sign language recognition. In B. Leibe, J. Matas, N. Sebe, & M. Welling (Eds.), *Computer vision—ECCV 2016* (vol. 9911, pp. 434–450). Springer International. https://doi.org/10.1007/978-3-319-46478-7_27

Zafrulla, Z., Brashear, H., Presti, P., Hamilton, H., & Starner, T. (2011b). CopyCat: An American Sign Language game for deaf children. *Face and Gesture 2011*, 647–647. https://doi.org/10.1109/FG.2011.5771325

Zafrulla, Z., Brashear, H., Starner, T., Hamilton, H., & Presti, P. (2011a). American Sign Language recognition with the Kinect. *Proceedings of the 13th International Conference on Multimodal Interfaces—ICMI '11*, 279. https://doi.org/10.1145/2070481.2070532

Zafrulla, Z., Brashear, H., Yin, P., Presti, P., Starner, T., & Hamilton, H. (2010). American Sign Language phrase verification in an educational game for deaf children. *Proceedings of the 2010 20th International Conference on Pattern Recognition* (pp. 3846–3849). Istanbul, Turkey: IEEE.

12.3

Discussion on New Technologies in Spoken and Signed Language Assessment

Sarah Ebling, Phuong Nguyen, Volker Hegelheimer, Necati Cihan Camgöz, and Richard Bowden

In this section, we discuss the implications that second language (L2) spoken assessment technologies and signed language assessment technologies have for the opposite field. Specifically, we discuss how signed language recognition (SLR) technology can be applied for the assessment of interactional competence in L2 spoken language assessment. Moreover, we outline assessment management systems and the improvement of signed language recognition and signed language animation technologies as important steps to support L2 signed language assessment. We also propose directions for future technological developments in both spoken language and signed language assessment.

THE USE OF SLR TECHNOLOGY IN THE ASSESSMENT AND TEACHING OF ADDITIONAL CONSTRUCTS OF SPOKEN LANGUAGE

Many language assessment experts have agreed that interactional competence, defined as the ability to comprehend spoken input and produce appropriate language in response to the input by using strategies such as negotiating meaning, taking turns, and providing visual cues, is an important aspect of oral proficiency (Louma, 2004; Ockey, 2018; Nakatsuhara et al., 2018). While current technologies for automated scoring of spoken responses have, to some extent, developed to assess test-takers' oral proficiency (see Chapter 9.1), they are not designed to take into account the assessment of interactional competence, especially the test-takers' use of facial expressions and body language. Therefore, the use of SLR technology could help score this aspect of oral proficiency automatically. The use of SLR technology is conceptually supported

Sarah Ebling, Phuong Nguyen, Volker Hegelheimer, Necati Cihan Camgöz, and Richard Bowden, *Discussion on New Technologies in Spoken and Signed Language Assessment* In: *The Handbook of Language Assessment Across Modalities*. Edited by: Tobias Haug, Wolfgang Mann, and Ute Knoch, Oxford University Press. © Oxford University Press 2022. DOI: 10.1093/oso/9780190885052.003.0037 by the fact that both spoken and signed language research make use of similar theoretical inventories when analyzing or producing facial and body movement, such as the Facial Action Coding System (FACS) (Ekman & Friesen, 1978).

In a classroom context, SLR technology could also be integrated with other learning tools that provide automated feedback to the learners' oral proficiency. In this way, learners are provided with feedback pertaining to not only traditional aspects of speaking ability, such as pronunciation, fluency, and grammatical accuracy, but also to appropriate nonverbal cues (a component of interactional competence), such as facial expressions, hand gestures, and shoulder movements.

As noted in Chapter 12.2 on the use of new technologies in L2 signed language assessment, current SLR technology needs to be improved to recognize more continuous sequences of manual and nonmanual features in addition to signs and manual features in isolation. When SLR systems become more robust in handling a variety of nonverbal features, they will become an invaluable tool to help assess test-takers' interactional competence and help learners improve in this area.

Assessment Management Systems for Signed Languages

As Haug et al. (2020) show, assessment management systems for signed language that allow the creation, administration, and analysis of signed language tests to date do not exist. The Signed Qualitative Usability Online Testing Environment (SignQUOTE) (Schnepp et al., 2011) represented an attempt at such a tool. Haug and Ebling (2019) used a popular survey environment, LimeSurvey, to implement a yes/no vocabulary test for Swiss German Sign Language (*Deutschschweizerische Gebärdensprache* [DSGS]). The comments provided by the learners on the suitability of the web-based DSGS vocabulary self-assessment instrument provided feedback toward improvement of the system.

IMPROVEMENT OF SLR TECHNOLOGY TO MATCH SPOKEN LANGUAGE TESTING SCENARIOS

The state of research in SLR technology previously described is precisely the reason why automatic scoring techniques in L2 signed language assessment still lag behind those of L2 spoken language assessment: to be able to score unrestricted signed discourse (comparable to the testing scenario of Speech-Rater outlined in Chapter 12.1), recognition above the isolated-sign level is needed. For this, an intermediate step will be supporting automatic assessment of sentence repetition tests that are available for signed languages (for DSGS, see, e.g., Haug et al., 2020). This will more closely resemble a signed language version of the Duolingo or the Versant testing scenarios described in the spoken language assessment section of Chapter 12.1.

What is more, to be able to automatically judge common aspects of L2 assessment (such as fluency, pronunciation, vocabulary, or grammatical accuracy) for signed languages, linguistic preprocessing tools such as tokenizers, part-of-speech [PoS] taggers, syntactic parsers, and so on are needed. While these exist for many spoken languages, they are largely lacking in the case of signed languages (for a noteworthy exception, see the PoS tagger for Swedish Sign Language developed by Östling et al., 2015). This is primarily due to the conceptual difficulty of determining the beginning and end of a sign (Hanke et al., 2012) as well as the immature state of signed language grammar writing: in 2015, Palfreyman et al. stated that "not a single reference grammar of a signed language has been published that meets the common standards set by spoken language reference grammars" (p. 179). More recently, such a reference grammar has been released for New Zealand Sign Language (McKee, 2015), and reference grammars for other signed languages are under way as a result of a COST Action that produced a blueprint for reference grammars (Quer et al., 2017) and a subsequent project that aims at implementing (fragments of) reference grammars using this blueprint framework. However, efforts in implementing syntactic parsers are still in their infancy.

It is worth noting that, different from the case of spoken languages, there is not a single signed language that is best resourced (that language being English in the case of spoken languages); while American Sign Language is certainly a very widespread signed language that is starting to influence the lexical inventory of other signed languages, in terms of language resources such as corpora, lexicons, and so on, it is not equipped markedly better than other signed languages. The emergence of resources for signed languages is heavily dependent on funding opportunities, and, with the recent efforts of funders targeting minority languages, such languages have often been able to create considerable resources. Such is the case, for example, for DSGS, a small language even in signed language terms, which features a lexicon of around 9,000 entries and several corpora (Boyes Braem & Ebling, 2016).

DRAWING ON VISUAL SPEECH ANIMATION TECHNIQUES FOR SIGNED LANGUAGE ANIMATION

As has been shown in the signed language portion of this chapter, the use of signed language animation in L2 assessment is still in its infancy. Partly, this is due to the state of the underlying animation technology. To create more faithful animations, work on the nonmanual aspects of signing has been emphasized most prominently in previous signed language avatar comprehensibility and acceptance studies (Kipp et al., 2011, and subsequent). This pertains, among other features, to *mouthings*, which are mouth movements related to spoken language words. To warrant faithful rendering of such mouthings, signed language animation has to draw on work in visual speech animation in the context of spoken languages (i.e., work in animating the speech of characters in movies, games, and so on). Here, signed language animation has yet to adopt the concept of *dynamic visemes* (Taylor et al., 2012) that are capable of capturing visual coarticulation.

FUTURE DIRECTIONS

Given the current development and potential of signed language technologies, the field of L2 spoken assessment is expected to integrate these technologies into various phases of the language testing cycle. For example, in the scoring phase, current automatic speech recognition systems could be used in combination with automatic SLR systems to more thoroughly assess various aspects of the oral communication construct. Once the integration of signed language technologies is implemented in L2 spoken tests, research could be undertaken to investigate how such tests can facilitate test authenticity, fairness, score reliability, the validity of test score interpretation and use, and, eventually, the impact they have on L2 instruction.

We have also demonstrated that the development of SLR systems that operate on a sentence or even a discourse level requires large amounts of data. Creating such data is incredibly time-consuming. Therefore, in analogy to current work in automatic processing of spoken languages, future automatic signed language processing approaches will have to pursue a two-step solution: training deep learning models on data that are available in comparatively large quantities (e.g., broadcast footage of signed language produced by hearing interpreters) and fine-tuning on data that are closer to the desired use case; namely signed language produced by native users/early learners of a signed language that ideally comes with rich linguistic annotation.

Research on signed language assessment in virtual environments is still in its infancy. An important aspect here is that the visual modality serves both as a means of conveying language and of setting the scene, while the two functions are distributed across two channels (acoustic and visual) in the case of speaking tests for spoken language.

REFERENCES

Boyes Braem, P., & Ebling, S. (2016). Preventing too many cooks from spoiling the broth: Some questions to consider for collaboration between projects in iLex. *Proceedings of the 7th LREC Workshop on the Representation and Processing of Sign Languages*, 25–28. Portorož, Slovenia.

Ekman, P., & Friesen, W. V. (1978). *Facial action coding system: A technique for the measurement of facial movement*. Consulting Psychologists Press.

Hanke, T., Matthes, S., Regen, A., & Worseck, S. (2012). Where does a sign start and end? Segmentation of continuous signing. *Proceedings of the 5th LREC Worksshop on the Representation and Processing of Sign Languages*, 69–74. Istanbul, Turkey.

Haug, T., Batty, A. O., Venetz, M., Notter, C., Girard-Groeber, S., Knoch, U., & Audeoud, M. (2020). Validity evidence for a sentence repetition test of Swiss German Sign Language. *Language Testing, 37*(3), 412–434. https://doi.org/10.1177/0265532219898382

Haug, T., & Ebling, S. (2019). Using open-source software for sign language learning and assessment: The case of a web-delivered yes/no vocabulary test for Swiss German Sign Language. *International Journal of Emerging Technologies in Learning (iJET), 14*(9), 188–196. https://doi.org/10.3991/ijet.v14i19.11123

Haug, T., Mann, W., Hoskin, J., Dumbrill, H. (2020). L1 sign language tests and assessment procedures and evaluation. In R. Rosen (Ed.), *The Routledge handbook of sign language pedagogy* (pp. 114–134). Routledge.

Kipp, M., Nguyen, Q., Heloir, A., & Matthes, S. (2011). Assessing the deaf user perspective on sign language avatars. *Proceedings of the 13th International ACM SIGACCESS Conference on Computers and Accessibility (ASSETS)*, 107–114. Dundee, Scotland.

Louma, S. (2004). *Assessing speaking*. Cambridge University Press.

McKee, R. (2015). *New Zealand Sign Language: A reference grammar*. Bridget Williams Books.

Nakatsuhara, F., May, L., Lam, D., & Galaczi, E. (2018). Learning-oriented feedback and interactional competence. *Cambridge Research Notes, 70*, 4–67.

Ockey, G. J. (2018). Oral language proficiency tests. In J. L. Liontas (Ed.), *The TESOL encyclopedia of English language teaching, 3*, 1–29. Wiley-Blackwell. https://doi.org/10.1002/9781118784235.eelt0234

Östling, R., Börstell, C., & Wallin, L. (2015). Enriching the Swedish Sign Language Corpus with part of speech tags using joint Bayesian word alignment and annotation transfer. *Proceedings of the 20th Nordic Conference of Computational Linguistics (NODALIDA 2015)*, 263–268. Vilnius, Lithuania.

Palfreyman, N., Sagara, K., & Zeshan, U. (2015). Methods in carrying out language typological research. In E. Orfanidou, B. Woll, & G. Morgan (Eds.), *Research methods in sign language studies: A practical guide* (pp. 173–192). Wiley-Blackwell.

Quer, J., Cecchetto, C., Donati, C., Geraci, C., Kelepir, M., Pfau, R., & Steinbach, M. (2017). *Signgram Blueprint. A guide to sign language grammar writing*. De Gruyter Mouton.

Schnepp, J., Wolfe, R., Shiver, B., McDonald, J., & Toro, J. (2011). Signquote: A remote testing facility for eliciting signed qualitative feedback. *Proceedings of the Sign Language Technology and Avatar Translation Workshop*, Dundee, Scotland. http://vhg.cmp.uea.ac.uk/demo/SLTAT2011Dundee/4.pdf

Taylor, S. L., Mahler, M., Theobald, B.-J., & Matthews, I. (2012). Dynamic units of visual speech. *Proceedings of the ACM SIGGRAPH/Eurographics Symposium on Computer Animation*, 275–284, Lausanne, Switzerland.

Epilogue

Finding Common Ground in Language Assessment of Signed and Spoken Language: So Far and Yet So Close

Wolfgang Mann, Tobias Haug, and Ute Knoch

Editing a book that involves contributions from multiple authors working in the same field is a challenge. Doing the same with 49 specialists from different fields—in our case spoken and signed language assessment with its many subareas (e.g., applied linguistics, psycholinguistics, deaf education, speech language therapy, computational linguistics)—is a mammoth task and has never been done before. In the case of this volume, it all started with a seemingly simple idea: to bring colleagues from two independent lines of research together to initiate a dialogue about issues linked to language assessment, share their experiences with one another, discuss similarities and differences, and explore the possible impact of one field on the other. One of the (many) challenges of such a project was to push the contributing authors from each field outside of their own comfort zones by asking them not only to compose an individual chapter in their area of expertise but also to jointly write a discussion chapter which draws on key issues that were highlighted in the individual chapters. This was met by many with some raised eyebrows and initial hesitation to commit to such a dual task but, in the end, 49 authors from different disciplines and backgrounds agreed to be a part of this project. While preparing this edition, we have learned much but also came to realize that this is just the first step in what we hope will serve as a starting point for many collaborative lines of research in the future that will benefit both fields and further our knowledge of language assessment. In assembling a collection as diverse and unique as this one, we have discovered that, aside from many differences between the fields of signed and spoken language assessment—and which includes at least one elephant in the room (i.e., the availability of relevant literature and tests in the area of signed language assessment)—there are also a surprising number of similarities. These similarities and differences became apparent

Wolfgang Mann, Tobias Haug, and Ute Knoch, *Epilogue* In: *The Handbook of Language Assessment Across Modalities*. Edited by: Tobias Haug, Wolfgang Mann, and Ute Knoch, Oxford University Press. © Oxford University Press 2022. DOI: 10.1093/oso/9780190885052.003.0038 throughout this volume and some resurfaced across chapters. For this reason, we feel that the following topics warrant closer attention in this epilogue: standardization samples, native speaker/signer norms, dynamic assessment, and use of the Common European Framework of Reference (CEFR).

STANDARDIZATION SAMPLE

Looking across the 12 themes of this volume, one aspect that keeps reappearing in multiple chapters is how the standardization sample size should be considered. Upon first glance, this issue seems to be inherently linked to signed language assessment, given the small and heterogeneous nature of the deaf and/or hard-of-hearing (D/HH), signing population, which makes developing norms for subgroups even more problematic. As Chiat, Herman, Rowley, and Roy (Chapter 1.3) point out, while standardized assessments of spoken language are normed on and predominantly intended for use with native speakers of that language, standardized assessments of signed language are intrinsically designed for use with a population of whom only a minority have the opportunity of learning signed language as their native language or from very early in life, in general before 2 or 3 years of age. Boudreault, Camilleri, and Enns (Chapter 2.3) add that this sets an adequately high benchmark of typical native signed language development but does not preclude the use of these assessments with children who have had limited exposure to the signed language in question. On the contrary, using native signers as a baseline is seen as an opportunity to measure the impact of signed language deprivation (Enns & Herman, 2011) and consequently identify the need for educational and other measures to be put in place. This links in with later discussions by Mann, Hoskin, Hasson, and Dumbrill (Chapter 3.3) and Murphy, Frizelle, McKean, and Quinto-Pozos (Chapter 5.3) and on how the use of standardized signed language assessments can render it hard to differentiate between test-takers' difficulties due to language delay or deprivation and difficulties due to language disorders or impairments, even if it means that all signing children can be assessed. As a consequence, test administrators need to incorporate a wider range of sources of information when interpreting the child's language performance—most importantly, an evaluation of the child's language history and exposure to signed language.

Extending the application of standardized assessments for spoken language (based on monolingual children) in a similar way with culturally and linguistically diverse children (CLD) may offer a way to advocate for additional services (including language therapy, enhanced peer interaction, placement in a signing educational environment), rather than taking a "wait and see" approach.

USE OF NATIVE SPEAKER/NATIVE SIGNER NORMS

The use of first language (L1) signer norms for describing achievement on assessments or assessment tasks is common in signed language assessment. Enns and Boudreault (Chapter 2.2) and others (e.g., Chapters 4.2, 4.3, and 5.3) describe the complexity of identifying and defining the L1 of deaf signers where the minority of children born deaf come from families with one or more deaf parents. Access to natural, quality interaction with highly proficient signers is varied for the others and usually depends on the availability of such communication in schooling or is determined by parental choices. For this reason, there is considerable variability of signed language skills within the Deaf community. Enns and Boudreault (Chapter 2.2) comment on the challenge arising from this for establishing assessment norms where the identification of norms requires the collection of data from children with access to signed language from birth or at least within the first 2–3 years of life. Their suggestion to accept native signers' norms for the use in assessment development and score interpretation in signed language assessments bears similarity to Camilleri's description of the use of norms in spoken language (Chapter 2.1).

The use of native speaker norms was also part and parcel of the applied linguistics and second language (L2) acquisition literature until the late 1990s. Mirroring this trend, native speaker norms were also common practice in L2 assessments at the time, most evident by the description of performance criteria in rating scales, where references to native speaker performances were common at the higher levels. In fact, in the late 1980s and early 1990s, almost all well-known scales used for L2 assessment (such as the Interagency Language Roundtable [ILR] scale, the Foreign Services Institute [FSI] scale, or the Australian Second Language Proficiency Scale [ASLPR]) all made references to native speakers at the higher levels. The reliance on native speaker norms in language learning and language assessment has since been criticized for a number of reasons (see, e.g., Davies, 1991, 2004, 2011, 2013; Piller, 2001, 2002). Davies (2013), for example, explores what it means to be a native speaker and how native speakers differ from native users (highly proficient non-native speakers who commonly live and work in English-speaking communities). He questions what the first group can do that the second cannot and arrives at the conclusion that there is often very little difference between the two groups. This is because native speakers are most commonly defined in what they can do with the standard language, and this definition does not automatically rule out native users. In fact, many people speaking and hearing English from birth as their only language are exposed to varieties, rather than standard language. Davies (2011) summarizes ways in which the native speaker has been characterized and argues that the native user, provided with the right conditions, is able to do anything that the native speaker can do, and the only characteristic that sets native speakers apart from native users is that they acquire the L1 in early childhood. This then, he argues, requires a classification based on background to identify a native speaker, rather than one based on language proficiency (see also Piller, 2001). Another challenge to the definition of the native speaker is multilingualism. The native speaker is most commonly defined as a monolingual (see, e.g., Crystal, 1997) who lives in a homogenous speech community. In reality, however, the majority of the world's population is multilingual, showing, as Piller (2001) argues, that the concept of the native speaker is "geared towards the exception, rather than the norm" (p. 4). Language development of children who learn a language from an early age is also often halted due to migration to a new country and subsequent schooling in a new language.

In language assessments scales, the native speaker was also commonly conceptualized as highly literate, able to produce many different text types with ease. Research on literacy levels in various countries has, perhaps unsurprisingly, cast doubt on this reality that all "native speakers" are able to reach such literacy levels (see, e.g., the results from the 2006 Adult Literacy and Life Skills Survey published by the Australian Bureau of Statistics, 2008). As a result, the performance of native speakers on language tests has been questioned (see, e.g., Hamilton et al., 1993). All these issues related to the concept of the native speaker led to Kramsch's (1997) definition of the native speaker as "an imaginary construct—a canonically literate monolingual middle-class member of a largely fictional national community whose citizens share a belief in a common history and a common destiny" (p. 363).

In spoken L2 assessment circles, the use of native speaker norms has generally been abandoned. There are other opportunities for benchmarking performance, as McKee and Frost (Chapter 10.3) point out. For example, in the case of an assessment for L2 signers training to become teachers of deaf children, performance criteria could be drawn up by examining closely (possibly by means of discourse analysis or the review of performance samples more broadly) what adult signers at different proficiency levels can actually do with the language. This can then form the basis of scale descriptions. An assessment that has a clear target language use domain, such as the example of teachers in deaf education, could also draw on the use of indigenous criteria (Jacoby, 1998; Jacoby & McNamara, 1999; Knoch & Macqueen, 2020), where domain insiders (e.g., experienced teachers working in a similar context) are asked to verbalize what they value at different proficiency levels. These verbalizations can then be used to directly feed into the assessment criteria (see, e.g., Elder et al., 2013; Pill, 2013).

DYNAMIC ASSESSMENT

Another aspect that keeps reappearing across chapter and themes is the need for alternatives to standardized assessments that are closely scripted and do not allow any assistance in the child's performance. These tests are based on the assumption that the testee is fully aware of what they are asked to do and, thus, perform to the best of their abilities. As pointed out by Mann and colleagues (Chapter 3.3), many D/HH children tend to perform low on standardized language assessments for reasons that are not always immediately apparent. Several chapters in this volume, including Chiat and colleagues (Chapter 1.3), Mann and colleagues (Chapter 3.3), Murphy and colleagues (Chapter 5.3), and Bedore and colleagues (Chapter 6.3) demonstrate that this is not limited to the D/HH population but also exist in spoken language assessment, with similar challenges arising from different profiles of subgroups of the population, including CLD children and children with special educational needs. In this context, Chiat and colleagues make reference to Gathercole, Kennedy, and Thomas (2016), who suggested a useful distinction between language proficiency and language ability and propose to differentiate tests to assess these populations. Chiat and colleagues (Chapter 1.3) call for caution that, while a combination of standardized tests to measure receptive and expressive language can provide a useful indication of the child's language knowledge and proficiency, and importantly, their readiness to meet the language demands of the classroom, test developers need to caution test users about the interpretation of scores that are below the normal range because tests do not reveal whether children's performance is low due to limited language experience or whether it is low due to a language disorder. This notion is echoed by Boudreault and colleagues (Chapter 2.3). It is important to bear in mind that the different sources of difficulty (e.g., language delay vs. language deprivation vs. language impairment) have different implications for the support that children need, but teasing them apart is no easy matter, particularly when assessing children who use signed language. For children who use a signed language to communicate, particularly careful consideration must be given to the timing, quality, and quantity of language exposure, and decisions about language disorder must be determined based on these factors and from comparisons with children who have similar language experiences. In light of the young state of signed language (assessment) research combined with the lack of knowledge regarding best practice in the assessment of signed languages, specifically in D/HH subpopulations (e.g., CLD, developmental language disorder [DLD]) Bedore and colleagues (Chapter 6.3) suggest that much can be learned from advances in knowledge of appropriate assessment of spoken languages for hearing children from these groups. One approach that has shown success in differentiating low test performances by bilingual children with a language impairment from their typically developing peers with equally low performance is dynamic assessment (DA). As described by Mann and colleagues (Chapter 3.1), DA combines teaching and assessment within a single assessment procedure that uses a mediated learning experience to evaluate children's language learning ability. Bedore and colleagues (Chapter 6.3) elaborated on its use to evaluate skills in domains such as vocabulary, macrostructure and microstructures in narratives, classifier use, and grammatical structures. In comparison, the more recent work with signing D/HH children has focused exclusively on assessing vocabulary knowledge (e.g., Mann et al., 2014, 2015). As pointed out by Mann and colleagues (Chapter 3.3), this situation bears similarity to the number and variety of available "static" assessment for signed language versus spoken language, leaving researchers, clinicians, and practitioners with limited resources appropriate for testing signing children. The recommendation by Mann and colleagues to further explore the potential of DA for use with signing D/HH children to address current gaps in our knowledge about different aspects of signed languages and their development finds support from other authors, including Chiat and colleagues (Chapter 1.3), Murphy and colleagues (Chapter 5.3), and Bedore and colleagues (Chapter 6.3).

USE OF THE COMMON EUROPEAN FRAMEWORK OF REFERENCE

One topic that has been addressed across a number of chapters is the use of the CEFR as a standards framework for both spoken and signed language assessment (e.g., Chapters 7.2, 9.2, 10.1, and 11.2). The 2020 version of the CEFR Companion Volume (Council of Europe, 2020) includes from the original CEFR adapted scales and descriptors for signed language (Leeson et al., 2016) and the development of signed language–specific descriptors (Keller et al., 2017) to make it modality-inclusive.

The document created by Leeson et al. (2016) is likely to be of use for teachers and test developers across various contexts because it is the first to set out a proficiency framework that can be used for the development of signed language assessments (as well as course planning). And, of course, the inclusion of descriptors for signed language sends a positive statement that signed language has equal status to other languages in Europe. Additionally, the CEFR has only been a topic in signed language education for a number of years, but it already had a considerable impact, for example, on signed language teaching and assessment and the training of signed language teachers and signed language interpreters. Nevertheless, in the future, it may face similar points of critique to those described for spoken language. (For a discussion on the counterarguments of the critique, see North, 2020).

Deygers (2019; Deygers et al., 2018) points out that the criticisms of the CEFR have been either related to its use or its scientific underpinnings (i.e., its development and content). In the case of the use of the CEFR for signed languages, the criticisms around the CEFR's development and content are probably more relevant here, as described next.

Fulcher (2004) argues that many of the flaws of the CEFR become clear when the development is closely scrutinized (see, e.g., North & Schneider, 1998). The CEFR was based on 30 preexisting proficiency scales which were deconstructed and then put back together by language teachers who were asked to judge their learners based on these descriptors. This was followed by a statistical scaling procedure and a repeat validation. While the approach followed was principled, the results depend on the original descriptors used, the teachers involved in the process, and the learners they were judging. The level descriptions and the distance between levels are therefore not based on empirical evidence, but on the intuition of what constitutes language development by a group of teachers and the content of the existing scales. This has led to calls that the CEFR is essentially atheoretical and ignores insights from L2 acquisition research (e.g., Deygers, 2019 Fulcher, 2004; Wisniewski, 2017) and that it instead represents a scale of teachers' perceptions of proficiency. The six levels are also very broad, contain impressionistic terminology, and are not useful for providing information on student progress within courses because the scale steps are too far apart. The learners involved in those validation activities were typically highly educated learners of foreign languages who may follow different language learning progressions than other test-taker populations, including presumably those learning signed languages for various purposes.

Another problem with the CEFR is that it is abstract by design to suit many different contexts. This generality is, of course, attractive, but it is also difficult to defend. There are dangers for score users who may consider that a score on Test X is the same as a score on Test Y once the tests are related to each other through the framework, which may, according to Taylor (2004), risk oversimplification and misinterpretation and create a sense of equivalence of different testing instruments that were developed for very different purposes. Alderson (2007) has also criticized the CEFR for being too vague to be useful for test development.

Most importantly for use with signed language, Alderson (2007) argues that the CEFR is deliberately language-independent and therefore assumes that "any communicative task requires a comparable level of proficiency from language to language" (p. 660; see also Little, 2007). This is intuitively difficult to defend for spoken languages, but is presumably even less likely to be valid for signed languages. There is a danger, therefore, that the modality-inclusive CEFR Companion

Volume for signed languages may be adopted as blindly as the original 2001 (Council of Europe, 2001) version for other languages, without users being familiar with its shortcomings or further critical validation. At this point, it is (still) not clear whether the development of signed language proficiency takes a different path compared to spoken languages and whether the generic descriptions of what learners can do hold for signed languages as well, given our limited knowledge about the process of learning a signed language as adults (e.g., Haug et al., 2021). As McKee and Frost (Chapter 10.3) point out, signed language interaction creates challenges not found in spoken language (e.g., visual turn-taking), and users of signed languages are often adept at drawing on multimodal communication with non-deaf people, aspects of competence possibly not documented.

While the scales for signed language in the Companion Volume will likely be readily adopted in various contexts, it is important that users understand the likely limitations of this document alongside its many advantages, remember that this does not fill the gap of empirical research in describing the development of signed language proficiency, and feed more directly into signed language curricula and assessment instruments (see McKee & Frost, Chapter 10.3).

CONCLUSION

Contrary to what many readers may think, there is a lot of common ground between the fields of signed language assessment and spoken language assessment. In the 36 chapters of this volume, we have tried to highlight these commonalities while at the same time acknowledging the differences that exists. It is our hope that reading this volume, specifically the discussions between specialists from both fields, will encourage and stimulate readers to engage in similar discussions with colleagues from the "opposite" field. As the volume has demonstrated, research on signed language assessment has a lot to offer to the much more established field of spoken language assessment, including new, exciting ways of approaching or revisiting familiar problems. Equally, the long experience of colleagues working in spoken language assessment can provide the field of signed language assessment with expertise and guidance to avoid making (some of) the same mistakes. In providing an objective and comprehensive analysis and discussion of relevant topics for both fields, the contributors have shown that there is a lot of promise in seeking a collaborative approach to tackling questions related to language assessment in child and adult learners. We close this work by extending our initial invitation to colleagues to partake in a dialogue between (two) different fields to you, the reader, in an effort to undertake similar collaborative efforts that draw you out of your comfort zone. The decision whether or not to accept lies with you.

REFERENCES

Alderson, C. (2007). The CEFR and the need for more research. *Modern Language Journal, 91*, 659–663. https://doi.org/10.1111/j.1540-4781.2007.00627_4.x

Australian Bureau of Statistics. (2008, September 1). *Adult literacy and life skills survey, summary results, Australia, 2006*. Australian Bureau of Statistics.

Council of Europe. (2001). *Common European Framework of Reference for Languages: Learning, teaching, assessment*. Council of Europe.

Council of Europe. (2020). *Common European framework of reference for languages: Learning, teaching, assessment. Companion volume with new descriptors*. Council of Europe.

Crystal, D. (1997). *English as a global language*. Cambridge University Press.

Davies, A. (1991). The notion of the native speaker. *Journal of Intercultural Studies, 12*(2), 35–45. https://doi.org/10.1080/07256868.1991.9963377

Davies, A. (2004). The native speaker in applied linguistics. In A. Davies & C. Elder (Eds.), *The handbook of applied linguistics* (pp. 431–450). John Wiley & Sons.

Davies, A. (2011). Does language testing need the native speaker? *Language Assessment Quarterly, 8*(3), 291–308. https://doi.org/10.1080/15434303.2011.570827

Davies, A. (2013). *Native speakers and native users*. Cambridge University Press.

Deygers, B. (2019). The CEFR companion volume: Between research-based policy and policy-based research. *Applied Linguistics*. https://doi.org/10.1093/applin/amz024

Deygers, B., Zeidler, B., Vilcu, D., & Hamnes Carlsen, C. (2018). One framework to unite them all? Use of the CEFR in European university entrance policies. *Language Assessment Quarterly, 15*(1), 3–15. https://doi.org/https://doi.org/10.1080/15434303.2016.1261350

Elder, C., McNamara, T., Woodward-Kron, R., Manias, E., McColl, G., Webb, G., & Pill, J. (2013). *Towards improved healthcare communication: Development and validation of language proficiency standards for non-native English speaking health professionals. Final report for the OET Centre*. (40 pp.) University of Melbourne.

Enns, C., & Herman, R. (2011). Adapting the assessing British Sign Language development: Receptive Skills Test into American Sign Language. *Journal of Deaf Studies and Deaf Education, 16*(3), 362–374. https://doi.org/10.1093/deafed/enr004

Fulcher, G. (2004). Deluded by artifices? The Common European Framework and harmonization. *Language Assessment Quarterly, 1*(4), 253–266. https://doi.org/10.1207/s15434311laq0104_4

Gathercole, V. C. M., Kennedy, I., & Thomas, E. M. (2016). Socioeconomic level and bilinguals' performance on language and cognitive measures. *Bilingualism: Language and Cognition, 19*(5), 1057–1078. https://doi.org/10.1017/S1366728915000504

Hamilton, J., Lopes, M., McNamara, T., & Sheridan, E. (1993). Rating scales and native speaker performance on a communicatively oriented EAP test. *Language Testing, 10*(3), 337–353. https://doi.org/10.1177/026553229301000307

Haug, T., Boers-Visker, E., & Van den Bogaerde, B. (2021). Testing sign language learners. In P. Winke & T. Brunfaut (Eds.), *The Routledge handbook of second language acquisition and language testing* (pp. 432–442). Routledge.

Jacoby, S. (1998). *Science as performance: Socializing scientific discourse through conference talk rehearsals* Unpublished doctoral dissertation. University of California, Los Angeles.
Jacoby, S., & McNamara, T. (1999). Locating competence. *English for Specific Purposes*, *18*(3), 213–241. https://doi.org/10.1080/15434300701623025
Keller, J., Meili, A., Bürgin, P., & Ni, D. (2017). Auf dem Weg zum Gemeinsamen Europäischen Referenzrahmen (GER) für Gebärdensprachen. *Das Zeichen*, *105*, 86–97.
Knoch, U., & Macqueen, S. (2020). *Assessing English for professional purposes: Language and the workplace*. Routledge.
Kramsch, C. (1997). The privilege of the nonnative speaker. *PMLA*, *112*(3), 359–369.
Leeson, L., van den Bogaerde, B., Rathmann, C., & Haug, T. (2016). *Sign languages and the Common European Framework of Reference for Languages*. Council of Europe. https://www.ecml.at/Portals/1/mtp4/pro-sign/documents/Common-Reference-Level-Descriptors-EN.pdf
Little, D. (2007). The Common European Framework of Reference for Languages: Perspectives on the making of supranational language education policy. *Modern Language Journal*, 91(4), 645–655. https://doi.org/10.1111/j.1540-4781.2007.00627_2.x
Mann, W., Peña, E. D., & Morgan, G. (2014). Exploring the use of dynamic language assessment with deaf children, who use American Sign Language: Two case studies. *Journal of Communication Disorders*, *52*, 16–30. https://doi.org/10.1016/j.jcomdis.2014.05.002
Mann, W., Peña, E. D., & Morgan, G. (2015). Child modifiability as a predictor of language abilities in deaf children who use American Sign Language. *American Journal of Speech-Language Pathology*, *24*(3), 374–385. https://doi.org/10.1044/2015_AJSLP-14-0072
North, B. (2020). Trolls, unicorns and the CEFR: Precision and professionalism in criticism of the CEFR. *CEFR Journal: Research and Practice*, *2*, 8–24.
North, B., & Schneider, G. (1998). Scaling descriptors for language proficiency scales. *Language Testing*, *15*(2), 217–263. https://doi.org/10.1177/026553229801500204
Pill, J. (2013). *What doctors value in consultations and the implications for specific-purpose language testing*. University of Melbourne Press.
Piller, I. (2001). Who, if anyone, is a native speaker? *Anglistic: Mitteilungen des Verbandes Deutscher Anglisten*, *12*(2), 109–121.
Piller, I. (2002). Passing for a native speaker: Identity and success in second language learning. *Journal of Sociolinguistics*, *6*(2), 179–206. https://doi.org/10.1111/1467-9481.00184
Taylor, L. (2004). Issues of test comparability. *Research Notes*, *15*, 2–5. http://www.cambridge-efl.org/rs_notes/rs_nts15.pdf
Wisniewski, K. (2017). Empirical learner language and the levels of the *Common European Framework of Reference*: The CEFR levels and learner language. *Language Learning*, *67*(S1), 232–253. https://doi.org/10.1111/lang.12223

Index

For the benefit of digital users, indexed terms that span two pages (e.g., 52–53) may, on occasion, appear on only one of those pages.

Tables and figures are indicated by *t* and *f* following the page number

www.ingramcontent.com/pod-product-compliance
Ingram Content Group UK Ltd.
Pitfield, Milton Keynes, MK11 3LW, UK
UKHW020850150926
475595UK00003B/109